www.harcourt-interna~~tional~~

Bringing you products from all Harcourt Health Sciences companies including Baillière Tindall, Churchill Livingstone, Mosby and W.B. Saunders

- **Browse** for latest information on new books, journals and electronic products

- **Search** for information on over 20 000 published titles with full product information including tables of contents and sample chapters

- **Keep up to date** with our extensive publishing programme in your field by registering with eAlert or requesting postal updates

- **Secure online ordering** with prompt delivery, as well as full contact details to order by phone, fax or post

- **News** of special features and promotions

If you are based in the following countries, please visit the country-specific site to receive full details of product availability and local ordering information

USA: www.harcourthealth.com

Canada: www.harcourtcanada.com

Australia: www.harcourt.com.au

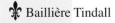 Baillière Tindall    CHURCHILL LIVINGSTONE   Mosby   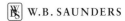 W.B. SAUNDERS

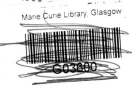

Evidence-based Healthcare

For Churchill Livingstone

Commissioning Editor: Michael Parkinson
Project Development Manager: Janice Urquhart
Project Manager: Nancy Arnott
Design direction: Sarah Russell
Illustrated by: Chartwell Illustrators

Evidence-based Healthcare

J. A. Muir Gray CBE

Project Director, National electronic Library for Health;
Programme Director, National Screening Committee;
Director, The Institute of Health Sciences, University of Oxford, UK

Appendices compiled by
Andrew and Sandra Booth

Creators of *Netting the Evidence*

Editor **Erica Ison**

Editorial Assistant **Rosemary Lees**

SECOND EDITION

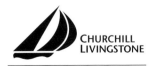

CHURCHILL
LIVINGSTONE

EDINBURGH LONDON NEW YORK PHILADELPHIA ST LOUIS SYDNEY TORONTO 2001

CHURCHILL LIVINGSTONE
An imprint of Harcourt Publishers Limited

© Harcourt Publishers Limited 2001

 is a registered trademark of Harcourt Publishers Limited

First published 1997
  Reprinted 1997
  Reprinted for AstraZeneca 1999
This edition 2001

ISBN 0 443 06288 9

British Library Cataloguing in Publication Data
A catalogue record for this book is available from the British
Library

Library of Congress Cataloging in Publication Data
A catalog record for this book is available from the Library of
Congress

Note
Medical knowledge is constantly changing. As
new information becomes available, changes in
treatment, procedures, equipment and the use of
drugs become necessary. The author and the
publishers have taken care to ensure that the
information given in this text is accurate and up
to date. However, readers are strongly advised
to confirm that the information, especially with
regard to drug usage, complies with the latest
legislation and standards of practice.

The
publisher's
policy is to use
**paper manufactured
from sustainable forests**

Typeset by IMH(Cartrif), Loanhead, Scotland
Printed in China

PREFACE TO SECOND EDITION

I have written this book for those who make decisions about groups of patients or populations. My overall purpose is twofold:

1. to improve the competence of health service decision-makers;
2. to strengthen the motivation of any health service decision-maker to use scientific methods when making a decision.

However, some opponents of this approach have characterised it as:

Arrogant, seductive and controversial

It must be admitted that the terms 'evidence-based medicine' and 'evidence-based healthcare' were chosen partly for their provocative nature. However, those of us involved in developing these initiatives had evidence that:

- the findings from research were not being put into practice quickly and systematically because the process of decision-making was based on a random cocktail of drivers – values, resources, and evidence;
- decision-makers were not aware which drivers were shaping their decisions, nor which of them was most important.

However, as proponents of an evidence-based approach, we may not have been as clear as we could have been in describing its development, partly because the ideas were continually evolving. This may be one reason why certain workers were critical. Many other people have found the concepts useful.

The approach advocated in this book is one that emphasises the need to apply logic to:

- the analysis of healthcare problems;
- the identification and appraisal of options for health improvement;
- decision-making about the delivery of healthcare for groups of patients or populations.

This approach of evidence-based decision-making could be given one of several different generic terms; for example, it could be called reductionist or positivist. However, proponents regard it as an essential component of providing modern healthcare, in the same way that we regard evidence-based medicine as an essential approach to clinical practice in the 21st century.

The preoccupation with productivity and quality that has dominated health service management towards the end of the 20th century has not necessarily led to the development of evidence-based policies, nor to the implementation of knowledge derived from research for the improvement of the effectiveness, safety, acceptability and cost-effectiveness of healthcare. There is now a general appreciation that decisions made about health services and clinical practice must be based on evidence to a much greater

degree than they have been in the past
such that the knowledge derived from
research can be used to improve the health
of patients and the public.

CONTENTS

CHAPTER 6
ASSESSING THE OUTCOMES FOUND 169

CHAPTER 7
THE EVIDENCE-BASED ORGANISATION 243

APPENDIX II
FILTERING THE EVIDENCE 405

II.1 Resource overview 405

II.2 Resources 406
II.2.1   PubMed Clinical Queries
         Interface
II.2.2   SUMSearch
II.2.3   Institute of Health Sciences
         (IHS) Library Filters

II.3 The Internet 407

Reference

Further reading
    How to harness MEDLINE
    Other items

APPENDIX III
APPRAISING THE EVIDENCE 409

III.1 Resource overview 409

III.2 Resources 409
III.2.1 ACP Journal Club
III.2.2 Bandolier
III.2.3 Clinical Evidence
III.2.4 Evidence-Based Health Care
         Workbook and CD-ROM
III.2.5 Evidence-based Healthcare
III.2.6 Evidence-Based Medicine
III.2.7 Evidence-Based Mental
         Health
III.2.8 Evidence-Based Nursing
III.2.9 CAT-Maker

HOW TO USE THIS BOOK

As the main aim in writing this book is to help those people who have to make decisions about groups of patients and/or populations base such decisions on a careful appraisal of the best evidence available, it has been structured in such a way as to increase the level of evidence-based decision-making in the provision of health services. The contents cover three main topics:

- finding and appraising evidence (Chapters 4–6);
- developing the capacity of organisations and individuals to use evidence (Chapters 7 and 9);
- implementation – getting research into practice.

Finding and appraising evidence

In Chapters 4–6, the focus is on the appraisal of evidence about three different dimensions (Fig. 0.1):

- different types of healthcare decision, such as decisions about new treatment services or management changes;
- different types of outcome, such as effectiveness, safety or quality;
- different types of research method, such as systematic reviews,

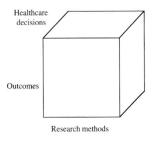

Fig. 0.1

randomised controlled trials, or cohort studies.

For any problem, all three dimensions must be considered.

Developing the capacity for evidence-based decision-making

In Chapter 7, the ways in which the level of evidence-based decision-making within an organisation can be increased are discussed. This is achieved by developing not only the skills of individuals (see Chapter 9) but also the culture, systems and structures within organisations. These two facets of development are inter-related (see Fig. 0.2).

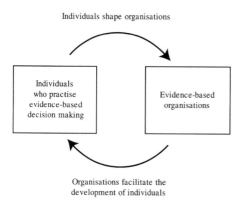

Individuals shape organisations

Organisations facilitate the development of individuals

Fig. 0.2

Getting research into practice

Throughout the book there is a focus on implementation, although it is recognised that it is often difficult to implement research evidence within clinical practice and health service management and policy.

The first step is to prepare a policy (see Fig. 0.3), i.e. a statement of what should happen; for example, that all women aged over 50 years should undergo mammography, or that all people who have had a myocardial infarction should receive a treatment regimen of aspirin and beta-blockers.

Once a policy has been developed, systems must be designed to ensure that the

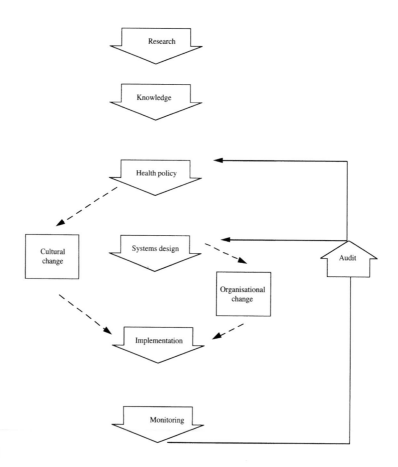

Fig. 0.3

policy is implemented. These systems must encompass organisational development and the education of both professionals and the public to improve healthcare, and the public health (Chapter 8).

Although a companion book on evidence-based medicine has been published, it is written primarily for clinicians. The essence of this discipline has been distilled in Chapter 10 for the benefit of health service managers because decisions about individual patients and those about groups are inter-related. Clinicians who are also managers, or involved in managing, will benefit from developing the skills described in both books because, although concepts such as appropriateness or effectiveness are the same, a different perspective needs to be brought to bear in each sphere.

DEFINING OUR TERMS

A rose is a rose is a rose.

Gertrude Stein

What's in a name? That which we
call a rose
By any other word would smell as
sweet;

William Shakespeare: Romeo and
Juliet, *Act II, Scene ii*

Gentle Reader,

*Visualise, if you will, Newcastle General
Hospital, the hub of hospital care in the
north-east for many years – solid,
Victorian and dependable. The hospital's
honest, uncompromising and practical
atmosphere might strike you as an
unlikely setting for the 20th century's
most influential philosopher, but Ludwig
Wittgenstein was employed as a
laboratory technician there during the
Second World War. He showed such
great promise as a laboratory investigator
that attempts were made to persuade him
to take up a scientific career. However, he
chose to return to philosophy, linguistic
philosophy in particular.*

Commentary

*One of Wittgenstein's central tenets was
that differences or arguments between
protagonists were often the result of a
simple failure to agree on the meaning of
the terms used.*

Throughout this book we have defined
certain terms and attempted to use those
definitions consistently. To this end, at the
beginning of some chapters, as relevant,
we have placed a box in the margin
entitled 'Jargon Soup'. In each box, we
show the key terms for that chapter; at the
end of each chapter, we present text
headed 'Defining our terms' in which our
definitions are given. However, it is
important to bear in mind, gentle reader,
that our definitions may not be the same as
yours.

Defining words with words

One of the ways of finding the meaning of
a word is to look it up in the dictionary.
Throughout this book, we have used the
Shorter Oxford English Dictionary, one of the
wonders of the English language.
However, dictionary definitions are not
always helpful. Take, for example, the term
'efficiency'; the definition of efficiency is
given as: 'efficient power, effectiveness,
efficacy'. If we then look up 'efficacy', we

find that it is 'the capacity to produce effects', and if we turn to 'effectiveness' it is 'the quality of being efficient'. There is a certain circularity here, of the first word being defined in terms of a second word which is defined in terms of the first.

Although it is true that more recent, official or specialised definitions of effectiveness and efficiency have been developed, meaning can change, particularly as a term becomes more widely used. Indeed, another of Wittgenstein's arguments was that the use of a term that had been clearly defined by a small committee as an aid to understanding and clarification could become counterproductive when employed in a wider arena where different people invest it with different meanings. This 'dissipation' of meaning could be said to have afflicted the term 'efficiency', now so widely used in so many different ways that it causes confusion and arguments.

Defining words by numbers

Vienna at the end of the Hapsburg empire was in the final stages of its glory, already turning a little rotten on the bough. Although rottenness implies decay, decay is necessary for the creation of new life forms. Wittgenstein was a product of Vienna or, to be more precise, of the intellectual and wealthy Jewish community living in Vienna; so too was Malinowski. Malinowski argued contrary to Wittgenstein that knowledge was created, not by the lonely intellectual sitting at his desk, as Wittgenstein did throughout the English winters, but by groups of people talking and using language to create new knowledge.

The Vienna School of Philosophy flourished as Wittgenstein left the city and became very influential, particularly in Britain, where it gave rise to what is known as 'logical positivism', the leading figure and most eloquent reporter of which was A. J. Ayer. In *Language, Truth and Logic*, Ayer took an approach to the definition of a term that did not rely on words at all. The logical positivists believe that no term should be examined in isolation – a study of the term 'efficiency' would be pointless – but investigated in the context of propositions, such as 'this hospital is more efficient than that hospital'. To define the meaning of this proposition, a logical positivist would not have recourse to a dictionary but instead seek to agree on the data that would need to be collected to confirm or refute it. Thus, for this particular proposition, the debate immediately becomes: 'How would you measure efficiency?'. Options include:

- cost per case;
- throughput per bed;
- percentage of costs spent on administration.

Indefinite definitions

Throughout this book, we have tried to give a clear definition of a term without implying that our definition is *the* definition; *caveat lector*, let the reader beware.

CONFESSIONS OF AN AMANUENSIS

Although famous for his work in electromagnetism, it is far from common knowledge that the young Michael Faraday acted as an amanuensis to Sir Humphrey Davy following an injury to Davy's eyes in a laboratory explosion.

The word 'amanuensis' was first recorded in 1619, derived from the Latin 'manu' for hand and 'ensis', a suffix meaning 'belonging to'. The definition in the *Shorter Oxford English Dictionary* is given as 'one who copies or writes from dictation'. This has been my function in the preparation of this book, which is a record of the work done during the 1990s, principally in Oxford, to promote 'evidence-based healthcare'. In the future, this work will be a focus for the Institute of Health Sciences (IHS), Oxford.

The idea of commissioning a multi-author book was rejected because of the problems inherent in such a project, particularly on a topic like evidence-based healthcare in which there is so much cross-cutting from one approach to another. As it would have been difficult to fuse several different contributions into a coherent whole, the decision was taken for one person to 'copy or write from dictation' from the work of a wide variety of people. Many of these people worked in the four counties that comprised the old Oxford Regional Health Authority, and built on the original ideas of the team at McMaster University, comprising Larry Chambers, Gordon Guyatt, Brian Haynes, Jonathan Lomas, Andy Oxman and Dave Sackett. Since then, Dave was a source of inspiration during the five years he spent in the UK, helping to change the culture and develop the skills of evidence-based decision-making.

Those whose work has been drawn upon for either the first or second edition are:

Clive Adams, Doug Altman, Chris Ball, Andrew Booth, Sandra Booth, Anne Brice, Catherine Brogan, Shaun Brogan, Chris Bulstrode, Iain Chalmers, Myles Chippendale, Andy Chivers, Martin Dawes, Anna Donald, Gordon Dooley, Jayne Edwards, Jim Elliott, Katie Enock, John Fletcher, John Geddes, David Gill, Michael Goldcare, Peter Gøtzsche, Sian Griffiths, Nick Hicks, Alison Hill, Richard Himsworth, Carol Lefebvre, Mark Lodge, Steve McDonald, Ian McKinnell, Henry McQuay, Theresa Marteau, Jill Meara, Ruairidh Milne, Andrew Moore, David Naylor, Gill Needham, Ian Owens, Judy Palmer, David Pencheon, Bob Phillips, W. Scott Richardson, William Rosenberg, Jill Sanders, Ken Schultz,

Valerie Seagroatt, Sasha Shepperd, Mark Starr, Barbara Stocking, Sharon Straus, Andre Tomlin, Ben Toth, Martin Vessey, and Chris Williams.

Many of these people have been supported by the NHS R&D Programme, the initial leadership of which by Sir Michael Peckham was very important in the evolution of evidence-based healthcare.

I am also indebted to those people, in various teams, with whom I have worked on the development of these ideas: the GRiPP team, the CASP team, the R&D team, and those in the Cochrane Collaboration and in the IHS Library.

Simply stringing words together is only part of the preparation of a text like this; the final product has been the combined work of a small team. The team is supported by Ann Southwell, who provided the business management skills that underpinned the creation of many of the projects that contributed to the development of evidence-based healthcare. Karen McKendry, a wizard with Powerpoint, created many of the diagrams that punctuate and enliven the prose. Without their contribution the book would have been of much poorer quality. The duo who hammered this book into its final form (not once but twice!), Rosemary Lees and Erica Ison, have continued to be endlessly good-humoured and hard-working and applied not only effort but also the highest level of skill to transform pig iron into steel, discursive prose into a text that is much briefer, clearer, and more powerful than it was when it left the hand of the amanuensis.

Finally, like another Scottish amanuensis – James Boswell – I must acknowledge the burden borne by my family – Jackie, Em, and Tat – who have put up with it all not once but twice!

The production of both editions of this book was supported by charitable trust funds, into which any income derived from publication has been and will continue to be returned. The objective in the disbursement of monies from these funds is the promotion of epidemiology as a practical tool for all healthcare decision-makers, working for what the President of the Royal Statistical Society in 1966 called the 'promotion of an evidence-based society'.[1]

Reference

1. SMITH, A.F.M. (1996) *Mad cows and Ecstasy: chance and choice in an evidence-based society.* J. R. Statist. Soc. A. 159: 367–83.

ELECTRONIC UPDATES

Important papers are published and new examples of evidence-based healthcare are identified continually. Although it is unlikely that any of these events will substantially change the text of this book, evidence-based healthcare is an evolving discipline and the reader will always require recent references and new tools for decision-making. For this reason, we have set up an Evidence-Based Healthcare Toolbox on the World Wide Web, an increasingly important source of information on healthcare, as described in the book *Medical Information on the Internet*.[1]

The website of the Evidence-Based Healthcare Toolbox is:

http://www.shef.ac.uk/~scharr/ebhc/Intro.html

It is linked to the Evidence-Based Medicine Toolbox, aimed primarily at clinicians, and a complementary tool to *Evidence-Based Medicine*, the companion volume to this book that has been written for those making decisions about individual patients.[2]

These Web pages allow you the opportunity to make comments and criticisms and we look forward to hearing from you.

References
1. KILEY, R. (1996) *Medical Information on the Internet*. Churchill Livingstone, London.
2. SACKETT, D.L., STRAUS, S., RICHARDSON, W.S., ROSENBERG, W. and HAYNES, R.B. (2000) *Evidence-Based Medicine: How to Practice and Teach EBM*. 2nd Edition. Churchill Livingstone, London.

THE GLOBALISATION OF HEALTHCARE PROBLEMS AND THEIR SOLUTIONS

Despite the differences in the ways in which health services around the world are funded and organised, many of the major problems in the delivery of healthcare are similar:

- the increasing costs of healthcare (see Fig. P.1);
- the lack of capacity in any country to pay for the totality of health services demanded by healthcare professionals and the general public;
- marked variation in the rates of delivery of health services within a country and among countries;
- delayed implementation of research findings into practice.

Jargon soup
- paying for healthcare
- purchasing healthcare
- commissioning health services

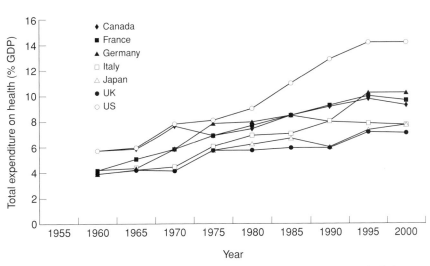

Fig. P.1 Expenditure on healthcare as a percentage of gross domestic product (GDP) in Canada, France, Germany, Italy, Japan, the UK, and the USA from 1960 to 1996 (Source: Hicks and Gray, ref. 1, Section 2.3.)

In addition, inflation in healthcare costs in most countries is greater than the growth of the economy. This rate of inflation is related to inefficiencies in the delivery of healthcare arising from:

- the supply-led nature of healthcare in which the professional tells the patient what is needed, thereby creating demand, or develops and advocates the use of a new service;
- the provision of inappropriate care.

Moreover, although the mode of health service provision appears to differ greatly from one country to another, there are certain common factors that are beginning to influence the evolution of systems of health service organisation and healthcare delivery in all countries irrespective of their geographical latitude:

- population ageing;
- rising patient expectations;
- the advent of new technology and new knowledge.

COMMON PROBLEMS: COMMON SOLUTIONS

As the problems associated with the delivery of healthcare world-wide begin to converge, the solutions being sought can be characterised by certain features that are not only evident within the health services of the post-industrial nations of the North but also important to the structural reforms of healthcare in the Third World:

- a preoccupation with cost control;
- the development of systems to prevent the burden of cost falling on the individual;
- an increasing authority being given to the function of purchasing healthcare either for people who live within a particular area or for those who are members of a health plan or insurance fund;
- a clearer definition and delineation of the purchasing function such that responsibility is being shifted from the heartland of government to an agency or agencies, the primary responsibility of which is to purchase healthcare and obtain value for money; in Germany, for example, there is now an increased emphasis on the power of insurance schemes;

- a growing appreciation of the need for the purchasers of healthcare to manage the evolution and development of clinical practice in partnership with clinical professions;
- increasing public and political interest in the evidence on which decisions about the effectiveness and safety of healthcare are based.

As a result of these common problems, pressures, and solutions, systems of health service organisation are also beginning to converge. In order to meet these powerful challenges, the principles of evidence-based healthcare can be applied to great effect, irrespective of whether a health service is organised nationally (as in the UK) or by province (as in Canada), whether it is tax-based or insurance-based (as in Japan), or whether the main source of funding is public or private (as in the USA).

However, it has emerged that there are two necessary pre-conditions to foster the practice of evidence-based healthcare:

1. a commitment to cover the whole population – where no such commitment exists, it is still possible to introduce any intervention that shows some evidence of effectiveness no matter how small;
2. a fixed budget for healthcare – as healthcare budgets were capped during the final years of the 20th century, there was a growing appreciation of the need for evidence-based decision-making as an essential element in the provision of healthcare for the 21st century. In France, for example, the Minister of Health in 1997, M. Jacques Richir, himself a doctor, challenged the medical profession when they were complaining about the introduction of tougher controls on healthcare spending.

> Le docteur Richir, qui continue à exercer la médecine, se lance: *'Pouvez-vous me dire avec certitude que chaque acte que vous effectuez a toujours une justification médicale?'*
>
> *'Oui!'*, s'écrient les internes en choeur, manifestement choqués qu'on puisse mettre en doute leur conscience professionnelle.
>
> *'Au moment de rédiger votre ordonnance'*, poursuit imperturbalement M. Richir, *'vous devez réfléchir quinze secondes et vous demander si votre acte est indispensable. C'est sur les actes redondants qu'on économisera un ou deux pour cents.'*
>
> Le Monde, *4 Avril 1997*

PROBLEMS AND SOLUTIONS IN POORER COUNTRIES

The challenges to the provision of healthcare may be obvious in post-industrial nations, but these challenges also affect developing countries. Thus, a Minister of Health in a developing economy is responsible for providing appropriate services to meet not only the typical health problems of the Third World, such as high infant mortality rates, and high mortality and morbidity rates as a result of the prevalence of infectious diseases – problems resolved in the 19th century in the industrial nations – but also the consequences of lifestyle habits, such as cigarette smoking, drug abuse, and dangerous driving, which became predominant in the post-industrial societies of the late 20th century.

New healthcare technologies may be introduced into a developing country by practitioners, or developed in teaching hospitals that have been built in emulation of famous centres in the USA or Europe. These technological developments, however, will be relevant to only a small proportion of the population, although they can consume a large proportion of healthcare resources. Thus, it is vital that health services in a developing economy are managed using an evidence-based approach, although it may prove more difficult to implement in this situation than within the context of a developed economy. In countries that have well-developed economies, private practice, which is much more difficult to influence, is relatively less important than care provided within formal managed systems. In developing countries, physicians can sometimes be so poorly paid that incentives other than conforming to the best evidence available may prevail.

Interventions that have been shown to do more good than harm at reasonable cost but which are not yet widely adopted in countries with developing economies include:

- the administration of aspirin, which reduces the health and economic burden resulting from stroke;
- vitamin A supplementation, which reduces all-cause mortality in children.[1]

Conversely, there are other interventions that have not yet been shown to be effective but which are in routine use; these interventions of unproven effectiveness consume resources that could be expended on interventions that do more good than harm at reasonable cost. Evidence-based decision-making has a role in the provision of healthcare in all countries, irrespective of the stage of their economic development (see Section 7.9.6).

THE USA AND THE REST OF THE DEVELOPED WORLD

The growing difference between healthcare decision-making in the USA and in the other developed countries was highlighted by the decision about which age-groups of women should undergo breast cancer screening, taken at the second attempt. This decision, elegantly analysed in a paper by Tannenbaum[2] and summarised in Box P.1, was a recommendation that breast cancer screening be undertaken in women *under* the age of 50 years.

Tannenbaum suggested that the main reason why the USA and Canada took different approaches (although the same argument could apply to any other developed country) was that in the USA decisions about health are individualistic, whereas in other developed countries they are primarily collective. In the USA, it is felt that government should recommend action if there is a possibility that the individual might benefit; it is then up to the individual to take the appropriate step – provided, of course, that they can afford to do so. In those countries in which healthcare is provided to the entire population, all decisions about health and healthcare have to be made taking into account finite resources and opportunity costs. Thus, people in other countries would not deny the possibility of a small benefit from universal screening for the population of women under 50 years, although they could point out that there will be a large number of women who would be harmed by the process and might be mindful of the other uses to which those resources could be put.

If the two preconditions for evidence-based healthcare – a fixed budget and a commitment to cover the entire population – are not present, as in the USA, those who pay for healthcare, for example, for-profit and not-for-profit health maintenance organisations and the insurance companies that back them, may seek to live within their resources either by increasing productivity or by excluding patients who are likely to be heavy users of the service, or both.

Box P.1 Summary of the paper by Tannenbaum (Source: Evidence-Based Health Policy and Management 1998; 2: 53.)

The epidemiological approach to the assessment of effectiveness in Canada and the United States is similar, although research results in Canada are expressed more often in terms of the population benefits that are likely to result but in the United States the results of research are seen as something not only for policy-makers and managers but also as a resource for consumers to make more informed decisions. Much of the debate in Canada takes place between the government and the organisations representing physicians who argue both that they should be involved in decision-making about resource allocation and that, having made broad decisions on the amount of resources available, individual clinicians should retain a high level of freedom in interpreting evidence and maximising effectiveness. The Canadian government, in paying and negotiating medical prices, represents not only Canadian patients but also population health interests and effectiveness research is used to obtain the best value for the population as a whole.

In the United States this type of negotiation does not take place at government level but is much more decentralised and dispersed, being interpreted by insurance companies and provider organisations on the one hand, and individual patients on the other. An analysis of who actually makes choices in the American health care system reveals that individual consumers do have choice but this is often determined, or constrained, by their employer.

Physicians have a different part to play in the interpretation of evidence about effectiveness or ineffectiveness in the two systems. In one system the physicians are very much involved in negotiation with the government about the total amount of resources available for health care, and therefore priorities, whereas in the United States physicians have a number of different types of relationships with those who pay for health care, depending on the type of organisation they work for and the patients they serve.

Author's conclusions

Both the United States and Canada have an explicit commitment to promote effective and to discourage ineffective care. However, the different cultures and the different decision-making processes mean that the knowledge about effectiveness and ineffectiveness, which is usually expressed in terms of probabilities, has a different contribution in decisions in both countries. The author's conclusion is that: 'Canadian policy-makers overstate the societal applicability and the US policy-makers the individual applicability of outcomes research findings'. The result of this is that different decisions may result from the same evidence.

Thus, decisions taken about healthcare, at a collective level, are different in the USA than in other countries. The Department of Health and Human Services and its related agencies, notably the Agency for Health Care Policy and Research, and the Veterans Administration, which has to cover a whole population on a fixed budget, do try to practise evidence-based healthcare but the majority of healthcare, paid for by insurance companies, is provided on a different set of principles.

References

1. GLASZIOU, P.T. and MACKERRAS, E.M. (1993) *Vitamin A supplementation in infectious diseases: a meta-analysis.* Br. Med. J. 306: 366–70.
2. TANNENBAUM, S.J. (1996) *'Medical effectiveness' in Canadian and U.S. Health Policy: the comparative policits of inferential ambiguity.* Health Services Research 31: 517–32.

DEFINING OUR TERMS: PAYING FOR, PURCHASING, AND COMMISSIONING HEALTHCARE

Although the person who buys a packet of aspirin can be said to be paying for healthcare, in the context of this book, the term 'paying for' implies third party payment, for example, by an insurance company, which pays for either the care of an individual or the care of a population covered by that insurance company.

In the UK, the term 'purchasing healthcare' was promoted by the Conservative government as part of its market reforms. The term 'purchasing' was intended to indicate a clear split between the purchaser and provider functions, with the purchaser being able to purchase the best quality healthcare at the most reasonable cost from among various providers of healthcare services. In practice, the market was relatively ineffective in transferring money from one part of the country to another because, in the UK at least, patients were reluctant to travel long distances to receive healthcare services such as elective surgery.

The Labour government introduced the term 'commissioning', the intention being to distinguish between the functions of identifying and prioritising the healthcare needs of a population and providing the health services for that population.

Gentle Reader,

Empathise with the walnut. You have put it into one of those nutcrackers in which the nut is held within a wooden cup and the pressure exerted by a wooden screw. The screw can be turned either to crack the shell and release the nut whole or to smash it to smithereens.

Commentary

Any health service is in the same situation as the walnut: existing within a fixed resource envelope that is subject to increasing pressure resulting from the population ageing, the advent of new technology and new knowledge, and rising patient expectations.

What do I mean when I refer to a health service? In this context, it can be represented by a decision-maker, that is, those like you who feel the increasing pressure as the screw tightens.

CHAPTER 1

EVIDENCE-BASED HEALTHCARE

1.1 EVIDENCE-BASED HEALTHCARE – A SCIENTIFIC APPROACH TO HEALTHCARE MANAGEMENT

Over the last two decades, tremendous advances have been made in the health sciences with the development of new technology and new knowledge. Hitherto these advances have principally been used to support clinical practice, with the result that clinical decision-making is now based on information derived from research to a much greater degree than it was. This approach is referred to as evidence-based medicine; a more generic term, evidence-based clinical practice, can also be used.

In this book, readers will be shown how some of the scientific advances and methods that have underpinned the development of this approach to clinical practice can also underpin decision-making involving the care of groups of patients, and populations. Evidence-based healthcare is a discipline centred upon evidence-based decision-making about groups of patients, or populations, which may be manifest as evidence-based policy-making, purchasing or management.

The science of most relevance to this approach to healthcare decision-making is epidemiology, that is, the study of disease in groups of patients and in populations. Although other sciences, such as occupational psychology, can be a source of information, epidemiology is the foundation of evidence-based healthcare.

In this chapter, the process and parameters of evidence-based decision-making in the provision of healthcare will be described; in Chapter 2, the evolution of an evidence-based approach will be discussed in relation to increasing constraints on the availability of resources for healthcare.

1.2 WHY FOCUS ON DECISION-MAKING?

There are two main reasons why it is important to focus on decision-making.

1. In the provision of healthcare, an enormous number of decisions is made. In the UK each year, for every million population, 40–50 million decisions are made about individual patients by clinicians, and thousands of decisions are made about groups of patients or populations by managers.
2. Decision-making in the provision of healthcare has a direct influence on the cost of delivering a health service. Changes in the volume and intensity of clinical practice constitute the major factor driving the increase in healthcare costs that it is possible to control.[1]

Although the changes in clinical practice that tend to receive prominence involve the introduction of a new treatment that is very expensive, it is the cumulative effect of small changes to clinical practice – such as the introduction of a new diagnostic test or an increase in the number of treatments for particular patients – across the service throughout the financial year (i.e. very large numbers of events) that substantially increases costs and has a massive impact on the healthcare budget.

Moreover, many of these small changes to clinical practice are those that:

- have no good evidence of doing more good than harm;
- have no good evidence of doing more good than harm at reasonable cost.

Furthermore, for some of these new interventions and procedures, there may be evidence of:

- doing more harm than good;
- doing more good than harm but at unreasonable cost.

Although in many countries systems for technology assessment have been set up, innovations may bypass those systems (see Fig. 7.3).

Reference

1. EDDY, D. M. (1993) *Three battles to watch in the 1990s.* JAMA 270: 520–6.

1.3   THE DRIVERS OF DECISION-MAKING: EVIDENCE, VALUES AND RESOURCES

> Now according to Dionysius, between man and angel there is this difference, that an angel perceives the truth by simple apprehension, whereas man becomes acquainted with a simple truth by a process from manifold data.
>
> *Thomas Aquinas*

Decisions about groups of patients or populations are based on a combination of three factors (see Margin Fig. 1.1):

1. evidence;
2. values;
3. resources

   At present, many healthcare decisions are driven principally by values and resources – a process that can be described as opinion-based decision-making. Little attention has been given or is paid to applying any evidence derived from research. However, as the pressure on the resources available for healthcare increases, decisions will have to be made explicitly and openly, a process that will be accelerated by demands from consumer groups, the media, and government for openness and accountability. Those who take decisions will be expected to present the evidence on which each decision was based. Even in cases for which the evidence is difficult to find or poor in quality, and the decision taken may ultimately be driven by values and resources, the decision-maker must search for, appraise and present the evidence. Thus, as the pressure on resources increases, there will be a transition from opinion-based decision-making to evidence-based decision-making (see Margin Fig. 1.2).

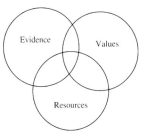

Margin Fig. 1.1

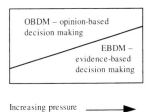

Margin Fig. 1.2

1.4   EVIDENCE-BASED DECISION-MAKING

During the 21st century, the healthcare decision-maker, that is, anyone who makes decisions about groups of patients or populations, will have to adopt an evidence-based approach. Indeed, to assume that healthcare decision-makers can operate in any other way in the hard times ahead is unrealistic. Every decision will have to be based on a systematic appraisal of the best evidence available in the context of the prevailing values and resources available. To accomplish this, the best available evidence relating to a particular decision must be found and applied (Fig. 1.1). This requires the development of evidence management skills, the promotion of circumstances conducive to the use of an evidence-based approach, and a recognition of the need to renew decisions in the light of new evidence.

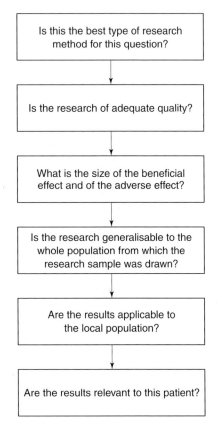

Fig. 1.1
The critical pathway of questions to help you find and apply the best evidence available

1.4.1   Skills for healthcare decision-makers

The skills necessary to practise evidence-based decision-making include being able:

- to ask the 'right' questions (Section 9.1);
- to define criteria such as effectiveness, safety and acceptability;
- to find articles on the effectiveness, safety and acceptability of a new test or treatment;
- to assess the quality of evidence from research findings;
- to assess whether the results of research are generalisable to the whole population from which the study sample was drawn;
- to assess whether the results of the research are applicable to the local population;
- to implement the changes indicated by the evidence.

The development of such skills may seem ambitious, but there is evidence that it can be done (see Section 7.5.2). Everyone involved in healthcare decision-making must have the skills to enable them to make decisions about 'doing the right things'.

- All chief executives should be able to discriminate between a good and a bad systematic review.
- All directors of finance should be able to find and appraise studies on health service cost-effectiveness.
- Every medical director should be able to determine whether a randomised controlled trial (RCT) in a specialty other than their own is biased.

These are the management skills necessary for the provision of healthcare in the 21st century.

1.4.2 Prerequisites for good decision-making

The performance (**P**) of an individual or team is a function of, i.e. determined by, three variables:

1. the level of motivation (**M**) of the individual/team (a direct relation);
2. the level of competency (**C**) of the individual/team (a direct relation);
3. the barriers (**B**) the individual/team has to overcome in order to perform well (an inverse relation).

$$P = \frac{M \times C}{B}$$

The resources every decision-maker requires in order to be able to overcome any barriers and practise evidence-based decision-making are shown in Box 1.1.

Box 1.1   Resources necessary to every decision-maker

- The support of a librarian
- Access to The Cochrane Library, MEDLINE, EMBASE and HealthSTAR (see Appendix I)
- Access to the World Wide Web
- Access to a personal computer with reference management software so that any articles identified as appropriate for use as evidence can be stored systematically

It is also vital for any decision-maker intent upon using the evidence to be working in an environment in which appropriate and effective decision-making is encouraged, that is, an organisation committed to evidence-based decision-making (see Chapter 7).

1.4.3   Reviewing decisions in the light of new evidence

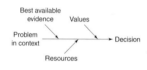

Margin Fig. 1.3

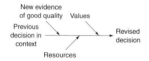

Margin Fig. 1.4

Having made a decision on the basis of evidence (Margin Fig. 1.3), it is essential to keep that decision under review as new evidence becomes available (Margin Fig. 1.4). To illustrate this point, a list of screening programmes that the National Screening Committee of the UK had deemed inappropriate for introduction in 1997 is shown in Table 1.1, together with the status of these screening programmes mid 2000. From this table, it can be seen how the publication of new evidence has altered the decisions being made about policy.

1.5   DEFINING THE SCOPE OF EVIDENCE-BASED HEALTHCARE

Evidence-based healthcare consists of three main stages (see also Fig. 1.2):

- producing evidence;
- making evidence available;
- using evidence.

Table 1.1 The effect of the publication of new evidence on evidence-based policy-making about screening

Screening programme	Status in 1997	Status mid 2000
Prostate cancer	Inappropriate for introduction	Inappropriate for introduction
Ovarian cancer	Inappropriate for introduction	New technology has been developed; an RCT is underway
Colorectal cancer	Inappropriate for introduction	2 RCTs published in which there is a reduction in mortality; pilot of colorectal cancer screening being undertaken to see if quality of service in a research setting can be reproduced in an ordinary service setting
Chlamydia	Inappropriate for introduction	Further research published; pilot of chlamydia screening being undertaken to see if quality of service in a research setting can be reproduced in an ordinary service setting
Human papilloma virus (HPV) testing as primary cervical screening test for cervical cancer	Inappropriate for introduction	Inappropriate for introduction; more research available, raising the possibility of using HPV tests during cervical screening to speed up and improve the management of some types of positive smear test results
Congenital biliary atresia in neonates	Inappropriate for introduction	Inappropriate for introduction
Cholesterol screening for whole population	Inappropriate for introduction	Inappropriate for introduction

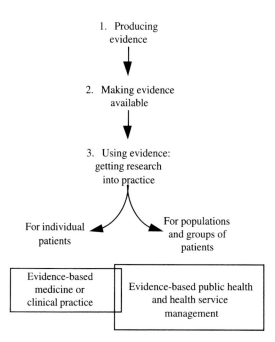

Fig. 1.2
The three main stages of evidence-based healthcare

1.5.1 Stage 1: Producing evidence

Producing evidence is the responsibility of research workers. In general, there are two main contexts within which research is conducted:

- in a framework set by policy-makers, in which research is commissioned by governments or research councils;
- in a subject area or on a topic that has been determined by the researcher(s), who actively seeks funding from a charity or other body; the funding body will provide the support if the research project is of good quality – this is known as responsive funding.

In every country, the trend is to reduce the amount of funding available to respond to the priorities of research workers and to transfer these funds into the commissioning of research to answer questions of importance to clinicians and patients, and to managers and policy-makers.

1.5.2 Stage 2: Making evidence available

Making the evidence derived from research available is vital, otherwise the potential value of new knowledge would never be realised. If research evidence has been made available, it is possible to gain access to it. In this book, examples are given of ways in which healthcare professionals can access information in libraries and from databases such as MEDLINE. However, better systems for gaining access to information at the time it is needed, for example, on a ward round, in a surgery or in a patient's home, must be developed.

For patients and carers, who are currently 'locked out' of medical libraries, the advent of the World Wide Web has provided unparalleled access to medical information.

1.5.3 Stage 3: Using evidence

There are three main ways in which research evidence can be used:

- to improve patient choice (see Section 1 5.3.1);
- to improve clinical practice (see Section 1.5.3.2);
- to improve health service management (see Section 1.5.3.3).

1.5.3.1 Evidence-based patient choice

Patients should be able to choose from treatment options, if they wish to, on the basis of best current knowledge.

1.5.3.2 Evidence-based clinical practice

Evidence-based clinical practice is an approach to decision-making in which the clinician uses the best evidence available, in consultation with the patient, to decide upon the option that suits the patient best. In Chapter 10, evidence-based clinical practice is described from the perspective of the health service manager, who can do much to promote both evidence-based clinical practice and evidence-based patient choice.

1.5.3.3 Evidence-based policy-making, purchasing and management for health services

Managers who are responsible for health services for groups of patients or populations have to make many decisions, all of which fall into one of three main categories:

1. policy;
2. purchasing or commissioning;
3. management.

As the number of constraints around decision-making increases, all three categories of decision will need to be based on evidence. The contents of this book will help health service personnel who make decisions about policy, purchasing (or commissioning) and management develop the skills necessary to base those decisions on the best evidence available.

1. Policy decisions

> Policy-making is a political process: it is based not solely on the evidence but also on the value politicians place upon different types of decision-making, for example, centralised as opposed to decentralised decision-making.

There are two main types of policy concerning health:

• health or public health policy – concerning public health;

- healthcare policy – concerning health service financing and organisation.

Healthcare policy decisions result in changes to the financing of a health service and to the way in which that service is organised to account for the resources used. The introduction of GP-fundholding changed the way in which finance flowed in the National Health Service (NHS), and thereby altered the authority and responsibility of those professionals working in any general practice that became fundholding.

In 1991, in the UK, what was known as the purchaser/provider split was introduced. The aim of implementing this was to alter the financial responsibility and authority of both purchasers and providers.

Although both these particular healthcare policy decisions have now been superseded, in the UK, and in almost every country, a clear distinction has been drawn between those who pay for or commission healthcare for populations or groups of patients and those who provide care, i.e. between the assessment of need in conjunction with the allocation of resources and the delivery of health services.

2. Purchasing or commissioning decisions

> Purchasing or commissioning is a process by which those responsible for expenditure on healthcare for a population or group of patients enter into a set of contracts with the providers of health services to obtain particular services at a specified level of quality and an agreed cost.

Purchasers or commissioners may be public bodies, such as a health authority, as is the case in the UK, or private organisations, such as insurance companies, as is the case in the Netherlands. (It should be noted that insurance companies in many countries are supported by the State, provided certain requirements have been met.) If finance is limited, purchasing is often linked to prioritisation (see Section 2.3).

(For a discussion of the difference between purchasing and commissioning, see Section 7.7.)

3. Management decisions

> Management is the process whereby the resources allocated to healthcare expenditure for a particular population or group of patients are utilised to best effect.

1.6 REALISING THE POTENTIAL OF EVIDENCE-BASED HEALTHCARE

The practice of evidence-based healthcare enables those managing a health service to determine the mix of services and procedures that will give the greatest benefit to the population served by that health service. However, there is no guarantee that any potential benefits identified within a research setting will be realised in practice, because one of the determinants of outcome is the quality of management. To ensure that a population/group of patients receives the maximum health benefit at the lowest possible risk and cost from the resources available, both evidence-based healthcare and quality management are essential practices (see Table 1.2).

Evidence-based healthcare + quality management = maximum health benefit at lowest risk and cost

Table 1.2 The responsibilities and concomitant skills necessary for healthcare managers to realise the potential of research findings

Managerial responsibility	Skills necessary
Offering only valuable services: ensure that all the services and procedures are supported by good-quality evidence that they do more good than harm	Technology assessment; critical appraisal
Getting the mix right: ensure that the mix of services and procedures provided is that which will give the greatest benefit for the population served	Needs assessment; priority setting; decision-making
Getting quality right: ensure that services and clinical practice are of sufficiently high quality to realise the potential for health improvement demonstrated in research settings	Professional education; public education; purchasing; quality management; clinical audit

1.7 STRATEGIC APPROACHES TO IMPLEMENTING EVIDENCE-BASED DECISION-MAKING IN HEALTHCARE SYSTEMS

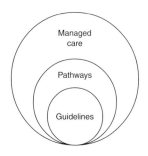

Margin Fig. 1.5

Several strategic approaches have been taken towards implementing evidence-based decision-making in healthcare systems (see Margin Fig. 1.5), including:

- the introduction of managed care – a high level approach which includes issues such as payment incentives and disincentives;
- the production of integrated care pathways;
- the development of clinical guidelines.

1.7.1 Managed care

In the past, it was possible to distinguish between two types of healthcare: clinical practice and public health (for the dichotomies between the two, see Table 1.3).

Table 1.3   The dichotomies between clinical practice and public health

Clinical practice	Public health
For individuals:	For populations:
Treatment for those who feel ill	Treatment of those who feel well
Low number needed to treat (NNT)	High NNT
Decisions unique to the individual	Decisions common to populations
Difficult to produce systems and guidelines	Easy to produce systems and guidelines
Paradigm problem: a patient who is feeling weak and tired	Paradigm problem: a population at risk of polio

Nowadays, however, this sharp distinction no longer obtains, as increasing effort is being invested into standardising care for patients who suffer from the same condition; this is known as managed care. Managed care lies between clinical practice and public health on the spectrum of healthcare (see Fig. 1.3).

Clinical care	Managed care	Public health

Fig. 1.3
The spectrum of healthcare provided to a population

In managed care, a systematic approach is taken to care management, whereby a predetermined care package is delivered to groups of patients who have certain common conditions for which it is possible to define a core set of interventions and services those suffering from the condition should receive. The application of managed care has sometimes resulted in a greater involvement of nurses in clinical decision-making, for example, when offering a point of primary contact or ensuring that a proposed referral to a specialist service is appropriate. This development has increased the need for care pathways in which the decision points are based on algorithms.

The trend towards the introduction of managed care is most marked in the USA,[1] where there is now a range of different approaches to regulating care. Indeed, in the USA, managed care has implications with respect to:

- the sources of funding for healthcare;
- the control of individual physicians;
- in cases where managed care is paid for by 'for-profit' health maintenance organisations, the amount of money made by those individuals who run such organisations at the expense of patients whose care is limited to provide those profits.

Kassirer, in his review of managed care and the morality of the market place, pointed out that transformation of the US healthcare system 'is producing corporate conglomerates with billions of dollars in assets that compensate their executives as grandly as basketball players'.[2] Patients and those who pay for healthcare are increasingly in direct conflict in the courts as patients challenge the right of payers to deny them treatment. These conflicts become highly charged when insurance companies or 'for-profit' health maintenance organisations are making very large profits.

At first sight, it may seem as if the introduction of managed care would counteract some of the vagaries in clinical practice and facilitate the introduction of evidence-based healthcare. However, although managed care has an important contribution to make, for instance, by reducing the duration of hospital stay or increasing the proportion of heart attack patients who are prescribed beta-blocker drugs, it should not be regarded as a universal panacea for healthcare problems for the following reasons.

- Some patients may present with conditions that will not allow them to be slotted into a managed care system.

- Patients whom it is theoretically possible to treat within a managed care system, because they are suffering from a disease such as diabetes or asthma, may have individual characteristics that make it difficult to apply the guidelines to all aspects of their care.
- The rigorous control of decision-making inherent in a managed care system may cause clinicians to become disaffected; as a consequence, they may perform less well in another sphere of clinical practice, such as communication with the patient.

The development of managed care does, however, offer important opportunities in the introduction of evidence-based healthcare because it allows those who pay for healthcare to be explicit about the interventions that should and should not be offered to patients.

1.7.2 Integrated care pathways

Integrated care pathways 'define the expected course of events in the care of a patient with a particular condition, within a set time-scale'.[3] Care pathways are structured according to time intervals during which specific goals and the progress expected are indicated, together with guidance on the optimal timing of appropriate investigations and treatment.[4] They are also known as:

- critical care paths;
- care maps;
- anticipated recovery paths.

Pathways are developed by members of a team involved in patient care. Multidisciplinary guidelines are used to develop and implement clinical plans that represent current local best practice for specific conditions.[5] Care pathways are a tool that can be used to facilitate the introduction of an evidence-based approach into routine clinical practice.

It is easier to introduce pathways for conditions in which there are established routines of practice and little variation among patients in the clinical course. Pathways have been produced for:

- hip and knee replacement;
- day case surgery;
- surgery for congenital heart disease;
- myocardial infarction;
- stroke;
- asthma;

- diabetes;
- leukaemia.

Although generic pathways can be constructed, any care pathway is usually unique to the particular institution in which it is developed because it will reflect details of care, which vary among institutions, and current practice.

There is evidence that the use of care pathways can improve outcome and thereby reduce the cost of healthcare. Holtzman et al.[6] investigated the effect of the introduction of care pathways on the length of stay and patient outcomes for two cohorts of patients undergoing renal transplantation, one of which received organs from cadavers ($n = 170$), the other from living donors ($n = 178$). After the development and implementation of a care pathway for those undergoing transplantation with organs from cadavers, it was found that:

- mean length of stay declined from 17.5 to 11.8 days ($P = 0.008$);
- the rate of complications fell from 38.1% to 14.8% ($P = 0.002$);
- the incidence of infection was reduced from 33.3% to 7.4% ($P < 0.001$).

However, the implementation of a care pathway for those undergoing transplantation with organs from living donors did not affect any of the outcomes or length of stay. Holtzman et al. identify three possible reasons that would explain the difference observed between the two cohorts.

1. The introduction of a care pathway for those undergoing renal transplantation using organs from cadavers did not confer any benefit – the improvements observed may have resulted from another, unknown, change.
2. The care pathway developed for those receiving kidneys from cadavers was superior to that for those receiving kidneys from living donors.
3. There was greater scope for improvement in the use of kidneys from cadavers which usually occurs in the context of unplanned emergency operations; in contrast, the use of a kidney from a living donor is usually carefully planned and organised.

Dowsey et al.[7] investigated the effectiveness of the use of care pathways for patients undergoing hip and knee arthroplasty. Patients were recruited over a two-year period, 92 being allocated to the intervention group and 71 being allocated to the control group (12 were excluded). For those patients in the intervention group, it was found that:

- mean length of stay was shorter (7.1 vs 8.6 days, $P = 0.011$);
- the readmission rate was lower (4.3% vs 13%, $P = 0.06$);
- the rate of complications was reduced (10.8% vs 28.1%, $P = 0.001$).

Dowsey et al. also concluded that the use of care pathways is 'an effective method of improving patient outcomes and decreasing the length of stay'.

The National Pathways Association, a UK organisation, has a website which is available at: http://www.thenpa.org.uk/

1.7.3 Clinical guidelines

Clinical guidelines can be defined as systematically developed statements to support healthcare professionals and patients when making decisions about the most appropriate healthcare in particular circumstances.

In the UK, within the NHS, the use of an evidence-based approach in general and of clinical guidelines in particular are viewed as ways to promote best practice; however, in the independent sector, guidelines are increasingly being used to authorise the type of care a patient should receive before it is given, or to contract with preferred providers.[8] The latter approach is a springboard for the introduction of managed care as in the USA.

Guidelines can be produced nationally or locally. The production of a set of guidelines should follow the well-established evidence about the factors determining success in development and implementation.[9] It is vital to obtain the best available evidence on which to develop clinical policy as expressed within guidelines or protocols (see Fig. 1.4) as opposed to justifying current practice post hoc. It is also important to ensure ownership of the guidelines by those professionals whom it is sought to influence.[10]

It is advisable not to 'import' or adopt guidelines, but rather to adapt them to local circumstances. Guidelines will be more effective on implementation if their development has involved all the relevant disciplines engaged in the care of a particular group of patients, including 'frontline staff' and the relevant managers.

Guidelines are more likely to be used if:

- a topic is chosen that clinicians believe to be important as opposed to well-researched areas of practice;
- acceptance is gained of the research evidence on which the guidelines are based;
- the implementation of the guidelines is linked to established audit groups (see Fig. 1.4).

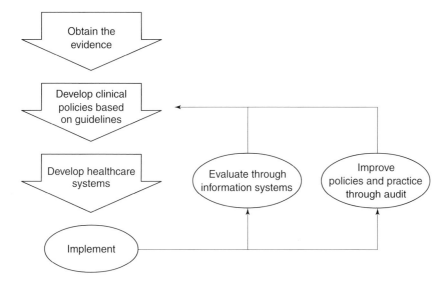

Fig. 1.4
From research to implementation and audit

1.7.3.1 Who's accountable for guidelines?

Gentle Reader,

Empathise with the relatives of people who were consumed by the Ravenous Bug-Eyed Monster of Traal. They tried to sue the publishers of the Hitch-Hiker's Guide to the Galaxy, *which claimed to be the definitive guide to the galaxy, because it contained a sentence that read 'The Ravenous Bug-Eyed Monster of Traal makes a good meal for visiting tourists', when the intention had been for it to read 'The Ravenous Bug-Eyed Monster of Traal makes a good meal of visiting tourists'.*

Commentary

In their defence, the publishers summoned a philosopher who claimed that the sentence as published was more beautiful than that originally intended and as beauty is truth then it was also true. The relatives' case collapsed.

When a clinician makes a decision, he or she is accountable for that decision, but when a doctor follows a guideline who is responsible when something goes wrong? At one point, it was thought that the introduction of guidelines would be followed by a wave of litigation directed at those who developed them, but this fear has never materialised. There is evidence, however, that guidelines can be used as evidence to defend clinicians in court, as well as to bring a case against them (see Section 7.10.3).

1.7.3.2   Clinical guidelines and the law

Ms Baxendale QC: *Some of the witnesses we have had have described these guidelines as a framework, within which to work ... Does that fit in with how you saw the guidelines?*

Lady Thatcher: *They are exactly what they say, guidelines, they are not the law. They are guidelines.*

Ms Baxendale QC: *Did they have to be followed?*

Lady Thatcher: *Of course they have to be followed, but they are not strict law. That is why they are guidelines and not law and, of course, they have to be applied according to the relevant circumstances.*

Ms Baxendale QC: *They are expected to be followed?*

Lady Thatcher: *Of course they have to be followed. They need to be followed for what they are, guidelines.*

> *Cross-examination of Lady Thatcher during the Scott Enquiry into the Arms for Iraq Affair quoted in Hurwitz*[11]

In a very important book, Brian Hurwitz reviewed the evidence available in 1998 about the relationship between clinical guidelines and the law,[11] and considered the legal status of clinical guidelines in negligence case law. The main principle Hurwitz defined is that any doctor acting *outside* the guideline could expose him- or herself to the possibility of being found negligent unless able to provide a specific justification why they had done so. Hurwitz's opinion is that 'In the UK, it is unlikely that authors or sponsors of faulty guidelines would be held liable for patient injury', principally because the court would expect the treating clinician to use appropriate discretion and judgement. This conclusion, however, emphasises the importance of developing good-quality guidelines.

1.7.3.3   Negligent authoring

There is increasing concern about the quality, reliability, and independence of practice guidelines. Grilli et al.[12] undertook a survey of practice guidelines that had been developed by specialty societies and published in English over a 10-year period from January 1988 to July 1998. Overall, 431 guidelines were identified through a search of MEDLINE that were considered eligible for the study. The quality of these guidelines was assessed against three criteria. The authors found that:

- for 67% of them, there was no description of the type of stakeholders involved in the production of the guideline;
- in 88% of cases, there was no information on the search strategy used to find evidence;
- in 82%, there was no explicit grading of the strength of the recommendations.

As commissioners and payers for healthcare promote the use of guidelines, great care must be exercised to ensure that is not replaced by what they believe to be negligent clinical practice with negligently prepared guidelines. It is also important to bear in mind that even when guidelines have been prepared to a high quality, they are valid only up until the point in time when they were sent to the printer.

1.7.3.4   Coping with the new Tower of Babel

Gentle Reader,

Empathise with Dr Hibble, one of the principals at the Sheep Market Surgery in Stamford, reputed to be the least changed town in England and frequently used for filming costume dramas. Despite the visions this conjures of an Arcadian past, in which sheep and their shepherds roamed the wolds, Dr Hibble's general practice epitomises modern healthcare at its best, utilising the power and potential of telecommunications while retaining the personal service valued by patients.

Commentary

Dr Hibble's situation sounds idyllic, but a blot on his landscape is the new Tower of Babel – i.e. the number of guidelines being sent to general practices. To determine the extent of the problem, Dr Hibble initiated a survey of 22 urban and rural general practices in Cambridge and Huntingdon Health Authority to unearth all the guidelines that had been retained for use. The results were astounding: a total of 855 guidelines weighing 28 kg were found.[13]

Hibble et al.[13] analysed various aspects of the 855 guidelines and found:

- the rate of increase in guideline production appeared to be exponential since 1989 (Fig. 1.5);
- 40% were produced nationally – of the 60% produced locally, 30% of them were produced by GPs, 50% by NHS Trusts; the local health authority had produced only 4%;
- 38% were undated;
- 75% covered clinical or disease management, and 12.5% related to referral pathways;
- the number of pages taken up by the text varied from 1 ($n = 243$), 2 ($n = 195$) to >10 ($n = 160$), including 25 presented as booklets or large folders.

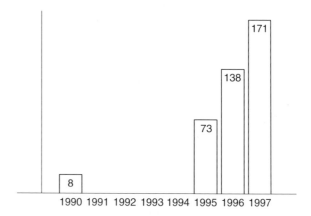

Fig. 1.5
The exponential increase in the production of guidelines for general practice. The figure for 1997 (171) is an estimate based on the finding that 57 were retained for use during the first third of that year. (Source: adapted from Hibble et al.[13])

In an observational study to determine which attributes of nationally produced clinical guidelines ($n = 10$) influence the use of guidelines during decision-making in general practice in the Netherlands, Grol et al.[14] found that overall recommendations were followed in 61% of decisions (7915/12 880). However, when the decisions were analysed in relation to specific guideline attributes, they found:

- controversial recommendations were followed in 35% of decisions (886/2947) whereas non-controversial recommendations were followed in 68% of decisions (7029/10 383);
- vague and non-specific recommendations were followed in 36% of decisions (826/2280) and clear recommendations in 67% (7089/10 600);
- recommendations that required a change in existing practice routines were followed in 44% of decisions (1278/2912) whereas those that did not were followed in 67% (6637/9968);
- recommendations based on research evidence were followed in 71% of decisions (2745/3841) whereas recommendations not based on research evidence were followed in 57% (5170/9039).

From these results, it would appear that evidence-based clinical guidelines are more likely to be used in clinical decision-making. However, other attributes of guidelines are also important and should be borne in mind by those who produce and disseminate them.

References

1. SWARTZ, K. and BRENNAN, T.A. (1996) *Integrated health care, capitated payment, and quality: the role of regulation.* Ann. Intern. Med. 124: 442–8.
2. KASSIRER, J.P. (1995) *Managed care and the morality of the marketplace [Editorial].* N. Engl. J. Med. 333: 50–2.
3. KITCHINER, D., DAVIDSON, D. and BUNDRED, P. (1996) *Integrated Care Pathways: effective tools for continuous evaluation of clinical practice.* J. Eval. Clin. Pract. 2: 65–9.
4. COFFEY, R.J., RICHARDS, J.S., REMMERT, C.S., LEROY, S.S., SCHOVILLE, R.R. and BALDWIN, P.J. (1992) *An introduction to critical paths.* Quality Management in Healthcare 1: 45–54.
5. KITCHINER, D. and BUNDRED, P. (1996) *Integrated care pathways.* Arch. Dis. Child. 75: 166–8.
6. HOLTZMAN, J., BJERKE, T. and KANE, R. (1998) *The effects of clinical pathways for renal transplantation on patient outcomes and length of stay.* Med. Care 36: 826–34.
7. DOWSEY, M.M., KILGOUR, M.L., SANATAMARIA, N.M. and CHOONG, P.F.M. (1999) *Clinical pathways in hip and knee arthroplasty: a prospective randomised controlled study.* Med. J. Aust. 170: 59–62.
8. FAIRFIELD, G. and WILLIAMS, R. (1996) *Clinical guidelines in the independent health care sector: An opportunity for the NHS to observe managed care in action [Editorial].* Br. Med. J. 312: 1554–5.
9. NHS CENTRE FOR REVIEWS AND DISSEMINATION and NUFFIELD INSTITUTE FOR HEALTH (1995) *Implementing Clinical Practice Guidelines.* Effective Health Care Bulletin No. 8, University of Leeds, Leeds.
10. GRIMSHAW, J.M. and RUSSELL, I.T. (1993) *Effect of clinical guidelines on medical practice: a systematic review of rigorous evaluations.* Lancet 342: 1317–22.
11. HURWITZ, B. (1998) *Clinical Guidelines and the Law: Negligence, Discretion and Judgement.* Radcliffe Medical Press, Abingdon, UK.

12. GRILLI, R., MAGRINI, N., PENNA, A., MURA, G. and LIBERATI, A. (2000) *Practice guidelines developed by specialty societies: the need for a critical appraisal.* Lancet 355: 103–6.
13. HIBBLE, A., KANKA, D., PENCHEON, D. and POOLES, F. (1998) *Guidelines in general practice: the new Tower of Babel.* Br. Med. J. 317: 862–3.
14. GROL, R., DALHUIJSEN, J., THOMAS, S., in t'VELD, C., RUTTEN, E. and MOKKINK, H. (1998) *Attributes of clinical practice guidelines that influence use of guidelines in general practice: observational study.* Br. Med. J. 317: 858–61.

1.8 EVIDENCE-BASED HEALTHCARE AND PROFESSIONAL LIBERTY

One of the fears of those in the medical profession is that evidence-based healthcare will be used as a means of removing individual professional liberty. This debate is most lively in the USA in response to the greater degree of control exerted there, but it is also beginning to be joined in other countries as different techniques, such as integrated care pathways, are introduced by those who manage or purchase healthcare.[1]

Although opportunities to influence the delivery of healthcare are tempting, their realisation must be tempered with the knowledge that most clinical decisions cannot be governed by strict rules; guidelines must remain as guidelines. The introduction of managed care is undoubtedly changing the role of the physician,[2] and although change is necessary it is vital that one of the most important, but under-valued and under-evaluated, aspects of medical care – the bond between clinician and patient – is not disrupted.

References

1. PEARSON, S.D., GOULART-FISHER, D. and LEE, T.H. (1995) *Critical pathways as a strategy for improving care: problems and potential.* Ann. Intern. Med. 123: 941–949.
2. SELKER, H.P. (1996) *Capitated payment for medical care and the role of the physician [Editorial].* Ann. Intern. Med. 124: 449–51.

1.9 THE LIMITS OF HEALTHCARE IN IMPROVING HEALTH

… three of the seven years' increase in life-expectancy since 1950 can be attributed to medical care. Medical care is also estimated to provide on average five years of partial or complete relief from the poor quality of life associated with chronic disease.

Bunker 1995[1]

1.9.1 Improving the health of populations

The best healthcare is that:

- from which, based on the best evidence available, all ineffective interventions have been eliminated;
- in which the interventions undertaken are of the highest possible effectiveness for those groups of patients within the population most likely to benefit;
- in which all services are delivered at the highest possible quality.

However, the health of a population is determined by four factors (see Margin Fig. 1.6), only one of which is healthcare. The other three factors are:

- physical and biological environment;
- social environment and lifestyle;
- genetics – an individual's genotype may confer a degree of protection or susceptibility to factors in the environment, whether physical or social, that trigger disease.

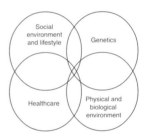

Margin Fig. 1.6

Thus, even the provision of the best healthcare will not necessarily ensure optimum levels of health in a population.

1.9.2 Improving the health of individual patients

Sick individuals present to clinicians with complicated problems which require an appreciation of the relationship between disease and illness.

The terms 'disease' and 'illness' are sometimes used interchangeably, but they have distinct meanings, as the definitions in the *Shorter Oxford English Dictionary* demonstrate.

- '**Disease:** a condition of the body, or of some part or organ of the body, in which its functions are disturbed or deranged.'
- '**Illness:** bad or unhealthy condition of the body (or, formerly, of a part); the condition of being ill.'
  A disease is a condition from which an individual suffers, like tuberculosis; an illness is a state of being, in which the individual enjoys the privileges of illness but must obey certain rules (see Table 1.4).

Table 1.4   The privileges and rules of illness

Privileges	Rules
Being excused normal social duties	The patient must be seen to be trying to get better
Extra sympathy and attention	The patient must give up many normal social pleasures, e.g. going out to parties

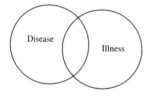

Margin Fig. 1.7

The relationship between disease and illness is best shown in a Venn diagram (see Margin Fig. 1.7). Most people who have a disease are also ill, although the degree to which any individual claims the privileges of illness varies considerably from one person to another.

1.9.2.1   Disease without illness

Some people have a disease but are not ill: an individual with undiagnosed diabetes has a disease but is unaware of the change in social status that will pertain when the diagnosis is known. Some people who have a disease do not wish to be ill or to be treated in a special way, for example, people who have disabilities do not wish to be discriminated against simply because of a disability resulting from disease.

1.9.2.2   Illness without disease

Some people feel ill but no causal disease can be found to explain their symptoms. This type of disorder has two common manifestations:

1. medically unexplained physical symptoms (MUPS), sometimes called somatoform disorders or somatisation, usually manifest as pain of various types;
2. hypochondriasis or excessive anxiety about a disease, usually cancer.

These disorders are very common. One estimate is that about half of all new referrals attending a general medical outpatient clinic have MUPS.[2] MUPS are reactions to various forms of external strain which may occur:

- as an alternative to constructive adaptive behaviour that will remove or reduce the causal strain;
- as an unproductive substitute for effective coping, as shown in Fig. 1.6.

There is, however, important evidence that MUPS can be treated effectively with cognitive therapy.[3] Indeed, as the pressure on resources increases, it will be necessary to treat this large group of patients in a more systematic manner. At present, a woman who presents with pelvic pain may be referred to as many as three different clinics and be subject to various investigations on separate occasions by doctors in training in different specialties in an attempt to cure the pain. In an RCT, Speckens et al.[3] evaluated the effect of additional cognitive behavioural therapy for patients with MUPS over optimised medical care. They found that the intervention group experienced a higher recovery rate at 6 months than the control subjects. This research is important: it shows that it is possible to apply the

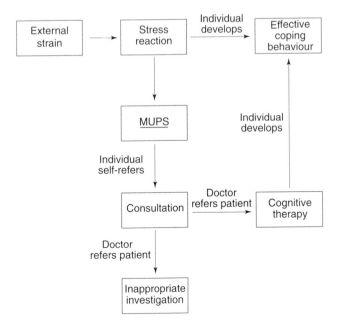

Fig. 1.6
Reactions to external strain

methodology of an RCT to such subtle and complex problems as MUPS.

Barsky and Borus, authors of a paper on somatisation and medicalisation in the era of managed care,[4] argue that the rate of presentation of MUPS in the USA will increase as managed care becomes more widespread. It is encouraging to note that some of the factors these authors identified as leading to increased referral rates are not relevant in the UK, where there has been a form of managed care, namely, capitation-based general practice, since the inception of the NHS. Nonetheless, MUPS is a common problem in primary care, and its prevalence may increase as society enters the post-modern era (see Epilogue).

The application of knowledge alone cannot solve all health problems, but without knowledge subtle disorders such as MUPS and subtle concepts such as the distinction between disease and illness will be overlooked in the drive towards increasing investment in medical technology to produce, at best, progressively less benefit or, at worst, more harm than good.

References

1. BUNKER, J.P. (1995) *Medicine matters after all.* J. Roy. Coll. Phys. Lond. 29: 105–12.
2. van HEMERT, A.M., HENGEVELD, M.W., BOLK, J.H. et al. (1993) *Psychiatric disorders in relation to medical illness among patients of a general medical out-patient clinic.* Psychol. Med. 23: 167–73.
3. SPECKENS, A.E.M., van HEMERT, A.M., SPINHOVEN, P. et al. (1995) *Cognitive behavioural therapy for medically unexplained physical symptoms: a randomised controlled trial.* Br. Med. J. 311: 1328–32.
4. BARSKY, A.J. and BORUS, J.F. (1995) *Somatization and medicalization in the era of managed care.* JAMA 274: 1931–4.

1.10 THE LINGUISTICS OF AN EVIDENCE-BASED APPROACH

In the UK and other countries in which English is the first language, one of the connotations of the term 'evidence' is that the information used is the product of research; evidence-based propositions therefore are those that can be supported by good-quality research, and contrast with propositions that depend only on the beliefs or intuition of the person making the proposition. One implication of evidence-based decision-making is that the decision-maker is being scientific and orientated towards applying the findings from research.

In other languages, however, the word 'evidence' – 'Evidenz' in German, 'evidencia' in Spanish or Italian – has a different connotation. The use of the term implies what in the UK would be understood as 'self-evident'. It is self-evident that night follows the day; no research is needed, no critical appraisal is required. As such, the promotion of 'evidence'-based medicine would be interpreted as the promotion of the traditional style of decision-making in which a decision-maker assumes that the proposition on which a decision is based is true because it is self-evident, and does not invite or require critical appraisal and evaluation.

In Italy, therefore, 'evidence-based medicine' has been translated as 'medicine based on proof of efficacy'. In German, the closest translation of 'evidence-based medicine' would be 'critische medizin' or 'critical medicine', but those who were involved in discussing the concept at the early workshops decided to adopt the term 'Evidenz Basiert Medizin', thereby boldly changing the German language.

Gentle Reader,

Empathise with the purchaser. He felt gutted. He had read with dismay the business case that the acute hospital Trust had put together to support the acquisition of spiral computed tomography (CT) which had revenue consequences of about £500 000 a year for several years. How could they? They knew their main purchaser faced a financial problem – a matter of a few millions. The Trust itself had a financial gap to close between their prices and the purchaser's position. Purchaser and provider had been discussing this gap 'maturely' for weeks, or so the purchaser thought, but of spiral CT nary a mention. Now it pops up like a jack-in-a-bloody-box.

Gentle Reader,

Empathise with the provider. She felt gutted. The purchaser had said they couldn't support the acquisition of new spiral CT kit. It was standard now; every Trust had it. They would be virtually the only Trust without it, and the business case was good. When compared with ordinary CT, the images are more accurate, disease can be diagnosed earlier and the scanning time is much faster, which makes it more acceptable to patients. It would increase the productivity of the Trust, and reduce waiting times; surely the purchaser had been demanding all these things from them for months. Now they turn round and say it's no go.

Commentary

The prologue presents a seemingly intractable situation of irreconcilable differences. To resolve the conflict, both parties need to find and appraise the evidence on which claim and counter-claim are based and then discuss the quality of the evidence, the size of the effect suggested by that evidence, and the applicability of those research findings to the population being served. This approach will be increasingly required as those who make decisions are subject to increasing pressure to 'do the right things right'.

CHAPTER 2

'DOING THE RIGHT THINGS RIGHT'

2.1 THE GROWING NEED FOR EVIDENCE-BASED HEALTHCARE

Jargon soup
- value for money
- reasonable cost

The need and the demand for healthcare are increasing. In almost every country, the rate of growth of both need and demand for healthcare is faster than the rate of increase in the resources available for providing it. There are four main reasons for this:

- population ageing;
- new technology and new knowledge;
- patient expectations;
- professional expectations.

The interaction of these factors is shown in Fig. 2.1.

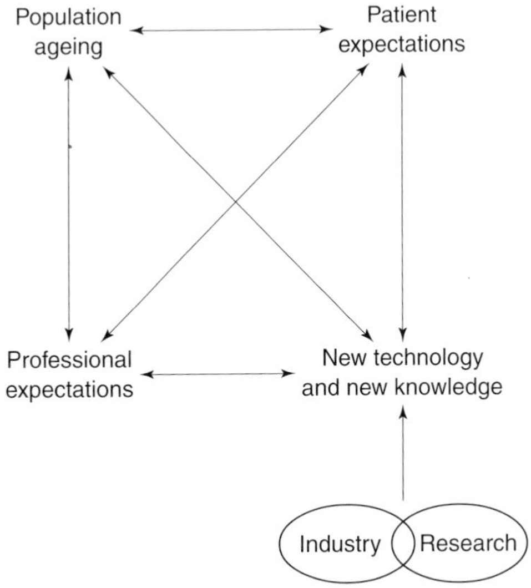

Fig. 2.1
The interaction of the four main factors that increase the need and demand for healthcare

2.1.1   Population ageing

Population ageing is the single most important factor increasing the need for healthcare. As the number of older people increases, so does the need for healthcare.

In addition, the interaction of an ageing population and rising patient expectations is significant. Cohorts of individuals currently approaching old age will have different expectations from those who are already old. In future, older people will be better organised, more assertive and have higher expectations of the quality of life that they wish to enjoy (75-year-olds will not accept chest pain as an inevitable consequence of biological ageing) and of the quality and volume of health services to which they feel entitled.

An ageing population will also have an impact on professional expectations and behaviour (see Section 2.1.4). Furthermore, professionals in some specialties may have to alter their orientation to reflect the changing demography and need for healthcare services. In dentistry, for example, the care of older people will become a major source of work.

Developments in new technology will also be influenced by population ageing. It is misguided to think of 'care of the elderly' and 'high-technology medicine' as mutually exclusive or alternatives competing for funding. Many new technological developments are beneficial to older people and will be used by them, for example, radiotherapy treatment for cancer. Consequently, the impact and cost of population ageing must be considered not only in the context of geriatric or social services but also in relation to the effects these factors will have on services using new and expensive technology. For example, coronary artery bypass grafting is a 'high-technology' intervention that is now commonly performed in older age-groups, and the average age of people receiving their first or follow-up grafts is increasing. Thus, the growing number of older people will mean an increase in the demand for coronary artery bypass grafting, irrespective of the trends in the incidence and prevalence of coronary heart disease.

2.1.2   New technology and new knowledge

The healthcare industry and those researchers working in health, health services and related disciplines will continue to develop new technologies. The nature of the technology may be 'high' – for instance, the development of biomaterials, sophisticated fundamental research on the human genome, or the development of computer systems, or a combination of all three – or 'low', such as effective simple interventions to prevent postnatal depression. Such research indicates what it is possible to achieve, which then influences both patient and professional expectations.

Moreover, *effective* new technology increases the need for healthcare, if 'need' is defined as a health problem for which there is an effective intervention. Once an effective intervention has been developed, a previously insoluble problem becomes transformed into a health need for which there is a consequent claim on resources. The knowledge that such an effective intervention exists leads to public and professional demand for that service to be provided. If a misleading impression of effectiveness is given, this may precipitate inappropriate demand. For example, the discovery of specific genes for the development of breast cancer has stimulated a demand for counselling services, but as yet there is no evidence to show that a woman's awareness of carrying a breast cancer gene or genes is beneficial unless that woman is willing to undergo bilateral mastectomy.

Sometimes, the application of a new technology will result in lower healthcare costs, or lower costs elsewhere in the economy, but even if healthcare costs are ultimately reduced by the use of a new technology there is often an increase in cost in the short term.

2.1.3 Patient expectations

Patient expectations of healthcare are rising, reflecting a societal change in attitude towards the provision of goods and services, a trend usually called 'consumerism'.

In most developed countries, the trend towards consumerism includes rising expectations of:

- the accessibility of health services;
- the quality of health services;
- the accountability of service providers, should there be any failure or perceived failure in the quality of healthcare.

There is general acceptance that the enjoyment of good health is a desirable and achievable objective; thus, if people have an expectation that their health should be better than it is, they will seek out services they believe will improve their health.

Changing attitudes in those approaching old age will mean that the sector of society which has the greatest need for healthcare will also make more demands in the future than it has in the past.

Rising patient expectations are also fuelled by the development of new technology.

2.1.4 Professional expectations

Professional expectations and attitudes are influenced by patient expectations. If patients who are 90 years old seek hip replacements, this will affect professional attitudes and expectations about the services that should be offered. Changing patient expectations about healthcare and the quality of healthcare can also influence professional attitudes and behaviour in a negative way: the threat of litigation may precipitate an increase in the practice of 'defensive medicine'.

Professional expectations are also influenced by developments in technology in that any new developments serve as a stimulus to increase expectations. Two important managerial challenges for the future are:

- to help professionals be more critical in their appraisal of new technology;
- to change the paradigm of healthcare such that a large proportion of the interventions offered to the population are those that have been shown by the performance of good-quality research to be effective.

2.1.5 The limits to demand for healthcare

In a recent article, Frankel et al.[1] have challenged the 'conventional assumptions' of an imbalance between demand and supply for healthcare in the UK, and argue that these assumptions are not supported by the evidence. They also challenge the 'pessimism' about future demands for healthcare arising from an ageing population, the costs of innovation, and rising public expectations, and state that these predictions are unsupported by good evidence. They suggest that perceived deficiencies in healthcare can be attributed to other factors such as the unwillingness of the public to accept the limits of effectiveness, and the self-interest of professionals. In conclusion, they propose that the limits to demand for key categories of healthcare lie within the capacity of a properly resourced NHS. A few months after this paper was published, the NHS Plan appeared (see Section 7.9.4.1), which provides an opportunity to test whether the arguments put forward by Frankel et al. are correct.

Reference
1. FRANKEL, S., EBRAHIM, S. and SMITH, G.D. (2000) *The limits to demand for health care.* Br. Med. J. 321: 40–5.

2.2 THE EVOLUTION OF EVIDENCE-BASED HEALTHCARE

The stages in the evolution of evidence-based healthcare from the early 1970s to the present day are described below and shown schematically in Fig. 2.2. During the 1970s and 1980s, the emphasis in the reform of health services or healthcare systems was on making structural changes or changes to the ways in which the systems were financed – 'doing things cheaper' (Section 2.2.1), 'doing things better' (Section 2.2.2) and 'doing things right' (Section 2.2.3).

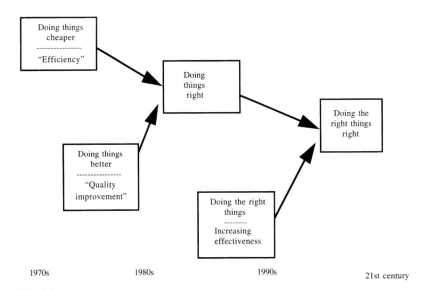

Fig. 2.2
The evolution of evidence-based healthcare

However, although structural reform is necessary, the impact it has is limited to:

- controlling the rate of cost increase;
- increasing productivity;
- increasing the quality of healthcare.

In order to gain the maximum value from the resources allocated to healthcare, it is necessary to 'do the right things' (Section 2.2.4) which requires a change in the way decisions within the health service are made.

2.2.1 Doing things cheaper

During the 1970s, financial pressure began to mount in the NHS after two decades during which investment in healthcare had increased steadily. The OPEC crisis and its financial consequences initiated an era in which healthcare decision-makers became more cost conscious. They were exhorted to increase efficiency, although this was actually manifest as an increase in productivity.

- **Productivity** is the relationship between inputs and outputs: number of bed days (therefore, the money necessary) per operation.
- **Efficiency** is the relationship between inputs and outcomes: number of bed days (therefore, the money necessary) to obtain 1 extra year of life.

Unfortunately, the two words are often used as if they were synonymous (see Section 6.7.1.1).

The impetus to increase efficiency was to reduce cost per case by ensuring that healthcare was delivered:

- for the shortest time;
- in the least expensive place;
- by the least expensive professional;
- using the cheapest possible drugs or equipment to provide an acceptable level of effectiveness and of safety.

2.2.2 Doing things better

During the 1980s, although the demand for increased efficiency was maintained, there was a new imperative, that of delivering quality improvement. As patients became better informed, more assertive and better organised, their expectations increased. Patients expected:

- easier access to services;

- more effective healthcare;
- safer care;
- more information;
- better communication.

These expectations for the provision of better healthcare reflected the general societal trend towards 'consumerism' (Section 2.1.3). The response within health services was 'to do things better' using the tools of quality assurance and clinical audit.

2.2.3 Doing things right

Doing things cheaper + Doing things better = Doing things right

During the 1970s and 1980s, health service managers concentrated on 'doing things right', a combination of focusing on cost, i.e. 'doing things cheaper', and quality, i.e. 'doing things better'. Indeed, a great deal of attention and money was invested to ensure that clinicians 'do things right', by encouraging the performance of clinical audit, for instance. Unfortunately, 'doing things right' is only one side of the old management adage; the other is 'doing the right things'.

2.2.4 Doing the right things

In the past, healthcare managers tended to leave 'doing the right things' to other forces such as commercial pressure and chance. During the 1990s, this position was no longer tenable, especially as clinicians do not necessarily always 'do the right things'. In the provision of healthcare, the overall objective is to do more good than harm. However, it is important to be mindful in this situation that virtually all interventions have the potential to harm, especially when those who champion the introduction of an innovation tend to emphasise the probability of benefit rather than that of harm occurring.

The interventions delivered within a health service can be categorised into three types according to their effect on patients:

1. doing more good than harm;
2. doing more harm than good;
3. of unknown effect or unproven efficacy.

The phrase 'more good than harm' encompasses four important concepts, three of which are embodied in the individual words whereas the fourth is unwritten:

'good' – in this context, the word implies effectiveness but also includes safety and acceptability (see Sections 6.5 and 6.6);

'harm' – this outcome of care should always be sought by decision-makers. The champions of a new service or intervention usually focus on the good the innovation will do, rather than the harm. Even when the possibility of harm is acknowledged, healthcare professionals may place a lower value on harm than the potential recipients of an intervention (see Section 10.3.1.2);

'more' – although the definition of 'more' may be self-evident, the *magnitude* of any difference described by the term is as important as the existence of a difference. The magnitude of any difference between the balance of good and harm observed in a research setting and the balance of good and harm in an ordinary service setting is determined by two main factors:

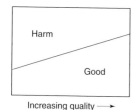

Margin Fig. 2.1

- the efficacy of the intervention as administered by the best hands in a research setting;
- the quality of the service in which the intervention is actually delivered (see Table 2.1 and Margin Fig. 2.1).

The degree of efficacy achieved in a research setting may not necessarily be reproducible in an ordinary service setting because the skills of the local healthcare professionals may not be of the same order as those of the researchers.

Table 2.1 The relationship between quality of service and the balance of good and harm conferred by an intervention

Quality of service	Balance
Very high	Good much greater than harm
Average	Good greater than harm
Below average	Good and harm equally balanced
Very low	Harm greater than good

The unwritten factor in this phrase is the **strength of the evidence**, which is determined by the quality of the research on which the evidence is based (see Chapter 5). The proposition that a therapy or test does more good than harm should be discarded if it is only an expression of personal opinion, but it should be used as evidence if it is a conclusion drawn from the conduct of high-quality research, the results of which showed that the intervention made a substantial difference with a low probability that the results were due to chance or biased findings.

Once the balance of good to harm has been established, decision-makers then need information on the costs of different options. This is because those interventions that do more good than harm can be subdivided into:

- those that do so at an affordable cost;
- those that do so at an unaffordable cost.

2.2.5 Doing the right things right

For all healthcare professionals, but particularly clinicians, the important question to address at the beginning of the 21st century is not simply 'Are we doing things right?' or 'Are we doing the right things?' but:

'Are we doing the right things right?'

The need to do the right things right sets a new management agenda (see Section 2.4).

2.3 DECISION RULES FOR RESOURCE ALLOCATION

In tandem with the evolution of evidence-based healthcare and the development of a new management agenda, the parameters used as a basis for decision-making about resource allocation have changed. A set of four decision rules for resource allocation[1] have been developed to illustrate the new paradigm.

Decision Rule I: The era of medical primacy

If resources are available, a healthcare intervention is provided, and thereby resources allocated, when a doctor is of the opinion that a particular intervention should be undertaken (see Margin Fig. 2.2).

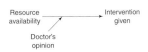

Margin Fig. 2.2

Decision Rule II: The era of effectiveness

If resources are available, a healthcare intervention is provided, and thereby resources allocated, if there is valid relevant evidence that a particular intervention will do more good than harm to a particular patient (see Margin Fig. 2.3).

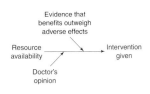

Margin Fig. 2.3

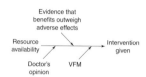

Margin Fig. 2.4

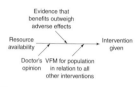

Margin Fig. 2.5

Decision Rule III: The era of cost-effectiveness

If resources are available, a healthcare intervention is provided, and thereby resources allocated, if there is valid relevant evidence that a particular intervention will do more good than harm to a particular patient *and* represents good value for money for the population (see Margin Fig. 2.4).

Decision Rule IV: The era of best value healthcare

If resources are available, a healthcare intervention is provided, and thereby resources allocated, if there is valid relevant evidence that a particular intervention will do more good than harm to a particular patient *and* represents value for money for the whole population in relation to all other interventions (see Margin Fig. 2.5).

Each of these decision rules can be described by a formula, all of which are given in Box 2.1.

Decision Rule I describes the situation that pertained 20–30 years ago in the health services of most countries when a healthcare intervention was provided on the basis of unsubstantiated opinion. Decision Rule II describes the situation that developed during the last decade when it was recognised that not all healthcare interventions confer a net benefit. Decision Rule III describes the situation that pertains at the beginning of the 21st century when it has been acknowledged that the resources for healthcare are finite and that cost and value for money must be considered in any system of resource allocation. Decision Rule IV describes the situation that is set to become the prevailing system of resource allocation in which those who pay for healthcare will require that interventions are provided only when their outcomes give greater benefits than any of the alternative uses of equivalent resources. The application of Decision Rule IV maximises value across a health service and provides a net benefit to the population as a whole, as opposed to maximising the benefit for each individual irrespective of cost (Decision Rule II).

Reference
1. HICKS, N.R. and GRAY, J.A.M. (1998) *Evidence-based Medicine*. Financial Times Healthcare, London.

Box 2.1 Formulae for describing the decision rules for resource allocation (Source: Hicks and Gray[1])

For all Decision Rules (I–IV):

$$Ralloc = \Sigma Iu + OH$$

        where   Ralloc = resources allocated

                      Iu = cost of intervention undertaken

                      OH = cost of overheads

Decision Rule I:

$$\Sigma Iu = \Sigma f(O.Ib{>}h) = Ravail$$

        where   O = doctor's opinion

                      b = benefit

                      h = harm

                      Ib>h = intervention confers net benefit

                      Ravail = resources available

Decision Rule II:

$$\Sigma Iu = \Sigma f(E.Ib{>}h) = Ravail$$

        where   E = evidence

Decision Rule III:

$$\Sigma Iu = \Sigma f(E.Ib{>}h.Ivfm) = Ravail$$

        where   vfm = value for money

                      Ivfm = intervention represents value for money

Decision Rule IV:

$$\Sigma Iu = \Sigma f(E.Ispecb{>}h > E.Iotherb{>}h) = Ravail$$

        where   Ispec = a specific intervention

                      Iother = all other interventions that could be

                      undertaken in that clinical situation

2.4 THE NEW MANAGEMENT AGENDA

The need to 'do the right things right' generates a new management agenda for those in any health service, the implementation of which requires an evidence-based approach, the focus of this book. However, few health service management texts or courses appear to address the specific context that pertains within a health service, namely, the nature of the provision of healthcare is driven not only by central policy-making but also by decentralised decision-making. Clinicians do make many of the decisions, thereby determining not only service provision but also resource expenditure (see Section 1.2). Given this context, it is of paramount importance that those who make decisions about healthcare provision base those decisions on good evidence, using as a framework the classification of healthcare interventions set out in Section 2.2.4 (see also Table 2.2).

The new management agenda for the delivery of health services comprises three main strategies:

- the initiation of strategies to increase the good:harm ratio (Table 2.2);
- the promotion of relevant research;
- the acceleration of change in clinical practice (see also Section 10.6).

Table 2.2 Strategies to increase the good:harm ratio in relation to the various types of intervention

Type of intervention	Strategies
Does more good than harm	• Promote use if it is affordable – starting starting right • Take steps to increase good and decrease harm to make ratio more favourable – quality improvement
Does more harm than good	• Stop them starting • Slow them starting • Start to stop them if it is not possible to increase good and decrease harm sufficiently to convert them into interventions that do more good than harm
Of unknown effect	• Stop them starting • Promote the conduct of RCTs both for new interventions and for interventions already in practice

In most health services operating today, the distribution of the various types of interventions administered probably follows the pattern shown in Fig. 2.3.

The *optimal* distribution of interventions administered is represented in Fig. 2.4.

Although quality improvement and cost reduction have been the imperatives in health service management since the 1980s, the other activities shown in Table 2.2, which will

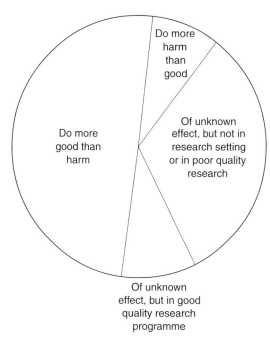

Fig. 2.3
Present distribution of the various types of intervention

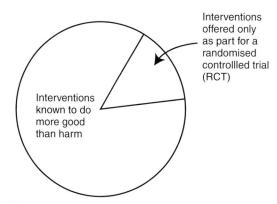

Fig. 2.4
Optimal distribution of interventions

have an influence on not only *how* clinicians practise but *what* they practise, are new items on the management agenda.

2.4.1 Strategies to increase the good:harm ratio

It may take years for an effective intervention to be described, much less promoted, in a textbook. The classic study of this phenomenon was conducted by Antman et al.[1] into the delay in recommending thrombolysis as an effective intervention following myocardial infarction (see Fig. 2.5). This example demonstrates that even when information is available, implementation is often slow and sporadic.

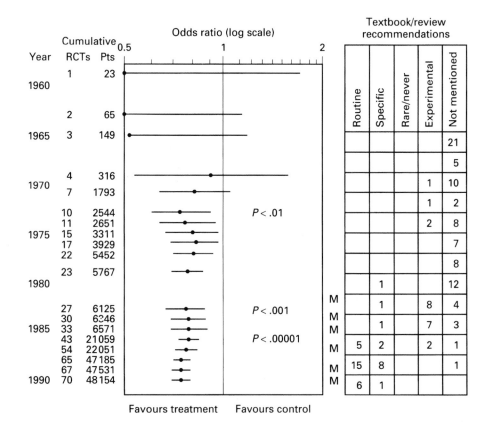

Fig. 2.5
Thrombolytic therapy: delay between evidence of effectiveness of the intervention becoming available and its inclusion in textbooks (Source: Antman et al,[1] Copyright 1992, American Medical Association)

A more pro-active approach to implementation is required to ensure that:

- patients are offered only those interventions that do more good than harm at reasonable cost;
- the right patients are offered those interventions;
- the interventions are delivered at a high standard.

As some of these management activities are new, managers need to combine several different approaches to ensure change takes place.

Some clinicians believe delay in implementation to be advantageous, often citing, as justification for their stance, the consequences of the administration of thalidomide as a hypnotic to pregnant women. However, the keys to control lie not in delaying the implementation of research findings but in the critical appraisal of the best research evidence available and sound decision-making based on that appraisal. In fact, the use of thalidomide is an example of the failure to base decisions on good evidence.

2.4.1.1 Starting starting right

If there is evidence that an intervention does more good than harm, and it is affordable, decision-makers must manage its introduction within the health service (see Section 7.7.3.1). This will require appropriate professional training, including communication skills, patient education to promote good decision-making, and the development of systems of care supported by quality standards and mechanisms for the detection and correction of quality failures. All these steps are necessary to ensure good clinical outcomes.

> Good clinical decision-making + good systems = good clinical outcomes

For example, to promote the use of aspirin as a treatment after acute myocardial infarction (AMI) the following approaches are required:

- public education about the benefits of aspirin after AMI;
- professional training, for instance, to promote the benefits of thrombolysis;
- changes in purchasing requirements, for instance, to specify in contracts the standard of delivery of

thrombolysis treatment expected for patients with AMI (door-to-needle time);
- audit, in which performance is measured against a specified standard.

2.4.1.2 Stopping starting and starting stopping

If interventions are doing more harm than good, decision-makers must ensure that either they are not introduced – 'stop them starting' – or, if they have already been introduced, that they are no longer practised – 'start stopping them'. However, starting stopping is much more difficult than stopping starting.

It is possible to stop an innovation completely and absolutely. For example, after consideration of the evidence on population screening for prostate cancer, the Department of Health in the UK issued guidance in 1997 that screening should *not* be introduced;[2] the guidance is shown in Box 2.2.

Similarly, the National Institute of Clinical Excellence (NICE) in the UK, in what was its first test since establishment in 1999, advised the Secretary of State for Health that Relenza, the new drug for the treatment of influenza, should *not* be prescribed. The Secretary of State stated that:

> In their own literature the company have acknowledged that they have as yet not a great deal of evidence of the impact of the drug on high risk groups, but there is more research under way. I believe that this decision is in the long term interests of patients, and NHS, and research based pharmaceutical companies.[3]

Indeed, a month earlier a Department of Health spokesperson had highlighted the need to increase the uptake of vaccination which is effective in high-risk groups in whom coverage is low.[4]

The decision-making process was described by Joe Collier, a member of the NICE rapid appraisal committee on Relenza, in the *Guardian* on 13 October 1999;[5] he pointed out that the drug had not been banned outright, and that the guidance to the service read 'should not' rather than 'must not'.[6] However, response to the guidance was mixed.

Richard Sykes, Chief Executive of Glaxo Welcome, said that this decision was a major blow to research-based pharmaceutical companies in the UK and that he would

Box 2.2 Population screening for prostate cancer (Source: EL(97)12[2])

Summary

1. Population screening for prostate cancer, including the use of prostate specific antigen (PSA) as a screening test, should not be provided by the NHS or offered to the public until there is new evidence of an effective screening technology for prostate cancer. Screening, for the purposes of this Executive Letter, is defined as the application of a test or inquiry to identify individuals at sufficient risk of a specific disorder to warrant medical attention on account of symptoms of that disorder (1).

Background

2. Two systematic reviews commissioned by the NHS Research and Development Health Technology Assessment Programme (2, 3) have concluded that current evidence does not support a national screening programme for prostate cancer in the United Kingdom.

3. Current screening technologies (including the PSA test) have a limited accuracy that could lead to a positive result for those without the disease. Follow up procedures could thus cause unnecessary harm to healthy individuals. The introduction of a prostatic cancer screening programme *at present* carries an unacceptable risk of more harm resulting than good.

4. The National Screening Committee has considered the evidence for introducing screening for prostate cancer and concluded that at this time and with current technology, there is no evidence of benefit resulting from population screening. This recommendation has been accepted by Department of Health Ministers.

5. Health Authority and General Practitioner Fund Holders are asked not to introduce or plan the purchase of population screening for prostate cancer until the National Screening Committee recommends an effective and reliable procedure.

6. This Executive Letter does not affect the clinical management of men presenting with symptoms of prostatic disease.

References

1. Adapted from: Wald NJ. Guidance on terminology. *Journal of Medical Screening 1994; 1: 76.*

2. Selley S, Donovan J, Faulkner A, Coast J, Gillatt D. Diagnosis, management and screening of early localised prostate cancer. *Health Technology Assessment 1997; 1: (2).*

3. Chamberlain J, Melia J, Moss S, Brown J. The diagnosis, management, treatment and costs of prostate cancer in England and Wales. *Health Technology Assessment 1997; 1 (3).*

resign from two Government Advisory Committees as a result. John Chisholm, Chairman of the British Medical Association's General Practitioners Committee, on the other hand, felt that the decision should have been given 'legislative force'; he favoured a complete ban (i.e. the use of the words 'must not') because it would make the position clear. He hoped that GPs would follow the guidance, but pointed out that 'the prospect remains of enormous patient demand' which might pose difficulties especially when trying to explain a decision not to prescribe to patients who request Relenza.[3]

The importance of stopping starting is heightened by the difficulty of starting stopping. Once an intervention is in routine use it can be very difficult to discontinue its use. The Cochrane Collaboration conducted a review of the effect of human albumin in critically ill patients.[7] The conclusion drawn was that:

> there is no evidence that albumin administration reduces mortality in critically ill patients with hypovolaemia, burns or hypoalbuminaemia, and a strong suggestion that it may increase mortality.[7]

This was published in the *British Medical Journal* of 25 July 1998. On 18 August that year, the Food and Drug Administration of the Department of Health and Human Services, USA, sent a letter to all doctors to draw their attention to the paper, to state that further research was needed, but

> the FDA urges treating physicians to exercise discretion in the use of albumin and plasma protein fraction based on their own assessment of these data.

The response in the UK to the findings of the review was slower and more hostile than that in the USA.

2.4.1.3 Slowing starting

Slowing starting may be a more readily achievable objective than starting stopping. For instance, the use of printed educational material may help to modify the prescribing habits of GPs. The results of a study in England showed that the distribution to all GPs in 1993 (at a total cost of £25 000) of an *Effective Health Care* bulletin in which the cost-effectiveness of prescribing selective serotonin reuptake inhibitors (SSRI) for the treatment of depression was questioned, potentially avoided about 138 000 person-years of SSRI treatment.[8] The acquisition cost of this SSRI treatment, which is more expensive than the conventional therapy of tricylic antidepressants, would have been nearly £40 million. Although the prescribing rate for SSRI did continue to increase, the rate of increase was less than that which would have occurred had the bulletin not been sent out.

2.4.2 Promoting relevant research

If an intervention is of unknown effect, it should not be introduced; if it is already in service, it should be withdrawn until its effects have been investigated within an RCT to determine the beneficial effects (Section 5.4) and within a case-control or cohort study to identify any adverse effects (Sections 5.5 and 5.6).

It is possible to promote the performance of trials by:

- creating a culture in which interventions of unknown effect have to be evaluated scientifically from the first patient;
- ensuring that those responsible for any health service invest in research and development.

However, there are two aspects to investing in research:

1. the investment required for the research itself;
2. the health service costs of the research – in the UK, the Department of Health identified 1.5% of the healthcare budget to cover such service costs, that is, the additional costs incurred by participating in multicentre RCTs funded by the Medical Research Council (MRC).

2.4.3 Managing the evolution of clinical practice

It is important to manage the introduction of any change in clinical practice; it is no longer sustainable to allow clinicians to make decisions about such changes in isolation. Although clinicians do implement changes in clinical practice that improve health, some of which will be achievable at a reasonable or reduced cost, they do not invariably choose 'the right things to do'. For example, during the 1980s, the surgical intervention laparoscopic cholecystectomy underwent rapid and widespread introduction in health services world-wide at the instigation of clinicians in the absence of good-quality evidence of its efficacy and despite concerns about its safety. The subsequent publication of the results of an RCT in which laparoscopic cholecystectomy was compared with conventional cholecystectomy showed there was no significant difference between the two study groups for hospital stay, time back to work for those employed, and time to full recovery, although laparoscopic cholecystectomy took significantly longer to perform.[9]

Sometimes changes to clinical practice can worsen outcomes overall; for instance, changes in the prescription of antibiotics have contributed to the genesis of a modern epidemic, the evolution of antibiotic-resistant bacteria, which has resulted not only in an increase in health service costs but also in mortality.

Until now, the evolution of clinical practice has been piecemeal, unco-ordinated, and driven by individual clinicians. This situation is no longer acceptable and those responsible for the management and funding of health services must develop a new relationship in which clinicians (collectively) and managers can work together to guide the course of the evolution of clinical practice. In the UK, this approach is being promoted with the introduction of clinical governance (see Section 10.4.4). Managing the evolution of clinical practice is probably the most challenging item on the new management agenda (see also Section 10.6).

References

1. ANTMAN, E.M., LAU, J., KUPELNICK, B. et al. (1992) *A comparison of results of meta-analysis of randomized control trials and recommendations of clinical experts.* JAMA 268: 240–8.
2. DEPARTMENT OF HEALTH (1997) *Population Screening for Prostate Cancer.* EL(97)12.
3. YAMEY, G. (1999) *Dobson backed NICE ruling on flu drug.* Br. Med. J. 319: 1024.
4. YAMEY, G. (1999) *Anti-flu drug may not reduce death rate.* Br. Med. J. 319: 659.
5. COLLIER, J. (1999) *Bonny bouncing baby.* The Guardian, Suppl., Wednesday 13 October, p. 9.
6. NATIONAL INSTITUTE FOR CLINICAL EXCELLENCE (2000) *Zanamivir (Relenza) guidance from NICE.* Available at: http://www.nice.org.uk/appraisals/rel_guide.htm *Fast Track Appraisal of Zanamivir (Relenza): Summary of Evidence.* Available at: http://www.nice.org.uk/appraisals/sum_evid.htm
7. COCHRANE INJURIES GROUP ALBUMIN REVIEWERS (1998) *Human albumin administration in critically ill patients: systematic review of randomised controlled trials.* Br. Med. J. 317: 235–40.
8. MASON, J., FREEMANTLE, N. and YOUNG, P. (1998/9) *The effect of the distribution of Effective Health Care Bulletins on prescribing selective serotonin reuptake inhibitors in primary care.* Health Trends 30: 120–2.
9. MAJEED, A.W., TROY, G., NICHOLL, J.P. et al. (1996) *Randomised, prospective, single-blind comparison of laparoscopic versus small-incision cholecystectomy.* Lancet 347: 989–94.

2.5 THE IMPACT OF SCIENCE ON CLINICAL PRACTICE AND HEALTHCARE COSTS

As a scientific approach to healthcare decision-making is championed in this book, it is appropriate to describe the impact that science, i.e. new technology and new knowledge, is having on clinical practice.

Sometimes, science may be put into practice by a well-considered national policy decision – for example, the introduction in the UK of breast cancer screening. However, most science is introduced into clinical practice by clinicians, who then seek the resources to fund the innovation from those who pay for the service to be delivered. The ways in which changes or innovations in clinical practice increase the cost of care are manifold (see Box 2.3).

Box 2.3 How innovations in clinical practice increase costs

- Treating conditions that were previously untreatable.
- Treating people who would previously have been untreated because of changing professional perceptions of need and appropriateness and changing public expectations. These may result from:
  - increasing safety of intervention;
  - more acceptable, less invasive, more pleasant interventions;
  - changing attitudes to chronological age as a reason for refusing treatment;
  - changing expectations about health and disease.
- Providing more expensive types of treatment:
  - more expensive drugs;
  - more expensive imaging;
  - more expensive tests;
  - more expensive staff.
- More intensive clinical practice:
  - longer duration of stay;
  - more tests per patient;
  - more professional interventions per patient;
  - more treatments per patient.

A study by Eddy in the USA showed that, in a healthcare system in which expenditure is not finite, changes in the 'volume and intensity' of clinical practice are the main factors driving increases in the cost of care that can be controlled by health service managers;[1] the other causes of increasing costs – population ageing, and medical and general price inflation – are beyond the power of health service managers to control (see Fig. 2.6). In other healthcare systems in which decisions are made within a context of finite resources, although expenditure does not spiral out of control, changes in the volume and intensity of clinical practice *will* generate financial and service pressures and can also drive the service in directions other than those that have been identified as priorities, for instance those on the new management agenda.

Reference
1. EDDY, D.M. (1993) *Three battles to watch in the 1990s.* JAMA 270: 520–6.

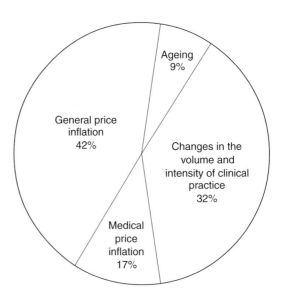

Fig. 2.6
Factors contributing to the increase in healthcare costs

2.6 EVIDENCE-BASED ALTRUISM

The need to control the costs of healthcare is accepted by all except the super-rich, and even they have an interest in controlling the cost of healthcare because of the effects that health insurance costs can have on corporate profitability and therefore on their super-richness. Furthermore, cost containment alone is not a policy that is likely to win friends or, even more important, votes. Those who are involved in cost containment have to accommodate two public desires (Fig. 2.7):

- the provision of high-quality healthcare;
- comprehensive coverage, that is, coverage of the whole population with a comprehensive range of services.

Different approaches to the control of healthcare costs have been used, often advocated on the basis of ideology:

- the free-market approach – it was anticipated that the market would have the capacity to control costs and improve quality, thereby allowing universal coverage to be offered, although perhaps there was an acceptance that coverage could not be assured in free-market healthcare;
- capitation – seen as the best way of controlling costs and ensuring comprehensive coverage. This approach was criticised by the free-market thinkers because of the effect it was claimed it would have on the quality of care.

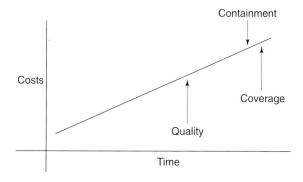

Fig. 2.7
Doing the right things right: achieving cost containment while providing good-quality healthcare and comprehensive coverage

2.6.1   Evidence of non-profit efficiency

One of the assertions made by those who believed that the free market could square the triangle depicted in Fig. 2.7 was that the involvement of highly skilled management personnel from the private sector would increase health service productivity and reduce costs. In a major study of the relationship between the type of ownership of a hospital and its Medicare spending,[1] Silverman et al. compared spending in 208 areas where all hospitals remained under 'for-profit' ownership during a six-year period with that in 2860 areas where all hospitals remained under 'not-for-profit' ownership. It was found that the rate per capita of Medicare spending and the increase in spending rate were greater in those areas served by for-profit hospitals when compared with those served by not-for-profit hospitals (Table 2.3).

Table 2.3   Adjusted total per capita Medicare spending in 'for-profit' and 'not-for-profit' hospitals (Source: Silverman et al.[1])

Year	For-profit	Not-for-profit	P value
1989	$4006	$3554	<0.001
1992	$4243	$3841	<0.001
1995	$5172	$4440	<0.001

In an accompanying editorial, it was stated that 'like blood, healthcare is too precious, intimate and corruptible to entrust to the market'.[2] This sentence makes reference to the classic study by Professor Titmuss on blood transfusion which, although published in 1971, remains as stimulating and relevant today as when it first appeared. Titmuss, one of the UK's great social policy thinkers in the second half of the 20th century, used evidence not only from economics but also from policy analysis to reach the conclusion that the best basis for funding a blood transfusion service was that of a gift and not that of a financial relationship.[3]

2.6.2   Quality of care under capitation schemes

In a review of the evidence about the relationship between capitation, a system of payment that allows cost containment, and comprehensive coverage, Berwick concluded that although 'capitation alone is only a weak instrument for improvement in the quality of care' it 'can encourage better decisions and facilitate the productive redesign of systems for the delivery of care'.[4]

References

1. SILVERMAN, E.M., SKINNER, J.S. and FISHER, E.S. (1999) *The association between for-profit hospital ownership and increased Medicare spending.* N. Engl. J. Med. 341: 420–6.
2. WOOLHANDLER, S. and HIMMELSTEIN, D.U. (1999) *When money is the mission – the high costs of investor-owned care [Editorial].* N. Engl. J. Med. 341: 444–6.
3. TITMUSS, R.M. (1971) *The Gift Relationship: From Human Blood to Social Policy.* Pantheon Books, New York.
4. BERWICK, D.M. (1996) *Quality of health care, Part 5: Payment by capitation and the quality of care.* N. Engl. J. Med. 335: 1227–31.

2.7   WHO CARRIES THE CAN?

As need and demand for healthcare outstrip resources, and patient expectations rise, an increase in the number of complaints about the limitations of healthcare is to be anticipated. At present, much of the opprobrium falls on clinicians; in future, it may be appropriate to give guidance to disaffected people about who should receive complaints concerning particular aspects of the provision of health services, that is, who should carry the can (Box 2.4).

Box 2.4   Checklist of who should carry the can in the UK

If concerned about a shortage of resources affecting either yourself or a member of your family, work through the questions below to identify who should carry the can.

- Has the government decided to limit the amount of resources available for public services? *Write to the Chancellor of the Exchequer.*
- Of the money allocated to public services, is insufficient going to health? *Write to the Prime Minister.*
- Of the money allocated to health, is insufficient allocated to the population in which you live? *Write to the Minister responsible for health services and ask that the formula used to distribute money geographically be reviewed.*
- Of the money allocated to your population, is insufficient allocated to people with your type of health problem? *Write to the insurance company or health authority responsible for allocating resources for the population in which you live.*
- Of the money allocated to people with your type of health problem, is insufficient being allocated to people with your particular diagnosis? *Write to the Chief Executive of the NHS Trust responsible for your service.*
- Is the clinician giving you insufficient time and resources? *Write to the clinician.*

DEFINING OUR TERMS: VALUE FOR MONEY (BANGS PER BUCK)

The value for money (VFM) of a health service can be measured directly by assessing the number of beneficial outcomes for the resources invested. In practice, value for money can be assessed by looking at the mix of services provided.

The factors that increase or decrease value for money are shown in Table 2.4.

Table 2.4   Factors influencing value for money (VFM)

Factors that increase VFM	Factors that decrease VFM
High productivity	Low productivity
Effective interventions	Ineffective interventions
Effective interventions that can be delivered at reasonable cost	Effective interventions that can be delivered only at unreasonable cost
Appropriate use of effective interventions, i.e. giving effective interventions only to patients most likely to benefit	Inappropriate use of effective interventions

The concept of reasonableness is subtle, and its application poses difficulties because it involves value judgement. QALYs have been used to assess reasonableness of cost. When QALYs are used to assess a range of new interventions, those interventions can usually be classified into one of three groups, as follows:

1. ridiculously cheap, a 'no-brainer decision' that should be implemented immediately, e.g. health workers giving brief advice to smokers to stop smoking at every consultation – excellent VFM;
2. unreasonable cost, i.e. ridiculously expensive and irresponsible to fund, e.g. annual cervical screening – poor VFM;
3. reasonable cost, i.e. gives a return on investment similar to that obtained for other interventions that are regarded as routine treatments, e.g. hip replacement or coronary artery bypass grafting – good VFM.

Gentle Reader,

Empathise with the young public health physician. He was walking past the Radcliffe Camera which stands in the middle of one of Oxford's most beautiful squares. As he passed by, he caught a whiff of musty paper. It came from the ventilation shafts of the government paper rooms that lie under the green sward around the Camera. These rooms house official documents which contain the deliberations of many experts and represent an accumulation of evidence, some of which has been used over the years to prevent disease and promote health.

He sighed heavily as the smell brought to mind the first report of The Royal Commission on Environmental Pollution, published in 1971. In it had been highlighted the problems of the illicit dumping of toxic waste – known as 'fly tipping' – on sites, such as waste ground, not registered to receive it. Although the problem had first been identified in 1963, the Government had not acted on this matter. Throughout 1971, the Royal Commission lobbied the Government to act, because of the potential danger to water supplies and the risk to public health. All to no avail, until one day a Midlands lorry driver called Lonnie Downes took the matter into his own hands. He had discovered that fellow drivers were being given a bonus of £20 a week to dump toxic waste (described as 'suds oil'). After complaining to the management, he was threatened with dismissal. Several weeks later, he was offered a promotion; Lonnie declined. He was offered £300 to leave the firm; again Lonnie declined. Instead, he went to the local branch of the Conservation Society, which sent a detailed report to the Secretary of State for the Environment. Despite this, the Government still did not want to act.

The Conservation Society then sent its findings to the press. The story was published in the Birmingham Sunday Mercury on 10 January 1972. On 24 February that same year, 36 drums of sodium cyanide were found on a derelict piece of ground near Nuneaton where children were known to play. The Government finally acted: a bill was drafted and passed into law by 30 March 1972.

Commentary

On this occasion, the evidence alone, even that contained within a scientifically respectable government report, was not enough to determine policy. Decisions taken by policy-makers and managers can be made either in response to public pressure or from an ideological position in which the scientific evidence may play a negligible part.

CHAPTER 3

MAKING DECISIONS ABOUT HEALTH SERVICES

When a proposal is made to introduce a new intervention, a healthcare decision-maker should:

- examine the evidence put forward by the proposer;
- find other evidence, if it exists;
- appraise the quality of the research evidence;
- estimate the outcomes, both beneficial and adverse, of the innovation;
- estimate the opportunity costs of introducing the innovation.

In general, there are two questions that must be asked when appraising the research evidence put forward to support the introduction of an innovation (see Box 3.1).

Box 3.1 General questions for the appraisal of research evidence

1. Is the design of this research study the most appropriate to answer my question?
2. How good is the quality of this particular research when compared with the best design of its type?

Detailed advice on appraising the quality of research, and the outcomes of studies is given in Chapters 5 and 6, respectively.

3.1   THE CONTEXT OF THE DECISION UNDER CONSIDERATION

The context of any decision a decision-maker may face can vary in complexity. Instances of the simplest type of decision to be made are those in which an enthusiast wishes to introduce a new therapy, test or service and the decision-maker has to consider the effects of the innovation proposed. There are, however, many other decisions that have to be made about more complex situations; for example, the need to find efficiency savings, or to reorganise a service because a lead consultant retires or some equipment needs to be replaced.

3.1.1   Dealing with difficult decisions

A common problem is faced by people who produce evidence that an intervention does not appear to be effective. While accepting that absence of evidence of effectiveness is not *ipso facto* evidence of ineffectiveness, in the competition for resources that pertains in the modern world, services for which there is no evidence of effectiveness are in a weak position when competing with other services for which the evidence base is strong.

One example of difficult decision-making followed the publication of the conclusions drawn from a systematic review of vision screening in children conducted by the Health Services Research Unit, University of Oxford, on behalf of the Health Technology Assessment Programme of the UK R&D Programme. Although no evidence of beneficial effects could be found, the proposal that the service be stopped was met with concern, indeed outrage. How can the decision-maker deal with situations such as these?

3.1.2   Battalions of difficult decisions

When sorrows come, they come not as single spies,
But in battalions.
William Shakespeare: Hamlet, *Act* IV, *Scene* v

For the decision-maker who wishes to manage change, the fact that troubles come not as single spies but as whole battalions can be advantageous. If a single service must be cut, for example, a community hospital has to be closed or an A&E Department has to be shut down, the public and press are able to focus on a single issue and present it negatively with potentially devastating consequences for the decision-maker. If, however, a decision to reduce investment in one particular service for which there is no evidence of effectiveness can be linked with five other options for increasing investment, three of which could be funded if the service currently provided could be scaled down, then this changes the context and enables the decision-maker to present the outcome in a positive way.

Thus, in making difficult decisions, the decision-maker should seek to avoid a situation in which a simple yes-or-no decision is required and instead identify various options, some of which could be funded by the limited resources available.

3.2 THERAPY

3.2.1 Dimensions and definitions

A therapy is any intervention given with the objective of improving the health status of patients or of populations. Drugs and surgical operations are obvious examples of a therapy, but preventive interventions, such as immunisation programmes or health promotion initiatives, are also therapies.

The criteria used to assess a therapy are:

- acceptability (Section 6.6.1.1);
- effectiveness (Section 6.4);
- safety (Section 6.5);
- patient satisfaction and patients' experience (Section 6.6);
- cost-effectiveness (Section 6.7);
- appropriateness (Section 6.9).

The term therapy usually refers to a single specific act that a professional undertakes or performs on either a single patient or all the individuals in a particular 'population'. However, it is also possible to apply the term to more complicated situations in which the effect of a series of therapeutic acts is tested, for example:

- a comparison of treatment by different professionals, e.g. doctor vs nurse, chiropractor vs orthopaedic surgeon;
- a comparison of treatment by different teams within a clinical service;

- a comparison of treatment by different types of clinical service.

This increasing complexity of therapeutic interventions, from the application of a single therapy to that of whole services, is shown in Fig. 3.1.

Screening, which is a combination of a diagnostic test and a therapy, is discussed in Section 3.4.

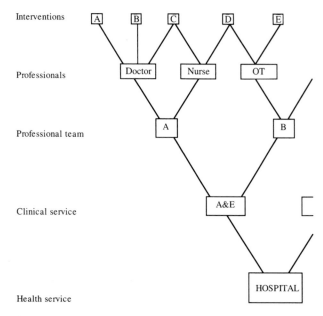

Fig. 3.1
The increasing complexity of therapeutic interventions, from the performance of a single therapeutic act to the introduction of a clinical service

3.2.2 Searching

Good advice on searching for research evidence pertaining to a therapy is given in the ACP Journal Club.[1]

A MEDLINE search for a therapy has four main components (see Table 3.1).

Table 3.1 Components of a MEDLINE search for a therapy

Component	Example
The clinical problem	Migraine
The therapy	Behaviour therapy
Study design	Review or RCT
The time frame	1985 to the present

The clinical problem is usually easy to specify.

The therapy itself is more difficult to specify because the handling of therapy by the indexers is not as well developed as that relating to clinical problems. It is sometimes helpful to 'explode' the term chosen to be more inclusive, and to group all the subtypes of therapy.

The study design can also be indexed under the publication type.

- The best single term to use when searching for publications from 1990 onwards is 'clinical trial'.
- As there is no specific term to search for systematic review, the term 'review' should be used.

See Appendix I for information on subject specialist databases (I.2.8).

3.2.3   Appraisal

3.2.3.1   Therapy: the balance of good and harm

The randomised controlled trial (RCT) is the best method for assessing the effectiveness of a therapy (Section 5.4), in the form of either an individual trial or a systematic review of trials. However, even this powerful research method may not answer the question: 'Does this intervention do more good than harm?'.

Adverse effects of therapy (side-effects) are usually rarer than beneficial effects. Thus, a study that has been designed with sufficient power to detect a 5% improvement in the effectiveness of a new therapy when compared with an existing therapy may not be sufficiently powerful to detect any side-effects that may occur with a frequency of 1 in 1000. If the side-effect is mild, a skin rash, for example, this matters little, but if the side-effect is death this is serious. As such, RCTs designed to assess effectiveness often need to be complemented by cohort studies to assess safety (see Section 5.6). Therefore, more than one type of evidence is necessary to enable a purchaser or clinician to assess the balance between good and harm conferred by a therapy.

A systematic review of RCTs in combination with a meta-analysis of adverse effects of these trials can identify both the beneficial and the adverse effects of treatment.

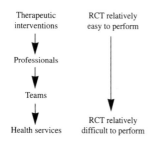

Therapeutic interventions

↓

Professionals

↓

Teams

↓

Health services

RCT relatively easy to perform

RCT relatively difficult to perform

Margin Fig. 3.1

3.2.3.2 *Assessing innovations in health service delivery*

Although the RCT is considered to be the 'gold standard' for evaluating the effects of a therapy, such trials are more difficult to organise with increasing complexity of therapeutic intervention (see Margin Fig. 3.1), either technically, because the number of services randomly allocated may be too few to ensure the trial has adequate power, or politically, because the politicians may be reluctant to admit that a new policy should be subject to a trial – trials indicate equipoise and uncertainty (see Box 5.7).

Consequently, studies of health service organisation and delivery are sometimes investigated using research methods other than the RCT, notably:

- the cohort study (see Section 5.6);
- the case-control study (see Section 5.5).

Often, these methods require the analysis of large databases of health service utilisation. The use of these methods allows the following types of question to be addressed.

- What is the total mortality resulting from an operation, as distinct from the mortality observed in hospital?
- Is the outcome of care observed at one hospital or one type of hospital better than that which would be expected by chance?

If the mortality rate observed at one type of hospital is greater than that at another type this may indicate the need to change policy or the management of the hospital system. If the mortality rate at one hospital is greater than that at other hospitals of the same type, this may indicate a problem with the quality of service delivery at that particular hospital (Section 6.8).

3.2.4 Getting research into practice

3.2.4.1 *Therapy*

Although there has been much discussion about the problems of implementing research evidence of the effectiveness of any new intervention within the health service, due to the difficulty of influencing professional practice, this type of change is relatively simple because good-quality evidence is available and should dominate decision-making.

3.2.4.2 Innovations in health service delivery

As the subject of the decision changes from simple interventions, such as the administration of new drugs, to more complex interventions, such as changing the patterns of skill mix or of hospital provision (see Fig. 3.1), the availability of evidence decreases, not only in absolute but also in relative terms, that is, relative to the two other factors decision-makers have to take into account:

1. 'local' circumstances; for example, it may not be possible to change an emergency service so that care is delivered by consultants due to the difficulties of recruiting and paying for the number of consultants required;
2. the political context in which the service is delivered; for example, the introduction of nurse practitioners may be opposed by the public, or the closure of a low-volume but much-loved local hospital service may be vigorously resisted by the community.

Resource constraints and political pressures do not, however, negate the need for evidence; on the contrary, the need for research-based knowledge is heightened even though these other factors may outweigh the scientific evidence when the final decision is taken.

Reference

1. McKIBBON, K.A. and WALKER, C.J. (1994) *Beyond ACP Journal Club: how to harness* MEDLINE *for therapy problems [Editorial].* ACP Journal Club Jul–Aug; 121 Suppl. 1: A10–2.

3.3   TESTS

Gus and Wes had succeeded in elevating medicine to an exact science. All men reporting on sick call with temperatures above 102 were rushed to hospital. All those except Yossarian reporting on sick call with temperatures below 102 had their gums and toes painted with gentian violet solution and were given a laxative to throw away into the bushes. All those reporting on sick call with temperatures of exactly 102 were asked to return in an hour to have their temperatures taken again.

Joseph Heller, Catch 22, *1962*

3.3.1 Dimensions and definitions

A test may be defined as any measurement (including an examination or investigation) used to identify individuals who could benefit from therapeutic intervention. These measurements may be:

- the presence or absence of a symptom – something a patient feels;
- the presence or absence of a sign – something a clinician can detect;
- laboratory results, expressed numerically;
- radiological images, interpreted perceptually;
- pathological specimens, interpreted perceptually.

The term 'test' is often used as a synonym for diagnostic test, but tests may have a function other than that of diagnosis, for example:

- to monitor the effect of treatment, and the results used to determine whether treatment should be continued, changed or stopped;
- to provide information about prognosis (the future course of a disease);
- to indicate the presence/absence or degree of risk.

Screening is discussed separately in Section 3.4 because the process involves more than the performance of a test: the beneficial effects of screening tests must be balanced against the adverse effects of any intervention resulting from those screening tests.

Some of the criteria used to assess the efficacy of tests are the same as those used to assess that of therapies, namely, effectiveness, safety, acceptability and cost. The criteria specific to the assessment of tests are:

- sensitivity;
- specificity;
- the relationship between sensitivity and specificity;
- predictive value;
- likelihood ratio.

3.3.1.1 Sensitivity and specificity

Diagnostic tests are used for many purposes, but in their simplest form the results are either positive or negative: an individual is identified as either having the disease or not having the disease. However, few tests are perfect. Most people who do not have the disease will have a negative result (true negatives), but some people with negative test results may actually have the disease (false negatives). Most people who do have the disease will have a positive test result (true positives), but some people with positive test results will not have the disease (false positives). Thus, four types of test result may be obtained as a combination of these two variables (Fig. 3.2).

The balance between true positives and false positives and between true negatives and false negatives is expressed by two criteria which are used to judge all diagnostic tests:

- sensitivity;
- specificity.

		Disease	
		Present	Absent
Test	Positive	True positive A | B	False positive
	Negative	C | D False negative	True negative

Fig. 3.2
The four types of test result

Sensitivity is the proportion of people with the disease who are identified as having it by a positive test result.

Specificity is the proportion of people without the disease who are correctly reassured by a negative test result.

A method for calculating the sensitivity and specificity of a diagnostic test is shown in Fig. 3.3.

Disease

	Present	Absent
Positive	A	B
Negative	C	D

Test

Sensitivity

$$\frac{A}{A + C}$$

Specificity

$$\frac{D}{B + D}$$

Fig. 3.3
Calculation of sensitivity and specificity of a diagnostic test

3.3.1.2 Sensitivity and predictive value

Sensitivity and specificity are constant criteria that can be applied to any diagnostic test irrespective of the characteristics of the population on which the test is used. However, the significance of a test result is determined not only by the sensitivity and the specificity of the test, but also by the prevalence of the condition in the population upon which the test is used, which can alter the predictive value.

The predictive value of a test is an expression of the probability that the test result indicates the presence or absence of disease, therefore:

- the positive predictive value is the probability that a person with a positive test result actually has the disease;
- the negative predictive value is the probability that a person with a negative test result does not actually have the disease.

Imagine conducting a diagnostic test that has a 90% sensitivity and a 90% specificity in two different populations of 1000 each, one in which there is a high prevalence of a disease and the other in which there is a low prevalence. The results in Matrix 3.1 reflect the situation in hospital practice, in which 50% of the patients have the disease (high prevalence), and 90% of the people who have a positive test result will have the disease, therefore the test is said to have a positive predictive value of 90%. The results in Matrix 3.2 reflect the situation in general practice, in which only 10% of patients have the disease (low prevalence); even though the sensitivity of the test is the same, the positive predictive value is only 50%.

This difference in the predictive value of a test despite the constancy of sensitivity and specificity is the main reason that:

- hospital doctors believe that GPs miss 'easy' diagnoses;
- GPs believe that hospital doctors over-investigate.

The criteria of sensitivity, specificity and predictive value are relevant for all tests whether numerical or perceptual.

Disease / Test	Present	Absent
Positive	450	50
Negative	50	450
Total	500	500

Matrix 3.1
Prevalence of disease 50%

Disease / Test	Present	Absent
Positive	90	90
Negative	10	810
Total	100	900

Matrix 3.2
Prevalence of disease 10%

1. Numerical tests
Some tests generate results in the form of numerical values, for example, biochemical tests. When test results are expressed numerically, the meaning of those results will vary depending on whether the test has been used to identify:

- certain individuals within the range of a single population, for example, those who have raised blood pressure (Fig. 3.4);
- the presence of two populations, for example, those who do and those who do not have spina bifida, where the test results of each population will fall within a range of values, and those two ranges will overlap (Fig. 3.5).

From Fig. 3.4, it can be seen how different test values can be chosen to distinguish between those identified as having 'normal' blood pressure and those identified as having 'high' blood pressure. From Fig. 3.5, it can be seen how the cut-off point between positive and negative can be varied. However, the choice of any numerical cut-off point within a data set, whether applied to a single population or to two populations, is arbitrary. The choice of a cut-off point is difficult because there is always a trade-off between sensitivity and specificity (see Section 3.3.1.3).

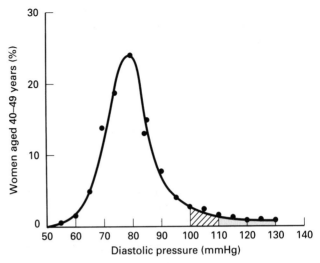

Fig. 3.4
Frequency distribution of diastolic pressure in females aged 40–49 years in a London population sample. The tinted area shows patients known to be at risk and known to have a high probability of receiving benefit from treatment. The hatched area, comprising pressures of 100–110 mmHg, represents subjects who are also at risk but have a lower probability of receiving benefit from hypotensive therapy. Subjects in the remaining white area are those with 'normal' blood pressures. (From Pickering, 1974, *Hypertension: Courses, Consequences and Management*, 2nd edition. Edinburgh, Churchill Livingstone, with permission.)

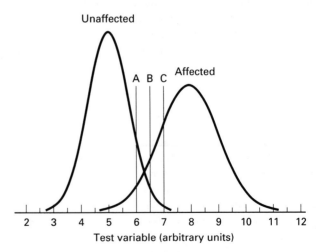

Fig. 3.5
Hypothetical example of the detection rate and false-positive rate of a screening test at three different cut-off levels: A, B and C (Source: Cuckle and Wald, 1984, in Wald, N.J. (ed.) Antenatal and Neonatal Screening. Oxford, Oxford University Press)

2. Perceptual tests
Some tests, known as perceptual tests, are dependent upon the use of a human being as the instrument of measurement. Human perception is used to distinguish positive from negative, by:

- seeing, e.g. the analysis of X-rays or histopathological specimens;
- hearing, e.g. the detection of heart murmurs;
- palpation, e.g. the detection of congenital dislocation of the hip.

Any test that involves human perception and judgement is bedevilled by variability of reporting on results. There are two forms of variability.

- Intra-observer variability – the phenomenon in which the same observer classifies the same test result differently on two separate occasions.
- Inter-observer variability – the phenomenon in which different observers classify the same test results differently.

Within epidemiology, the phenomenon of inter-observer variability is widely accepted; it is also gaining acceptance by healthcare professionals. Indeed, this phenomenon should be recognised as an inevitable consequence of the use of perceptual tests. Unfortunately, within the legal system where 'expert' witnesses can be called by both the prosecution and the defence, inter-observer variability is interpreted categorically as one observer being 'right' and another being 'wrong'.

3.3.1.3 Between a rock and a hard place

As any threshold is an arbitrarily selected value, it is possible to change the threshold and therefore the balance between positive and negative results. At any particular threshold, the balance of false positives and false negatives will be different. This illustrates one of the central principles of testing, namely, that any increase in sensitivity is usually accompanied by a decrease in specificity (Margin Fig. 3.2) and vice versa. The greater the degree to which a service is designed never to miss a diagnosis, the greater will be the number of false-positive results generated. As sensitivity increases, a point is reached at which very small increases in sensitivity are accompanied by very large

Sensitivity increases

↓

Specificity decreases

↓

Costs, risk and patient anxiety increase

Margin Fig. 3.2

decreases in specificity, i.e. the number of false-positive results increases.

An increase in the number of false-positive test results increases:

- patient anxiety;
- the costs of treatment;
- the risk associated with unnecessary treatment (see Margin Fig. 3.2).

The results of two studies demonstrate the disadvantage of increasing sensitivity; both examples illustrate the outcome of increasing the sensitivity of imaging tests.

The sensitivity of magnetic resonance imaging (MRI) in the detection of pituitary adenoma (tumour) can be increased by the administration of certain chemicals to those undergoing imaging: in this study, the images from 100 healthy volunteers were mixed with those from 57 patients who had pituitary adenoma; the images were read by three experts independently. Ten per cent of the healthy volunteers were diagnosed as having adenoma, which is a very rare disease.[1]

In another study, the MR images of 98 asymptomatic people were mixed with those of 27 people who had back pain; the images were read by two experts independently. Sixty-four per cent of the asymptomatic individuals were classified as 'abnormal'.[2] In the accompanying editorial,[3] it was stated that: 'The recent increase in the rates of lumbar spine surgery may be related in part to the availability of new imaging techniques'.

3.3.1.4 Tests: the producer's perspective

The number of new tests developed, particularly biochemical tests, is increasing each year, and the rate of increase will accelerate as new genetic tests become available.

To the developer of a test, increased test precision is often sufficient to justify the introduction of a new product.

Manufacturers rarely evaluate new tests or new versions of tests against such criteria as sensitivity or predictive value. The manufacturer is usually satisfied if:

- the chemical specification of the test has been improved: for example, if proteins can be separated with increased precision;
- the performance of the test is easier and requires a lower level of skill from laboratory staff;

- the cost of the test has been reduced.

Those clinicians responsible for developing tests focus primarily on increasing sensitivity, but this strategy carries a concomitant decrease in specificity (see Section 3.3.1.3).

3.3.1.5 *Tests: the purchaser's perspective*

For the decision-maker in any health service, however, the perspective is different: although the manufacturers' criteria are relevant, other criteria are also important. Purchasers need to know whether a marginal increase in sensitivity leads to better outcomes for the population as a whole or for individual patients only.

For the clinician wishing to introduce a new test, changes in sensitivity and specificity may provide sufficient justification. However, the purchaser responsible for the health of a population must take into account the impact that a new test, or an expansion of testing, has on the health of that population in terms not only of sensitivity but also of specificity and the number of false-positive diagnoses made. Any increase in the number of individuals having tests will result in an increase in the number of positive test results; some individuals with positive test results will have the disease, others will not (false positives; see Fig. 3.6). However, even if the false positives are excluded and all the people who have a positive test actually have the

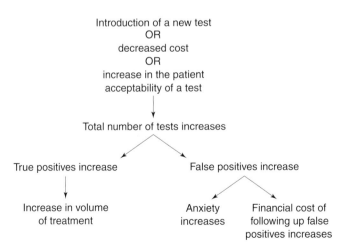

Fig. 3.6
The relationship between an increase in the volume of testing
(for various reasons) and the outcomes of that increase

disease, the effects of increasing the number of people tested may be simply to detect people with less severe disease (see Fig. 3.6).

Research conducted in the USA has demonstrated that an increase in the number of tests performed increases the volume of treatment. In a cohort study of 12 coronary angiography service areas in New England in which the intensity of investigation by stress test of individuals with chest pain varied,[4] a positive relationship was found between total stress test rates and the rates of subsequent coronary angiography; a strong relationship was also shown between coronary angiography and revascularisation. Furthermore, in an analysis of the Medicare National Claims History files, which cover 30 million elderly Americans, it was found that investigation rates increased markedly over a 7-year period – from 50% to 300%.[5] These increases in the rates of diagnostic testing were associated with an increase in the rates of administration of relevant treatments (see Table 3.2). One explanation could be that the increased rate of testing revealed exactly the same type of cases as had been diagnosed previously, but this explanation is not based on evidence. Another possibility is that an increase in testing, or an increase in test sensitivity, merely detects less severe cases, and the benefits obtained from increased expenditure on testing may decline as the volume of testing increases.

Table 3.2   Investigations and the associated treatments: increased rates of testing lead to an increase in rates of intervention (Source: Verrilli and Welch[5])

Investigation	Treatment
Cardiac catheterisation	Cardiac revascularisation (CABG and PTCA)
Spinal imaging (CT and MRI)	Back surgery
Swallowing studies	Percutaneous gastrostomy
Mammography	Breast biopsy and excision
Prostate biopsy	Prostatectomy

It is clear that increased diagnostic testing is one of the major factors leading to an increase in the volume of treatment. Any attempt to control the volume of treatment that does not include the control of the development of diagnostic services is doomed to failure.

3.3.2 Searching

Good advice on searching for evidence about tests is given in the ACP *Journal Club*.[6]

A MEDLINE search for a test has five components (see Table 3.3).

Table 3.3   Components of a MEDLINE search for a test

Component	Example
The clinical problem	Coeliac disease
The test	Gliadin antibody test
The characteristics of the test	Sensitivity and specificity
Study design	Review
The time frame	1985–1995

In terms of study design, the first step is to look for meta-analysis of studies using:

- the term 'meta-analysis';
- text word 'meta';
- any word starting with 'analy'.

In addition to text words, MeSH headings can be used when searching for papers on tests. The relevant MeSH headings are:

- sensitivity and specificity;
- predictive value of tests;
- false-negative reactions;
- false-positive reactions;
- diagnosis, differential;
- diagnostic test;
- diagnostic service;
- routine diagnostic test;
- diagnosis.

If you wish to limit the number of MeSH headings, use:

- sensitivity;
- diagnosis (NB: 'explode' the term 'diagnosis' if asked).

3.3.3 Appraisal

Appraisal is a two-stage procedure.

1. What is the best research method for appraising a test?
2. How good is any of the research found?

The best method for appraising a test is a large well-designed RCT that has patient outcomes, such as survival or quality of life, as end-points. Unfortunately, RCTs of tests are scarce. As a compromise, it is probably necessary to accept results from research studies designed to have better test performance as an end-point, for example, greater sensitivity of a test for a disease for which it has been shown in an RCT that intervention is effective.

As large trials are rarely feasible, it is essential to find reviews of small studies in which meta-analysis of the data from the individual studies has been undertaken irrespective of whether the test results are presented as dichotomous (i.e. 'positive' or 'negative') or continuous. Irwig et al.[7] have developed Guidelines for Meta-analyses Evaluating Diagnostic Tests; their checklist for evaluating meta-analyses of diagnostic tests is shown in Box 3.2, which can be used to supplement the general guidance on appraising systematic reviews (see Section 5.3.3).

Box 3.2 Checklist for evaluating meta-analyses of diagnostic tests (Source: Irwig et al.[7])

- Is there a clear statement about:
  - the test of interest?
  - the disease of interest and the reference standard by which it is measured?
  - the clinical question and context?
- Is the objective to evaluate a single test or to compare the accuracy of different tests?
- Is the literature retrieval procedure described with search and link terms given?
- Are inclusion and exclusion criteria stated?
- Are studies assessed by two or more readers?
  - Do the authors explain how disagreements between readers were resolved?
- Is a full listing of diagnostic accuracy and study characteristics given for each primary study?
- Does the method of pooling sensitivity and specificity take account of their interdependence?
- When multiple test categories are available, are they used in the summary?
- Is the relation examined between estimates of diagnostic accuracy and study validity of the primary studies for each of the following design characteristics:
  - appropriate reference standard?
  - independent assessment of the test or tests and reference standard?
- In comparative studies, were all of the tests of interest applied to each patient or were patients randomly allocated to the tests?
- Are analytic methods used that estimated whether study design flaws affect diagnostic accuracy rather than just test threshold?
- Is the relation examined between estimates of diagnostic accuracy and characteristics of the patients and test?
- Are analytic methods used which differentiate whether characteristics affect diagnostic accuracy or test threshold?

If there are no meta-analyses available, individual studies must be appraised. For this type of appraisal, the McMaster checklist can be used (see Box 3.3).

Box 3.3 Methodological questions for appraising journal articles about diagnostic tests (Source: McMaster University[8])

The best articles evaluating diagnostic tests will meet most or all of the following eight criteria.

1. Was there an independent, 'blind' comparison with a 'gold standard' of diagnosis?
2. Was the setting for the study, as well as the filter through which study patients passed, adequately described?
3. Did the patient sample include an appropriate spectrum of mild and severe, treated and untreated disease, plus individuals with different but commonly confused disorders?
4. Were the tactics for carrying out the test described in sufficient detail to permit their exact replication?
5. Was the reproducibility of the test (precision) and its interpretation (observer variation) determined?
6. Was the term 'normal' defined sensibly? (Gaussian, percentile, risk factor, culturally desirable, diagnostic or therapeutic?)
7. If the test is advocated as part of a cluster or sequence of tests, was its contribution to the overall validity of the cluster or sequence determined?
8. Was the 'utility' of the test determined? (Were patients really better off for it?)

3.3.4 Getting research into practice

New tests, particularly biochemical tests, flood into clinical practice because there are no controls to restrict their introduction; it is rarely necessary therefore to promote the use of any new test. To compound the situation, there is very little evidence of effectiveness for new tests that become available. The main challenge, therefore, is stopping starting (see Sections 2.4.1.2 and 7.7.3.2), that is, controlling the introduction of new tests.

References

1. HALL, W.A., LUCIANO, M.G., DOPPMAN, J.L. et al. (1994) *Pituitary magnetic resonance imaging in normal human volunteers: occult adenomas in the general population.* Ann. Intern. Med. 120: 817–20.
2. JENSEN, M.C., BRANT-ZAWADKI, M.N., OBUCHOWSKI, N. et al. (1994) *Magnetic resonance imaging of the lumbar spine in people without back pain.* N. Engl. J. Med. 331: 69–73.
3. *Magnetic resonance imaging of the lumbar spine. Terrific test or tar baby?* [Editorial]. N. Engl. J. Med. 331: 115–16.

4. WENNBERG, D.E., KELLETT, M.A., DICKENS, J.D. Jr et al. (1996) *The association between local diagnostic testing intensity and invasive cardiac procedures.* JAMA 275: 1161–4.
5. VERRILLI, D. and WELCH, H.G. (1996) *The impact of diagnostic testing on therapeutic interventions.* JAMA 275: 1189–91.
6. McKIBBON, K.A. and WALKER-DILKS, C.J. (1994) *Beyond ACP Journal Club: how to harness MEDLINE for diagnostic problems [Editorial].* ACP Journal Club Sept–Oct; 121 Suppl. 2: A10–2.
7. IRWIG, L., TOSTESON, A.N.A., GATSONIS, C. et al. (1994) *Guidelines for meta-analyses evaluating diagnostic tests.* Ann. Intern. Med. 120: 667–76.
8. McMASTER UNIVERSITY *Critical Appraisal Card from Department of Clinical Epidemiology and Biostatistics.* McMaster University, Hamilton, Ontario, Canada.

3.4 SCREENING

Screen: an apparatus used in the sifting of grain, coal, etc. 1573.

Shorter Oxford English Dictionary

Gentle Reader,

Empathise with Jock Armstrong and Will Taggart. They glared at one another across the row of straw which had been spewed forth from the Claas combine harvester, a massive mechanical monument, now still in the blackening wheat of a Scottish harvest field.

'Look at the wheat on the ground, man,' roared Jock, 'You've set the holes in the screen too big so that you could hash on for the next job.'

'Ach, away man,' growled Will, his eyes shining forth in a face almost black with stour.

'I'm due at Balanin the night and she's blocked solid with chaff because the screen's set as small as they'll go.'

The peewit cried in the Galloway sky, its whooping call like a referee's whistle keeping the two opposing forces on either side of the line of straw: the farmer wanting the screen set so that not a single grain falls to earth; the contractor knowing that the smaller the holes, the more often will chaff, grain, stones and straw build up and cause first colic then complete obstruction in his combine harvester. And with him wanting to drive as fast as he can to the next farm to combine barley before the rain curtails harvesting (and income).

Commentary

Farmer or contractor; saving of grain or saving of time; sensitivity or specificity – the eternal tensions in any screening programme.

3.4.1 Dimensions and definitions

Screening is a health service in which members of a defined population, who do not necessarily perceive they are at risk of a disease or its complications, are asked a question or offered a test to identify those individuals who are more likely to be helped than harmed by further tests or treatment to reduce the risk of disease or its complications.

Screening may be organised proactively, by inviting members of the population at risk to attend for testing, as is the case in breast cancer screening, or opportunistically, for example, blood pressure measurement performed during the course of a patient's visit to the general practitioner about another unrelated health problem. The evaluation is the same for both types of programme management.

In contrast, case-finding is a process of identifying individuals who are asymptomatic but who are at risk of disease because they are related to a symptomatic individual: for example, contacting all the first-degree relatives of an individual who has had a myocardial infarction at the age of 42 years and who has been diagnosed as having familial hypercholesterolaemia.

When screening is discussed, the term is usually taken to refer to a single test, for example, a cervical smear within a cervical screening programme. However, screening actually consists of all the steps in a programme from the identification of the population at risk to the diagnosis of the disease or its precursor in certain individuals to the treatment of those individuals. In the case of cervical screening, the steps range from the identification of women in the age-group 24–64 years (the group that will benefit) to the accurate histopathological diagnosis and effective treatment of cervical cancer (Fig. 3.7).

Thus, the effectiveness of any screening programme is determined by:

- the sensitivity of the series of tests applied to the population;
- the effectiveness of the therapy offered to those individuals identified as having the condition.

Screening effectiveness =
test accuracy + therapeutic effectiveness

It is the involvement of a subset of the entire population
that distinguishes screening from clinical practice. In
clinical practice, a person concerned about a health

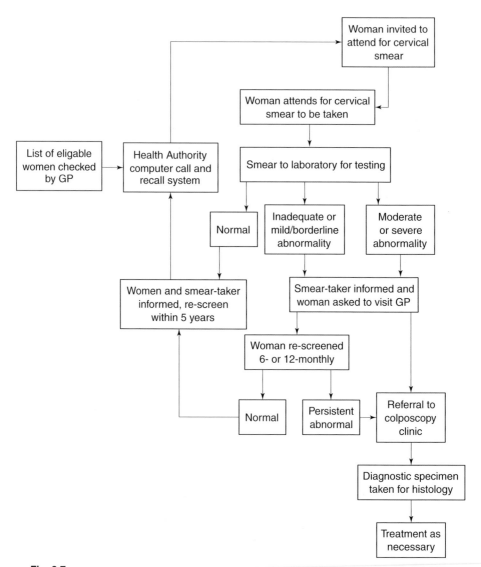

Fig. 3.7
The cervical screening programme in the UK (Source: NHS Cervical Screening
Programme)

problem seeks help knowing that not every patient benefits and some people experience side-effects; in screening, healthy individuals are drawn into a health service, only a small proportion of whom will benefit, and those diagnosed as false positives will suffer harm, having previously been well. Thus, the balance of good to harm is of particular importance in decisions about screening.

3.4.1.1 The changing balance of good and harm

Screening programmes, like any other intervention, have the potential to do both good and harm. However, the balance between good and harm will change with the frequency of testing and the quality of the programme. The beneficial effects of screening illustrate the law of diminishing returns (Fig. 3.8A): in women aged 20–64 years, cervical screening at a frequency of once every 3 years reduces the incidence rate of cervical cancer by 91.2% compared with a reduction of 83.6% when the screening frequency is once every 5 years – an increase of only 7% in effectiveness. The adverse effects of screening, or of any other intervention, usually follow a straight line (Fig. 3.8B): the greater the number of individuals involved in a screening programme, the greater the number experiencing side-effects (Fig. 3.8C). Thus, the ratio of good to harm changes as the number of screening tests performed increases.

If the quality of the screening programme is low, the benefits are reduced and adverse effects increase (Fig. 3.9); if an adequate level of quality is not achieved, there may be a point at which the harm done by screening is greater than the good. Thus, the decision to introduce screening must be taken with the greatest of care.

3.4.2 Searching

A MEDLINE search for a screening programme has five useful components (see Table 3.4).

Table 3.4 Components of a MEDLINE search for a screening programme

Component	Example
The health problem	Breast cancer
The principal test	Mammography
The type of intervention	Screening
Study design	Review or RCT
The time frame	1985–1995

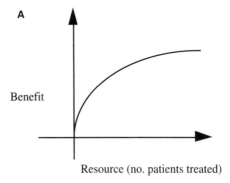

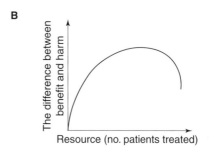

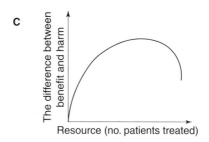

Fig. 3.8
A The beneficial effects of screening; B the adverse effects of screening; C the relationship between the beneficial and adverse effects of screening (Source: Donabedian; see ref. 2, p. 221)

3.4.3 Appraisal

The first step is to identify the research design most likely to be helpful. In screening, it is the RCT or a systematic review of RCTs. Difficult as they may be to organise, RCTs of public health interventions such as screening should be subjected to the same rigorous appraisal as is applied to

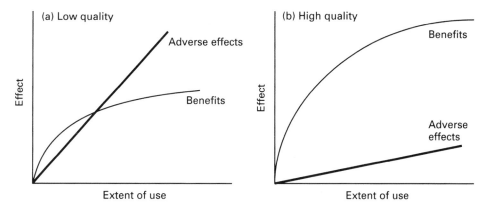

Fig. 3.9
The beneficial and adverse effects of a screening programme that is of (a) low quality, and (b)
high quality

clinical interventions. Indeed, it could be argued that there is a need for stronger evidence to support the introduction of screening as a public health intervention because it is offered to healthy populations. As no intervention is without risk, some of the people who are subject to it – a proportion of whom would not have developed the disease even if the intervention had not been introduced – will be put at risk.

Proponents of the introduction of any screening programme sometimes base their argument on cohort studies, which are designed to follow a series of people who have had a screening test and compare their survival with that of the general population. However, this is a poor method of evaluating screening, principally because of what is termed lead-time bias.

Imagine a disease that has a natural history of 10 years and causes symptoms after 5 years, which usually prompt the sufferer to visit a doctor; the survival time from the point of symptomatic diagnosis is 5 years (Fig. 3.10A). A test that enables a diagnosis to be made at an earlier, presymptomatic stage, for example at 3 years, will apparently increase survival time by 2 years (Fig. 3.10B). This apparent increase in survival time does not necessarily mean that screening is effective; it may simply mean that the person with the presymptomatic disease identified by screening is aware of the condition for 7 years as opposed to 5 – this is referred to as lead-time bias. It is essential that any screening programme is evaluated within an RCT that

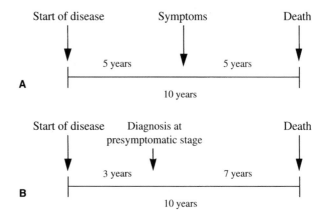

Fig. 3.10
The phenomenon of lead-time bias in screening

has been designed with death as the outcome in order to control for lead-time bias.

The classic set of criteria for appraising screening tests was developed by Wilson and Jungner[2] in 1968 (see Box 3.4).

Box 3.4   Criteria for appraising screening developed in the 1960s (Source: Wilson and Jungner[2])

- The condition sought should be an important health problem.
- There should be an accepted treatment for patients with recognized disease.
- Facilities for diagnosis and treatment should be available.
- There should be a recognizable latent or early symptomatic stage.
- There should be a suitable test or examination.
- The test should be acceptable to the population.
- The natural history of the condition, including development from latent to declared disease, should be adequately understood.
- There should be an agreed policy on whom to treat as patients.
- The cost of case-finding (including diagnosis and treatment of patients diagnosed) should be economically balanced in relation to possible expenditure on medical care as a whole.
- Case-finding should be a continuing process and not a 'once and for all' project.

Although these criteria have been useful, they are weak for several reasons.

- There is insufficient emphasis on the adverse effects of screening and on the need to ensure that a programme does more good than harm. Although these considerations were important in the 1960s, in the context of a general public which is nowadays better informed, more assertive and more likely to sue if harm is done, it is essential to attend fully to these considerations.

- Wilson and Jungner state that an 'accepted treatment' should be available, but some 'accepted' treatments are either ineffective or of unproven efficacy.
- There is no discussion of the quality of the evidence upon which the decision to screen should be made.

A more suitable set of criteria for current use has been developed by the National Screening Committee in the UK (see Box 3.5).[3] These criteria are based on those

---

Box 3.5 Criteria for appraising the viability, effectiveness and appropriateness of a screening programme (Source: National Screening Committee[3])

The condition

- The condition should be an important health problem.
- The epidemiology and natural history of the condition, including development from latent to declared disease, should be adequately understood and there should be a detectable risk factor, disease marker, latent period or early symptomatic stage.
- All the cost-effective primary prevention interventions should have been implemented as far as practicable.

The test

- There should be a simple, safe, precise and validated screening test.
- The distribution of test values in the target population should be known and a suitable cut-off level defined and agreed.
- The test should be acceptable to the population.
- There should be an agreed policy on the further diagnostic investigation of individuals with a positive test result and on the choices available to those individuals.

The treatment

- There should be an effective treatment or intervention for patients identified through early detection, with evidence of early treatment leading to better outcomes than late treatment.

- There should be agreed evidence-based policies covering which individuals should be offered treatment and the appropriate treatment to be offered.
- Clinical management of the condition and patient outcomes should be optimised by all health care providers prior to participation in a screening programme.

The screening programme

- There should be evidence from high quality Randomised Controlled Trials that the screening programme is effective in reducing mortality or morbidity.
- There should be evidence that the complete screening programme (test, diagnostic procedures, treatment/intervention) is clinically, socially and ethically acceptable to health professionals and the public.
- The benefit from the screening programme should outweigh the physical and psychological harm (caused by the test, diagnostic procedures and treatment).
- The opportunity cost of the screening programme (including testing, diagnosis and treatment) should be economically balanced in relation to expenditure on medical care as a whole.
- There should be a plan for managing and monitoring the screening programme and an agreed set of quality assurance standards.
- Adequate staffing and facilities for testing, diagnosis, treatment and programme management should be available prior to the commencement of the screening programme.
- All other options for managing the condition should have been considered (e.g. improving treatment, providing other services).

developed by Wilson and Jungner, but have been prepared taking into account international work on the appraisal of screening programmes, particularly that in the USA[4] and in Canada.[5]

3.4.4 Getting research into practice

Getting research into practice for a screening programme is a major undertaking, perhaps more so than for any other type of healthcare intervention. This is because the introduction of a new screening programme requires the concomitant introduction of a wide range of clinical interventions, together with the management and information support systems that will enable quality to be assured. Any quality assurance programme must include:

- explicit agreed standards of good practice;
- an information system that enables performance against those standards to be measured;

- the authority to take action if standards are not achieved.

For a screening programme to do more good than harm requires not simply the demonstration that it is possible to achieve this outcome in a research setting, but also an emphasis on quality in practice that will allow the potential to be realised in any setting.

3.4.5 Aphoristic warnings

The decision to introduce screening is relatively easy; resolving the problems that may result from it can be much more difficult. For this reason, some aphorisms on screening are provided for the reader to ponder before succumbing to the temptations of screening.

- ➤ A stitch in time does not necessarily save nine.
- ➤ The decision to introduce a new screening programme should be taken as carefully as the decision to build a new hospital.
- ➤ Never think about screening tests, only about screening programmes.
- ➤ Screening programmes shown to be efficacious in a research setting require an obsession with quality to be effective in a service setting.
- ➤ The public are overoptimistic about screening; professionals are overpessimistic.
- ➤ Finding 'asymptomatic' disease by means of screening always increases the length of time a person knows s/he has the disease; this increased period of awareness should not be confused with increased survival.
- ➤ All screening programmes do harm; some can do good as well.
- ➤ The harm from a screening programme starts immediately; the good takes longer to appear. Therefore, the first observable effect of any programme, albeit an effective one, is to impair the health of the population.
- ➤ A screening programme without false positives will miss too many cases to be effective.
- ➤ Like the tightrope walker above Niagara Falls, any screening programme must balance false negatives and false positives.
- ➤ A screening programme without false negatives will cause unnecessary harm to the healthy population.

➤ For the distressed patient seeking help, the clinician does what s/he can; for the healthy person recruited to screening, only the best possible service will suffice.

➤ Screening programmes should be run with firm management. If quality falls, a screening programme that was doing more good than harm may then do more harm than good.

➤ Though insignificant to the population, a single false positive can be of devastating significance to the individual.

➤ If a screening programme is *not* supported by a quality assurance system comprising standards, information and authority to act, it should be stopped.

➤ If a quality assurance programme is not generating at least one major public enquiry every 3 years, it is ineffective.

➤ At best, screening is a zero-gratitude business.

References

1. EDDY, D.M. (1990) *Screening for cervical cancer.* Ann. Intern. Med. 113: 214–26.
2. WILSON, J.M.G. and JUNGNER, G. (1968) *Principles and Practice of Screening for Disease.* World Health Organization, Geneva.
3. NATIONAL SCREENING COMMITTEE (1998) *First Report of the National Screening Committee.* Health Departments of the United Kingdom. A version of this report is available on the Department of Health (England) website: http://www.open.gov.uk./doh/nsch.htm
4. U.S. PREVENTIVE SERVICES TASK FORCE (1996) *Guide to Clinical Preventive Services: Report of the U.S. Preventive Services Task Force,* 2nd Edition. Williams & Wilkins, Baltimore.
5. CANADIAN MEDICAL ASSOCIATION (1994) *Canadian Guide to Clinical Preventive Health Care.* Ministry of Supply and Services, Canada.

3.5   HEALTH POLICY

3.5.1   DIMENSIONS AND DEFINITIONS

> **Policy:** 5. a course of action adopted and pursued by
> a government, party, ruler, statesman, etc.; any
> course of action adopted as advantageous or
> expedient. (The chief living sense).
> *Shorter Oxford English Dictionary*

In classifying health policy, the usual approach is to use the
determinants of health over which it is possible to exert an
influence (see Fig. 8.1):

- the physical environment;
- the biological environment;
- the social environment;
- health services.

There are two main reasons why health policy may be
formulated and introduced:

1. to change the way in which health services are funded,
   organised or held accountable – healthcare policies;
2. to improve health through changes in the physical,
   biological and/or social environments – health or public
   health policies.

3.5.1.1   Healthcare policy

If health services are effective, it is possible to prevent or
reduce (by curing it) the prevalence of a disease or to
alleviate its burden by minimising the disability that
disease causes. Increasing the level of effectiveness within a
health service is governed by healthcare policy.

Changes to health services that might be introduced
through healthcare policy include:

- the delegation of responsibility for decision-making
  about the use of resources;
- increasing the number of people involved in decisions
  about resources;
- increasing incentives to achieve better value for money;
- clarifying and strengthening accountability;
- improving performance against targets;
- improving patient care.

Although such changes are often political, that is, decided upon by politicians, they always have managerial consequences; managers must ensure that policy objectives are met using the resources available.

Managers can also introduce changes to health services to improve:

- efficiency;
- quality;
- accountability;
- acceptability.

For example, managers may:

- introduce schemes of quality improvement;
- increase investment in training;
- change managerial structures to increase professional involvement, to decrease the amount of time wasted by professionals in management, or both;
- change the financial computing system;
- introduce measures to involve patients in the process of care;
- externalise certain services, such as cleaning or pathology.

However, such managerial changes have only indirect effects on clinical decision-making, whereas politicians make policy decisions that affect clinical practice directly. In the UK, one such decision has been to influence GP prescribing habits by excluding certain drugs from the list from which doctors can choose; another such decision has been the introduction of case management (a US term) or care management (a UK term) to improve the quality of care for severely mentally ill people.

3.5.1.2 Health or public health policy

The primary focus of health or public health policies is change in the physical, biological and/or or social environments.

Changes in the physical, biological and/or social environments are the main factors influencing:

- the incidence of disease, i.e. the number of new cases of a disease in the population.
- the prevalence of the disease, i.e. the number of cases of a disease in the population at any one point in time.

3.5.2 Searching

To find articles on health policy, use the MeSH term 'health policy'.

It may be productive to search HealthSTAR, a specialist database (see Appendix I, I.2.8.2).

3.5.3 Appraisal

3.5.3.1 Appropriate study designs

For healthcare policy, it may be possible to find evidence from RCTs, such as the one that failed to demonstrate a beneficial effect of case management in people who had severe mental illness.[1,2] However, for healthcare policies that influence the finance and organisation of a health service, the evidence most easily available is that derived from descriptive studies of other comparable health services.

For health or public health policies, the evidence may be available from more conventional scientific study designs, such as:

- the case-control study (Section 5.5);
- the cohort study (Section 5.6);
- cluster analysis (Section 7.9.5.1).

3.5.3.2 Natural experiments

There is a common belief that research on health policy or approaches to health service management is difficult to translate from one country to another because of the myriad social, cultural, and political differences. Although it is true that it is often not possible to transfer a policy or managerial option directly from one country to another, research on health policy and management conducted in different countries can be illuminating.

If the healthcare systems are similar, any initiatives or innovations are of interest; if the healthcare systems are different, it is useful to regard the difference as a 'natural' experiment. In a 'natural' experiment, differing approaches to the same problem can be compared despite the fact that those approaches were not planned in a research setting but arose by reason of different circumstances.

Even when the social, cultural, and political circumstances of a country are very different to those of one's own, there is much to be learned. Anthropological studies, such as that by Frankel described in *The Huli Response to Illness*,[3] can provide many insights into the human response to disease, illness and treatment, which may be helpful to policy-makers and managers. Indeed, managers and policy-makers may have underestimated the potential for learning from research conducted in other countries and within different cultures.

3.5.3.3   Appraising research on health policies

When appraising research evidence on a policy, there are two key questions to ask.

- How valid is the evaluation?
- How relevant is the policy to the local service?

If the evaluation of a policy was carried out in a different country, the issue of relevance is important.

There are two aspects to relevance in this situation:

1. the feasibility of introducing a particular policy into one's own country;
2. the practicability of introducing the intervention associated with the implementation of that policy into one's own country.

For example, legislation passed in the USA is of limited relevance elsewhere in the world, and vice versa, but the potential effects of legislation on professional behaviour or managerial decision-making are relevant and it may be possible to reproduce those in other countries, albeit through different legislation or by other means.

A checklist of useful questions for the appraisal of research designed to evaluate health or healthcare policy is shown in Box 3.6.

3.5.4 Getting research into practice

As individuals usually have strong views about what is right in terms of policy or management, there may be greater exception to implementing knowledge derived from research into policy-making and management than that encountered when promoting the adoption of research findings in clinical practice. If a policy has been based primarily on an ideology, or if a management change stems from the conviction of an individual manager, then evidence that such a policy or management change is

---

Box 3.6 Checklist for the appraisal of research designed to evaluate health or healthcare policy

- Were the explicit policy objectives clearly stated?
- Did the research workers identify and articulate any implicit objectives of the policy under investigation?
- Were valid outcome measures identified for each of the explicit and implicit objectives?
- Was data collection complete?
- Were data collected before and after the introduction of the new policy?
- Was the follow-up of sufficient length to allow the effects of policy change to become evident?
- Were any other factors that could have produced the changes (other than the policy) identified in the key criteria and discussed?
- Were possible sources of bias in the research workers acknowledged in the paper or in any accompanying editorial?

---

ineffective or counterproductive is likely to meet with resistance. A policy-maker may be defensive about challenges to his/her ideology, and the manager may regard any challenges as a personal affront. It is important, however, that a double standard is not introduced, namely, that policy-makers and managers exhort clinicians to implement research findings in clinical practice when they themselves are either not actively searching for evidence or failing to implement knowledge derived from research when it is presented to them.

References

1. MARSHALL, M. (1996) *Case management: a dubious practice [Editorial].* Br. Med. J. 312: 523–4.
2. MARSHALL, M., GRAY, A., LOCKWOOD, A. and GREEN, R. (2000) *Case management for people with severe mental disorders.* (Cochrane Review) In: The Cochrane Library, Issue 3 2000: Update Software, Oxford.
3. FRANKEL, S. (1986) *The Huli Response to Illness.* Cambridge University Press, Cambridge.

Gentle Reader,

Empathise with Jair de Jesus Mari, Professor of Psychiatry in São Paulo. September is hot in São Paulo, sometimes oppressively so. However, it was not the heat that bothered Jair in 1994. He was frustrated with the process of publishing scientific papers. For more than a year, he had laboured to summarise all the trials of psychosocial family interventions in schizophrenia that could be found by hand-searching psychiatric journals. His review, based on six trials, was submitted to a prestigious journal in August 1993 and published in August 1994,[1] after a delay that was torment to him. He had received praise from colleagues, and felt satisfied when he finally saw his review in print.

One month later it was out of date; two further trials, both from China, had been published in another journal. He swore (the equivalent of 'bloody hell' in Portuguese). What should he do now? Write a letter to the first journal? Perhaps, but what he really wanted was to revise the meta-analysis and base the revision on all eight trials. Anyway, readers who saw the letter would not necessarily have the original article to hand; what's more, letters are not peer-reviewed so they're not necessarily taken seriously by readers. Jair de Jesus Mari faced an insoluble dilemma.

Commentary

Jair's dilemma cannot be solved on paper, but it is possible to resolve electronically.

All decision-makers should have computer access to the best information about the effectiveness of any intervention, that is, a systematic review of trials based on a complete search of the literature, which also:

- *can be quickly updated when new evidence appears;*
- *has summaries of the original trials available;*
- *includes practical implications, as well as scientific conclusions;*
- *has a responsive 'letters' column in which all comments/criticisms and the author's replies are available instantaneously.*

The Cochrane Library, available on compact disk, now provides such a facility; the review by Pharoah, Mari and Streiner[2] meets all of the above criteria.

References
1. MARI, J.J. and STREINER, D. (1994) An *overview of family interventions and relapse in schizophrenia.* Psychol. Med. 23: 565–78.
2. PHAROAH, F.M., MARI, J.J. and STREINER, D. (2000) *Family intervention for schizophrenia.* (Cochrane Review) In: The Cochrane Library, Issue 3 2000. Update Software, Oxford.

SEARCHING FOR EVIDENCE

4.1   THE SEARCHER'S PROBLEMS

The decision-maker wishing to find evidence upon which
to base a decision is confronted by many obstacles, shown
in Fig. 4.1 and discussed below. The steps that can be taken

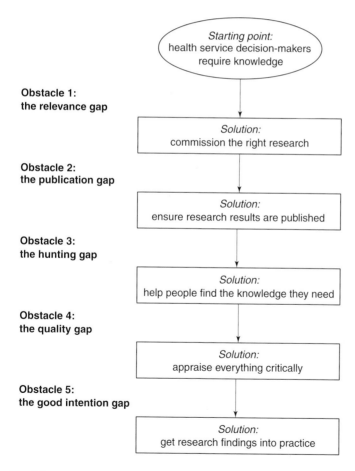

Obstacle 1:
the relevance gap

Obstacle 2:
the publication gap

Obstacle 3:
the hunting gap

Obstacle 4:
the quality gap

Obstacle 5:
the good intention gap

Starting point:
health service decision-makers
require knowledge

Solution:
commission the right research

Solution:
ensure research results are published

Solution:
help people find the knowledge they need

Solution:
appraise everything critically

Solution:
get research findings into practice

Fig. 4.1
The evidence gaps

collectively to overcome these obstacles are also shown in Fig. 4.1; however, the individual searcher can also take action to negotiate these obstacles.

4.1.1 The relevance gap – absence of high-quality evidence

Despite years of research, the available evidence is not best suited to the needs of healthcare decision-makers. This is illustrated by the analysis of Frankel and West presented in Table 4.1;[1] relatively few papers are published about common conditions whereas there are numerous papers about relatively uncommon conditions. However, this finding should not be used as a reason to challenge investigator-driven research. To take a case in point, the papers on slow virus diseases of the central nervous system (CNS) may now be of greater relevance to decision-makers given the explosion of interest in bovine spongiform encephalopathy (BSE).

Table 4.1 The index of interest (number of papers listed in Index Medicus 1986 in English/discharges and deaths from Hospital In-patient Enquiry x 1000) in various diagnoses (Source: Frankel and West[1])

Diagnoses	Discharges and deaths (D&D)	Index of interest (Papers/D&D × 1000)
Slow virus disease of CNS	40	2000
Myasthenia gravis	930	156
Crohn's disease	6670	44
Carcinoma of the breast	41 220	33
Rheumatoid arthritis	26 060	27
Carcinoma of the bronchus	54 440	20
Myocardial infarction	102 720	10
Cerebrovascular disease	111 250	7.7
Irritable bowel syndrome, etc.*	19 840	6.7
Cataract	54 990	6.5
Hip replacement	37 400	5.0
Haemorrhoids	20 700	1.0
Inguinal hernia	64 400	0.8
Tonsils and adenoids	76 600	0.7
Varicose veins	47 160	0.6

* Includes irritable bowel syndrome, dumping syndrome, constipation and other functional bowel disease

The research agenda, however, is also dictated by those who invest in R&D. In a thoughtful article in *The Lancet*, David Melzer argued that owing to the possibility of a return on capital investment, pharmaceutical companies are willing to invest in the research and development of new drugs.[2] One of the outcomes of this strategy is that in evidence-based decision-making priority is increasingly being given to drugs rather than, for example, psychological treatments or group therapy because there is better evidence available about drugs. As Melzer points out, 'methods of treatment of the human or animal body by surgery or therapy or of diagnosis practised in the human or animal body' are excluded from patent protection, therefore there is no incentive for companies to invest in research to develop and evaluate them. He argues that the extension of patent protection to such procedures would lead to increased investment in research, leaving 'governments to review the results and fund areas that are inherently unpatentable such as basic research and old technology'.

Knowledge management solution
In the UK, one of the main functions of the NHS R&D Programme is the identification of NHS requirements for research-based knowledge. The intention is to narrow the 'relevance gap' and correct the imbalance by commissioning specific research that will provide answers to the questions healthcare decision-makers, and patients, want answered. At present, however, many healthcare decisions must be made for which there is no high-quality evidence.

The searcher's solution
The absence of high-quality evidence does not make evidence-based decision-making impossible; in this situation, what is required is the *best evidence available*, not the best evidence possible, using the classification shown in Table 4.2.

4.1.2 The publication gap – failure to publish research results

Any searcher must find the sources of evidence. Although much is made of the 'grey literature', that is, the results of studies not published in scientific journals, the main source of evidence is the published literature. However, this is incomplete for several reasons:

• the 'sloppy' researcher – too many researchers fail to write up and submit their findings for publication;

- the 'disheartened' researcher, less motivated to complete and submit for publication negative results – known as submission bias;
- the 'coy' pharmaceutical company, nervous of revealing results that may not show the company's products in the most advantageous light – another example of submission bias;
- the 'biased' editor, keener to publish positive than negative results – known as publication bias;[3]
- the influence of language – positive findings are more likely to be published in English language journals, and negative findings more likely to be found in other language journals – known as language bias.

Three of the reasons for the non-publication of research results produce a positive bias in the published literature as a whole; the last-mentioned reason produces a positive bias in the English language literature.

Knowledge management solutions
The compulsory registration of all research studies at their commencement would begin to counteract the incompleteness of the published literature because it would then be possible to trace unpublished studies.

In 1998, Glaxo Wellcome, and Schering pharmaceutical companies voluntarily agreed to publish *all* research relevant to their licensed products – an agreement welcomed by the academic and clinical communities, and one which should begin to counteract one of the sources of submission bias.

The development and application of guidelines for journal editors may help to counteract publication bias.

Table 4.2 Classification of the strengths of evidence (Source: *Bandolier* 1995; 12;1)

Type	Strength of evidence
I	Strong evidence from at least 1 systematic review of multiple well-designed randomised controlled trials
II	Strong evidence from at least 1 well-designed randomised controlled trial of appropriate size
III	Evidence from well-designed trials without randomisation, single group pre-post, cohort, time series or matched case-control studies
IV	Evidence from well-designed non-experimental studies from more than 1 centre or research group
V	Opinions of respected authorities, based on clinical evidence, descriptive studies or reports of expert committees

The searcher's solutions

It is appropriate to search for unpublished data if one is a research worker, but if one is a busy decision-maker it is not an effective use of time. It is difficult for the searcher to compensate for publication bias; the best solution is to search for a systematic review, and to be aware of the phenomenon of positive bias in its various guises when appraising research articles (see Table 6.2). To compensate for language bias, a MEDLINE search should be complemented by searches of other databases that include articles from journals published in other languages, e.g. EMBASE.

4.1.3 The hunting gap – difficulties in finding published research

4.1.3.1 *The limitations of electronic databases*

There are many electronic databases, but the two principal sources are MEDLINE (see Appendix I, I.2.6) and EMBASE (see Appendix I, I.2.7). However, database coverage is limited:

- only about 6000 of the biomedical journals currently published world-wide (estimated at 15 000–17 000) are scanned;
- by no means all of the papers in these journals are included;
- primarily English language journals are scanned.

Knowledge management solutions

One of the objectives of The Cochrane Collaboration is to make the results of more trials available to searchers. This objective is fulfilled in two main ways:

- by compiling The Cochrane Library (see Appendix I, I.2.1);
- by hand-searching journals and incorporating any trials found into MEDLINE.

Hand-searching of the *British Medical Journal* and *The Lancet* has added greatly to the number of trials available on MEDLINE (Fig. 4.2).[4]

In the UK, one of the aims in the establishment of the National electronic Library for Health (NeLH) was to provide easy access to the best current knowledge for clinicians, managers, and patients (see Section 4.4.2).

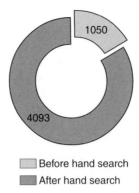

Before hand search
After hand search

Fig. 4.2
British Medical Journal and *Lancet* trials (1966–1994)
identifiable in MEDLINE before and after the hand-search
(Source: McDonald et al.[4] with permission, BMJ Publishing
Group)

The searcher's solution
The use of specialist databases (see Appendix I, I.2.8) can
minimise but not resolve the problems posed by the
limitations of electronic databases. Access to The Cochrane
Library diminishes the problems of searching for RCTs;
users should consult the Cochrane Database of Systematic
Reviews (CDSR; see Appendix I, I.2.1.1) and the Cochrane
Controlled Trials Register (CCTR; see Appendix I, I.2.1.3).

4.1.3.2   Inadequate indexing

Owing to inadequacies in the indexing of research papers,
not only within journals but also within the electronic
databases, many papers cannot be found. In general, only
about half of the trials in MEDLINE can be found by even
the best electronic searcher[5] and the experienced clinical
searcher will find less than half of those found by the
expert (see Table 4.3).

Table 4.3   The percentage of RCTs in MEDLINE found by an
experienced clinical searcher and an expert searcher in
comparison with that found by hand-searching journals (Source:
Adapted from Adams et al.[5])

	Experienced clinical searching		Optimal skilled MEDLINE searching		Hand-searching
% of RCTs found	18	Skills gap	52	Hunting gap	94
95% CI	15–21		48–56		93–95

Knowledge management solution
The continuing development of The Cochrane Library, and other sources of bibliographic information, such as *Clinical Evidence*, will enable searchers to access relevant knowledge despite inadequate indexing.

The searcher's solution
The use of good search strategies will minimise the impact of inadequate indexing. The best strategy is to have an expert searcher on hand, but often one has to cope alone and improve one's searching skills (see Sections 4.3.2 and 9.2). It is advisable to search the CDSR (I.2.1.1) and CCTR (I.2.1.3), and to consult *Clinical Evidence*.

General advice on finding evidence is given in Appendix I.

4.1.4 The quality gap – the need for critical appraisal

4.1.4.1 Misleading abstracts

A search produces papers. The quality of any search is measured by two criteria:

- accuracy – the proportion of findable articles that are found;
- precision – the proportion of articles found that are useful; the rest are 'junk'.

> Precision = 1 – 'junk'

Although good searching increases accuracy, it almost invariably decreases precision, i.e. it uncovers 'junk'. Once articles have been found, it is necessary to identify and discard the 'junk'.

The simplest way to identify 'junk' is to read the abstract, but abstracts tend to be written with a bias towards highlighting the most positive aspects of a paper.[6] Moreover, a review of abstracts in the world's best medical journals showed that between 18% and 68% of the abstracts were inaccurate, that is, either they were inconsistent with the data in the main text or they contained data not given in the main text.[7]

Knowledge management solutions
In 1996, The CONSORT Statement[8] was published, in which are set out standards for the reporting of trials,

including instruction for the structure of abstracts. In 1999, the QUOROM Statement[9] was published, in which standards for the reporting of meta-analyses are set out, again including instruction for the structure of abstracts. These developments should facilitate an improvement in the quality of abstracts of trials and meta-analyses.

The continuing development of good-quality databases of systematic reviews, such as CDSR and *Clinical Evidence*, will provide searchers with sources of information that are not subject to the problem of misleading abstracts.

The searcher's solution
Every research article found requires critical appraisal. There are two guidelines for reading abstracts.

- If the abstract is unstructured, be suspicious.[10]
- If the abstract highlights negative findings, it may not be biased; if it highlights positive findings, appraise the methods section carefully before accepting the results as good-quality evidence.

4.1.4.2 Bias in published papers

There are two sources of bias in published papers:

- flaws in the methodology of the research, such as in randomisation, introduce a positive bias known as methodological bias;[11]
- the way in which the results are presented – the use of relative risk data introduces a positive bias – known as the framing effect.[12]

Knowledge management solution
In recent years, as the deficiencies in the design, analysis and reporting of trials have been documented, the need to develop standards for the practice and documentation of trials has been recognised. As discussed above, in 1996 the CONSORT Statement was published,[8] followed by the QUOROM Statement in 1999.[9] These guidelines, if widely implemented, should help to improve the quality of reporting of research findings and minimise the positive bias that currently hinders decision-makers and others who must interpret research results.

The searcher's solutions
It is important for the searcher to be aware of sources of bias within research articles, and to appraise critically both

the study design and the mode of presentation of the results. It is also important when making a decision that the evidence used to support it is not based solely on an analysis in terms of relative risk reduction.

The searcher should also consult the CDSR (I.2.1.1) and the Database of Reviews of Effectiveness (DARE; I.2.1.2).

References

1. FRANKEL, S. and WEST, R. (1993) *Rationing and Rationality in the National Health Service.* Macmillan, Basingstoke, p. 11.
2. MELZER, D. (1998) *Patent protection for medical technologies: why some and not others?* Lancet 351: 518–19.
3. EASTERBROOK, P.J., BERLIN, J.A., GOPALAN, R. and MATTHEWS, D.R. (1991) *Publication bias in clinical research.* Lancet 337: 867–72.
4. McDONALD, S.J., LEFEBVRE, C. and CLARKE, M.J. (1996) *Identifying reports of controlled trials in the BMJ and the Lancet.* Br. Med. J. 313: 1116–17.
5. ADAMS, C.E., POWER, A., FREDERICK, K. and LEFEBVRE, C. (1994) *An investigation of the adequacy of MEDLINE searches for randomized controlled trials (RCTs) of the effects of mental health care.* Psychol. Med. 24: 741–8.
6. GØTZSCHE, P. (1989) *Methodology and overt and hidden bias in reports of 196 double-blind trials of nonsteroidal anti-inflammatory drugs in rheumatoid arthritis.* Control. Clin. Trials 10: 31–56.
7. PITKIN, R.M., BRANAGAN, M.A. and BURMEISTER, L.F. (1999) *Accuracy of data in abstracts of published research articles.* JAMA 281: 1110–11.
8. BEGG, A., CHO, M., EASTWOOD, S. et al. (1996) Improving the quality of randomised controlled trials. The CONSORT Statement. JAMA 276: 637–9.
9. MOHER, D., COOK, D.J., EASTWOOD, S., OLKIN, I., RENNIE, D., STROUP, D.F. for the QUOROM Group (1999) *Improving the quality of reports of meta-analyses of randomised controlled trials: the QUOROM Statement.* Lancet 354: 1896–900.
10. AD HOC WORKING GROUP FOR CRITICAL APPRAISAL OF THE MEDICAL LITERATURE (1987) *A proposal for more informative abstracts of clinical articles.* Ann. Intern. Med. 106: 598–604.
11. SCHULZ, K.F., CHALMERS, I., GRIMES, D.A. and ALTMAN, D. (1994) *Assessing the quality of randomization from reports of controlled trials published in obstetrics and gynecology journals.* JAMA 272: 125–8.
12. FAHEY, T., GRIFFITHS, S. and PETERS, T.J. (1995) *Evidence-based purchasing: understanding results of clinical trials and systematic reviews.* Br. Med. J. 311: 1056–60.

4.2 THE INFORMATION BROKER

The traditional role of the librarian is changing. As the 21st century begins, the librarian will become an information broker, facilitating the interchange between those who need and those who provide information.

A fine example of the benefits of having a good librarian is presented in Box 4.1. A searcher had contacted the evidence-based health mailbase stating that he wanted to find evidence about mental health nursing but did not think there was much that could be used. The reply from Robin Snowball, a librarian at the Cairns Library in Oxford, is reproduced in Box 4.1, a constructive rebuttal to the speculation that there was not much evidence available (although it must be admitted that the average searcher has about as much chance as a snowball in hell of finding some of the evidence required – see Section 4.1). For those who wish to consult Snowball further about a structured approach to developing a search strategy from your clinical or other search question and refining it to alter search sensitivity and specificity as required, see Further Reading below (Snowball's chapter also includes a list of useful information resources).

Further reading

SNOWBALL, R. (1999) *Finding the evidence: an information skills approach.* In Dawes, M. (Ed.) *Evidence-based Practice: a Primer for Health Professionals.* Churchill Livingstone.

Box 4.1   The benefits of a good librarian, or Snowball's six-minute search

Subject: Evidence on mental health nursing

Date: 20 January 1999 11.15

Results of a quick (6 mins.) MEDLINE search (WinSpirs from 1991, updated 4.9.2000), using Thesaurus/Subject search, limited Free Text/Textword searching – and Publication Type Limits to isolate trials with a control group or high-quality (including systematic) reviews and meta-analyses:

(1) explode Mental-Disorders/all subheadings: 6243 Randomised Controlled Trials (RCTs), 1481 Controlled Clinical Trials (CCTs), 2867 Academic or Literature Reviews, 514 Meta-analyses

(2) explode Mental-Disorders/nursing: 57 RCTs, 31 CCTs, 67 Ac/Lit Reviews, 2 Meta-analyses

(3) explode Mental-Disorders/all subheadings AND nurs*: 209 RCTs, 56 CCTs, 131 Ac/Lit Reviews, 13 Meta-analyses

(2) may be a little narrow ('nursing' may not be a wholly reliable subheading), and (3) a little too wide (although it might also have missed papers where terms other or more specific than 'nurse, nurses, nursing' are used). But isn't some of (1) – a very high-sensitivity search which could be widened even further with some fancy Free Text/Textword searching, or turned into a higher specificity search by writing a strategy for a more specific question, as one would normally do in practice – also likely to be relevant to mental health nursing: however defined, and if only for some question types?

(Didn't check Embase, Cinahl, PsycLit or Cochrane Library etc. – and PubMed may produce some more recent references than other versions of MEDLINE).

4.3 COPING ALONE

In managing the acquisition of knowledge there are two principal modes:

- proactive;
- reactive.

A proactive style of knowledge management is to scan the literature regularly and thereby search for potentially relevant knowledge (predominantly a scanning activity). A reactive style of knowledge management is based on the principle that no decision-maker will ever be able to anticipate all the questions that are likely to arise and therefore it is more effective to develop good searching skills and use them as and when required (predominantly a searching activity). Each decision-maker must strike a balance between the two types of activities and define a mode of knowledge management most appropriate to needs and circumstances (see Margin Fig. 4.1).

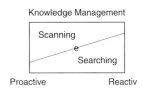

Margin Fig. 4.1

4.3.1 Becoming a better scanner

When preparing a scanning strategy, use the checklist of questions shown in Box 4.2.

Box 4.2 Useful prompts in the preparation of a scanning strategy

- How many hours each week do I want to spend scanning for new knowledge?
- What sources of knowledge do I want to scan regularly?
- What sources of information will I exclude?
- How can I ensure that I do not miss important new knowledge using this strategy?
- What checklists can I use to ensure that I stick to my scanning objectives? (A weekly checklist is useful.)
- Is there anyone else who could develop, or has developed already, a scanning strategy with whom I could share the load?
- How can I review the benefits and weaknesses of this strategy at the end of the year?

4.3.2   Becoming a better searcher

There are two steps that can be taken to improve searching skills (see also Section 9.2).

1. Undertake formal training; ask the librarian if there are any searching training courses available.
2. Elicit the support of a librarian; first enrol for an induction session, then search with the librarian, and finally ask the librarian to review some searches completed without support to obtain feedback on sensitivity and precision.

4.3.3   Becoming better at critical appraisal

Formal training in critical appraisal is becoming increasingly available (see Section 9.3). If there is no access to formal training, take the following steps.

- Collect the series of articles on critical appraisal entitled 'Users' guides to the medical literature' (see Further Reading in Appendix III).
- Download the information from the book's website: http://www.shef.ac.uk/~scharr/ebhc/Intro.html
- Set up a problem-based journal club in order to work with colleagues to find and appraise articles relating to decisions that have to be made.

4.3.4   Becoming a better storekeeper

Information can be stored in many ways, but the most appropriate storing strategy is to use reference management software and store the articles on it using keywords (see Section 9.4). The paper copies can be filed alphabetically by first author.

4.3.5   Use it or lose it

Any decision-makers within a health service who find, appraise and use evidence will contribute to changing the culture of the organisation in which they work (see Section 7.3). This course of action provides an example to other people who will discuss the evidence found and begin to search for evidence themselves. As such, the skills of searching for, appraising and storing evidence will be strengthened, not only within individuals but also throughout the organisation.

4.4 DEVELOPING LIBRARIES FOR THE 21st CENTURY

Gentle Reader,

Visualise the Radcliffe Camera (the one our young public health physician walked past in Chapter 3), which rises like a giant pannetone at the heart of one of Oxford's most beautiful squares. It is part of the Bodleian Library, to which it is connected by an underground railway (large enough only for small goblins). Deep underground are the stacks which house not only many treasures but also, as the Bodleian is a copyright library and receives every book published in Britain, an odd miscellany. For instance, on emerging from the underground passage through which one can walk from the New Bodleian to the Radcliffe Camera, one is greeted by the sight of the entire output of Mills & Boon, a publisher of romantic novels known in the trade as 'bodice-rippers'.

Commentary

The Bodleian Library epitomises the library of the 20th century; however, with the advent of the World Wide Web, a completely different type of library is developing to serve the needs of those seeking for knowledge in the 21st century – the e-library.

4.4.1 Defining features of the e-library

The e-library is founded on hypertext, i.e. text that can be prepared with the software used to run the World Wide Web, which allows any bit of information on the Web to be connected to any other bit of information on the Web. This power to link information allows those who have access to the World Wide Web to gain rapid access to a wide range of different sources and resources. As the Web will soon be made available through digital television, the potential exists for anyone to access any computer from their own home (although there may be a charge associated with access and use).

The defining features of the e-library for those seeking knowledge about health and healthcare are shown in Box 4.3.

Box 4.3 The defining features of the e-library

- The stock available is not limited by shelf space: small organisations can have as big an e-library as big organisations.
- Access is not limited to opening hours.
- The skills of librarians can be made available to a much wider range of users.
- Knowledge can be provided where and when it is needed.
- Knowledge can be kept up to date quickly and easily.
- The methods used to produce the knowledge can be displayed easily and completely so that the reader can appraise its quality.

4.4.2 The National electronic Library for Health

In their strategy, *Information for Health*, the UK government announced that a National electronic Library for Health (NeLH) would be set up with the following aims:

- to provide easy access to best current knowledge;
- to help improve health and healthcare, clinical practice and patient choice.

The principles underpinning the development of the NeLH are shown in Box 4.4. Operational definitions for each of these objectives are given on the Web page at www.nelh.nhs.uk; the standards for user ease of access to knowledge are shown in Table 4.4.

Box 4.4 The principles underpinning the development of the NeLH

- It will be obsessed with the quality of knowledge and not merely its quantity.
- It will be equally open to patients, clinicians and managers.
- It will be available only electronically.
- It will contain knowledge and know-how.
- It will facilitate action and interaction as well as providing knowledge.
- It will enhance and build on existing libraries.

Table 4.4 Standards for user ease of access to knowledge in the NeLH

When knowledge is needed	How quickly
Speaking with a patient, e.g.: • in a consultation • on a ward round	Within 15 seconds
Reflecting on a patient, e.g.: • over coffee when discussing a case with colleagues • when writing to a colleague	Within 2 minutes
During training or professional development	Within 1 week

Further reading

HAYNES, R.B. (1995) *Current awareness and current access: ACP Journal Club goes electronic.* ACP Journal Club Jul–Aug; 123(1): A14.
McKIBBON, K.A. et al. (1995) *Beyond ACP Journal Club: how to harness MEDLINE for prognosis problems.* ACP Journal Club Jul–Aug; 123(1): A12–14.

Gentle Reader,

Empathise with the epidemiologist. He stood in the dock, cool, calm and collected. The judge entered, adjusted her robes, peered over her half-moon spectacles, and imposed, by all the non-verbal signals commonly used in that particular form of theatre, her presence on the court.

> *'How do you plead?' she said, 'Guilty or not guilty?'*

The epidemiologist replied, 'How should I know until I have heard the evidence?'

Commentary

This story, the only prologue intended to be humorous which can be found by the editorial team despite exhaustive searching, highlights the appropriate question that should always be asked when any proposition is made: 'How do I know until I have heard the evidence?'. However, hearing the evidence alone is insufficient. It is always important to make judgements about quality. A witness may be able to recount an impressive version of what happened but if s/he is not reliable then the evidence will be of little use.

CHAPTER 5

APPRAISING THE QUALITY OF RESEARCH

5.1 WHAT IS RESEARCH?

Research is a process of enquiry that produces knowledge. It is related to other activities, such as audit, but has several distinguishing features (see Box 5.1).

Box 5.1 The distinguishing features of research as defined in the NHS R&D Programme in the UK

- To provide **new knowledge** necessary for the improvement of the performance of the NHS in enhancing the health of the nation.
- To generate results that are **generalisable**, i.e. that will be of value to those in the NHS who face similar problems but who are outwith the particular locality or context of the research project.
- To have been designed to follow a clear, well-defined study **protocol**.
- To have had the study protocol **peer reviewed**.
- To have obtained the approval, where necessary, of the relevant **ethics committee**.
- To have defined arrangements for **project management**.
- To report findings such that they are open to critical examination and accessible to all who could benefit from them – this will normally involve **publication**.

Research can be classified into one of two categories:

1. that which increases the understanding of health, ill health, and the process of healthcare;
2. that which enables an assessment of interventions that could be used to try to promote health, to prevent ill health, or to improve the process of healthcare.

These two categories of research are linked. The former provides a base of knowledge from which ideas can be generated for preventing ill health or managing disease more effectively and efficiently – sometimes called hypothesis-generating research; the latter is used to evaluate the effects of putting such ideas into practice – sometimes called hypothesis-testing research. In this book, the focus is primarily on hypothesis-testing research because it is of greatest use to decision-makers.

5.1.1 Hypothesis-testing research

There are two methods for testing a hypothesis:

1. observational;
2. experimental.

1. Observational research
In observational research, the researcher observes a population or group of patients or manipulates data about those subjects. The nature of the subject data used by the researcher can be:

- those that are already available;
- those collected additionally, from interviews either with patients or with healthcare professionals, or from datasets such as cancer registries and death certificates.

Qualitative research (Section 5.9), surveys (Section 5.7) and case-control studies (Section 5.5) are all forms of observational research. An observational study can be conducted:

- on variations already known to exist among different types of healthcare professional or service – sometimes called a 'natural experiment';
- as part of an evaluation of a change in health service delivery that has been introduced as a result of policy, managerial innovation or by a commercial company.

2. Experimental research
In experimental research, the intervention under investigation is performed at the instigation of the researcher. The most powerful type of experimental study is the RCT (Section 5.4).
    It should be noted that:

- cohort studies (Section 5.6) can be either observational or experimental;
- although systematic reviews can be performed on any type of research, the term is most often used to describe reviews of RCTs.

An economic appraisal can be built into both methods of testing an hypothesis (see Section 6.7).

Frequently, there are disputes between the proponents of experimental research ('trialists') and the proponents of observational or qualitative research; however, the focus on areas of disagreement has hidden the fact that there are many areas of agreement. A letter published in the *British Medical Journal*, written in response to an editorial,[1] contains a useful summary of the contribution of observational research (Box 5.2),[2] which should be seen as complementary to experimental research trials and not presented falsely as a dichotomy.

Box 5.2   Important roles for observational methods (Source: Black[2])

1. Some interventions, such as defibrillation for ventricular fibrillation, have an impact so large that observational data are sufficient to show it.
2. Infrequent adverse outcomes would be detected only by RCTs so large that they are rarely conducted. Observational methods such as post-marketing surveillance of medicines are the only alternative.
3. Observational data provide a realistic means of assessing the long-term outcome of interventions beyond the time-scale of many trials. An example is long-term experience with different hip joint prostheses.
4. Whatever those who question the value of healthcare interventions might think, many clinicians often will not share their concern and will be opposed to an RCT; observational approaches can then be used to show clinical uncertainty and pave the way for such a trial.
5. Despite the claims of some enthusiasts for RCTs, some important aspects of healthcare cannot be subjected to a randomised trial for practical and ethical reasons. Examples include the effect of volume on outcome, the regionalisation of services, a control of infection policy in a hospital, and admission to an intensive care unit. To argue that these topics could theoretically be evaluated by an RCT is of little practical help in advancing knowledge.

Indeed, for the Christmas 1997 edition of the *British Medical Journal*, the Editor asked the world's two leading researchers, in a spirit of peace and goodwill, to write a joint leader which was entitled 'Choosing the best research design for each question. It's time to stop squabbling over the "best" methods'.[3] Sackett and Wennberg[3] wrote:

Each method should flourish, because each has features that overcome the limitations of the others when confronted with questions they cannot reliably answer …

But focusing on the shortcomings of somebody else's research approach misses the point. The argument is not about the inherent value of the different approaches and the worthiness of the investigators who use them. The issue is which way of answering the specific question before us provides the most valid, useful answer. Health and health care would be better served if investigators redirected the energy they currently spend bashing the research approaches they don't use into increasing the validity, power, and productivity of ones they do.

5.1.2 Fraud in medical research

The underlying assumption in this chapter is that any research published is genuine. However, it is now recognised that fraud in medical research is more common than was previously imagined. Lock and Wells cover this topic comprehensively.[4] Fraud has been defined by the US Food and Drugs Administration (FDA) as follows:

… the deliberate reporting of false or misleading data or the withholding of reportable data. There are three general types of fraud:

Altered Data – generating biased data or changing data that are otherwise legitimately obtained. Examples are changing laboratory clinical data, altering animal weights, breaking the study blind and/or study randomization.

Omitted Data – not reporting data that have an impact on study outcomes. Examples include removing subjects from the study for bogus reasons, not reporting or disguising adverse effects (events/experiences), and replacing animals on trial.

Manufactured Data – fabricating information or creating results without performing the work. Examples are filling in values in the case report form (e.g. blood pressure, lab values, X-ray reports) for which no data were obtained, photocopying data from one patient for another, and creating fictitious patients (as cited in Schwarz, 1997[5]).

References

1. SHELDON, T.A. (1994) *Please bypass the PORT*. Br. Med. J. 309: 142–3.
2. BLACK, N. (1994) *Experimental and observational methods of evaluation*. Br. Med. J. 309: 540.
3. SACKETT, D.L. and WENNBERG, J.E. (1997) *Choosing the best research design for each question. It's time to stop squabbling over the 'best' methods [Editorial]*. Br. Med. J. 315: 1636.
4. LOCK, S. and WELLS, F. (Eds) (1997) *Fraud and Misconduct in Medical Research*. 2nd Edition. BMJ Books, London.
5. SCHWARZ, J.A. (1997) *Detection, handling and prevention of fraud in clinical studies in Europe*. Drugs Made in Germany 40: 8–15.

5.2 CHOOSING THE RIGHT RESEARCH METHOD

This chapter has been designed to help decision-makers within any health service to appraise information arising from research. In this context, there are two fundamental categories of research:

- primary research, in which the focus is on patients or populations;
- secondary research, in which the focus is on *reviewing* primary research.

The suitability of various research methodologies for evaluating different types of intervention is summarised in Matrix 5.1, and that for evaluating different outcomes in Matrix 5.2. Often, for a complete evaluation, the results from more than one type of research method need to be used.

Matrix 5.1

Intervention	Type of research				
	Qualitative research	Case control	Cohort	RCT	Systematic review
Diagnosis			✓	✓✓	✓✓✓
Treatment			✓	✓✓	✓✓✓
Screening				✓✓	✓✓✓
Managerial innovation	✓	✓	✓	✓✓	✓✓✓

Matrix 5.2

Outcome	Type of research					
	Qualitative research	Survey	Case control	Cohort	RCT	Systematic review
Effectiveness of an intervention					✓✓	✓✓✓
Effectiveness of health service delivery	✓	✓	✓	✓	✓✓	✓✓✓
Safety	✓	✓			✓✓	✓✓✓
Acceptability	✓	✓			✓✓	✓✓✓
Cost-effectiveness					✓✓	✓✓✓
Appropriateness	✓	✓				✓✓✓
Quality	✓	✓	✓	✓		✓✓✓

5.3 SYSTEMATIC REVIEWS

Secondary research has long been viewed as 'second class'. In the UK, work done to produce reviews was not recognised as a legitimate activity in the Research Assessment Exercise until 1995. The consequence was that a research worker who might devote hours to polishing an article describing primary research to be read by other researchers would, when preparing a review, take a handful of articles from a filing cabinet and throw them into a weekend bag. Sadly, this attitude has been detrimental, not only to science but also to the public health.

However, there is now a growing body of evidence that highlights numerous flaws in the design and reporting of primary research, most of which result in an exaggeration of the beneficial effects of an intervention (see Table 6.2). To improve the quality of reporting of controlled trials, the CONSORT Statement recommended that the results of any single trial should be discussed and appraised in the context of all available research evidence on that particular topic. To investigate whether this recommendation was being acted upon, Clarke and Chalmers[1] analysed the discussion section of 26 trials that had been published in the following five general medical journals – *The Lancet*, the *British Medical Journal*, the *Annals of Internal Medicine*, the *Journal of the American Medical Association* and the *New England Journal of Medicine*. They found that in only two of the articles was the RCT discussed in the context of an updated systematic review of earlier trials (Fig. 5.1); in four articles, although reference was made to a relevant systematic review, no attempt was made to integrate the results of the new trial into an updated version of the review; for 19 articles, there was no evidence that a systematic attempt had been made to set the new trial's results in the context of those of previous trials. Of the six studies for which the researchers made the claim that it was the first to address a particular question, only one appeared to be a genuine first trial – Clarke and Chalmers were able to identify similar studies that had been published previously by searching the Cochrane Controlled Trials Register and holding discussions with the relevant Cochrane Collaborative Review Groups. Clarke and Chalmers concluded that there was little evidence that the results of an RCT are discussed in the context of the totality of available evidence.

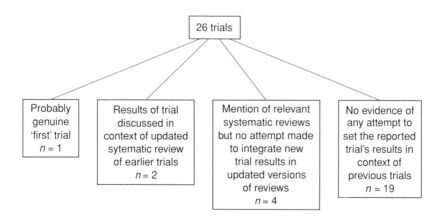

Fig. 5.1
The validity of claims of 'breakthroughs' in peer-reviewed articles (Source: Clarke and Chalmers[1])

5.3.1 Dimensions and definitions

A review of primary research, i.e. secondary research, may cover:

- only one type of research method – for example, a review of surveys or of RCTs;
- a combination of different research methods – for example, a review of the literature on the relationship between abuse (sexual and physical) and gastrointestinal illness that included surveys, and case-control and cohort studies, revealed an association between these two problems.[2]

There are four kinds of review:

- traditional or unsystematic reviews, a category that includes editorials;
- systematic reviews;
- systematic reviews that include meta-analysis;
- Cochrane Collaboration Reviews.

The main differences between traditional and systematic reviews are highlighted in Table 5.1, and those between systematic reviews and Cochrane Collaboration Reviews are shown in Table 5.2. Although traditional or unsystematic reviews may be readable and convenient to obtain, they can often be misleading, principally because they are unscientific.[3]

Table 5.1 The main differences between traditional or unsystematic reviews and systematic reviews

Characteristics	Traditional or unsystematic review	Systematic review
Strategy used to search for primary sources	Limited, usually to 1 electronic database, e.g. MEDLINE	Well-defined search of published and unpublished literature
Explicit description of search strategy	Not included	Included
Abstraction of data from primary sources	Subjective and haphazard choice	Systematic appraisal of quality of all papers identified using explicit quality criteria
Analysis of results from primary sources	Variety of techniques used	Systematic analysis using validated methods, e.g. correcting for heterogeneity

Table 5.2   The main differences between systematic reviews and Cochrane Collaboration Reviews

Characteristics	Systematic review	Cochrane Collaboration review
Strategy used to search for primary sources	Search of published literature, which might include hand-searching	Search of published and unpublished literature by hand
Dynamics of review process	Singular – limited to within a certain time frame, i.e. no updating	Iterative – regular updating as further studies published
Degree of consumer involvement	None	Consumers participate in all stages of the process

Economic evaluation can be a component of any of the types of review described above (see Section 6.7), but it is not necessarily included in a traditional or unsystematic review.

5.3.3.1 Meta-analysis

In a systematic review, the data from individual studies may be pooled and re-analysed using established statistical methods. This technique is called meta-analysis, but a systematic review in which this technique is employed is sometimes also called a 'meta-analysis'. Ioannidis and Lau have characterised the potential of meta-analysis as an:

> ... objective methodological engine, which enables information to be prospectively incorporated into a continuum of a large body of evidence.[4]

There are two types of meta-analysis, categorised according to the source of the data analysed.

- MAL meta-analysis, in which the data analysed are abstracted from published papers in the literature, i.e. it is data concerning groups of patients;
- MAP meta-analysis, in which the data analysed are individual patient data obtained directly from the authors of published papers; a MAP meta-analysis may also include unpublished data obtained from drug companies.

Stewart and Clarke found MAP meta-analyses to be more accurate than MAL meta-analyses;[5] however, in this comparison, the patients included in the individual patient data analysis were followed for a longer period of time. As MAP meta-analysis is a laborious and time-consuming process, it is probably more cost-effective to undertake MAL meta-analysis, and then, in exceptional cases, decide whether it is necessary or appropriate to undertake MAP meta-analysis.

5.3.2 Searching

When searching for a systematic review, there is a simple sequence of steps to follow.

Step 1: Is there a review in the Cochrane Database of Systematic Reviews (CDSR; see Appendix I, I.2.1.1)? If not, proceed to Step 2.

Step 2: Is there a review in the Database of Abstracts of Reviews of Effectiveness (DARE; see Appendix I, I.2.1.2)? If not, proceed to Step 3.

Step 3: Search MEDLINE (see Appendix I, I.2.6), EMBASE (see Appendix I, I.2.7) and other specialist databases (see Appendix I, I.2.8).

To search for systematic reviews in MEDLINE, Hunt and McKibbon[6] advocate the use of either a simple or comprehensive search strategy, as set out below.

Simple
1. meta-analysis (pt)
2. meta-anal: (textword)
3. review (pt) AND medline (textword)

Comprehensive
1. meta-analysis (pt)
2. meta-anal: (textword)
3. metaanal: (textword)
4. quantitative: review: OR quantitative: overview: (textword)
5. systematic: review: OR systematic: overview: (textword)
6. methodologic: review: OR methodologic: overview: (textword)
7. review (pt) AND medline (textword)

1 OR 2 OR 3 OR 4 OR 5 OR 6 OR 7

Next, add content terms to narrow the search to the particular clinical topic.

5.3.3 Appraisal

As healthcare decision-makers increasingly make use of the findings from systematic reviews as a source of evidence, it is vital to appraise their methodological quality. The two examples given below demonstrate the need for critical appraisal before accepting the findings from a systematic review or meta-analysis as reliable evidence.

Jadad et al.[7] used the Oxman and Guyatt Index to evaluate the quality of reporting and of the review for 50 systematic reviews and meta-analyses on the treatment of asthma, 12 of which were published in The Cochrane Library and 38 in peer-review journals. Using this index, they found that:

- 40 of the reviews had 'serious or extensive flaws';
- all 6 reviews associated with industry had 'serious or extensive flaws';
- of the 10 most rigorous reviews, 7 were published in The Cochrane Library.

McAlister et al.[8] followed up Cindy Mulrow's work of almost a decade earlier, in which she had highlighted the lack of scientific soundness in summarising evidence for review articles,[3] and they assessed the methodological quality of all reviews of clinical topics published in six general medical journals during 1996. Of 158 review articles, they found that:

- only 2 satisfied all 10 methodological criteria of good quality;
- less than one-quarter described how evidence was identified, evaluated or integrated.

In addition, of the 111 reviews in which treatment recommendations were made, only 45% cited randomised controlled clinical trials to support their recommendations.

5.3.3.1 Systematic reviews

A systematic review of all the evidence available is always more reliable than any single piece of evidence; a review of the relationship between abuse and gastrointestinal illness demonstrates this.[2] However, as systematic reviews can vary in quality, each one must be carefully appraised. A checklist of questions that can be used for the appraisal of systematic reviews is given in Box 5.3.

> **Box 5.3**   Checklist for the appraisal of systematic reviews (Source: Hunt and McKibbon [6])
>
> 1. Did the review article address a focused question?
> 2. Is it likely that important, relevant studies were missed?
> 3. Were the inclusion criteria to select articles appropriate?
> 4. Was the validity of the included studies assessed?
> 5. Were the assessments of studies reproducible?
> 6. Were the results similar from study to study?
> 7. What are the overall results and how precise are they?
> 8. Will the results help in caring for patients?

A source of bias in systematic reviews has been found by Misakian and Bero,[9] which arises from delays in the publication of, and failure to publish, non-significant results. These authors assert that this time-lag in publication provides an argument for the regular updating of reviews as practised by The Cochrane Collaboration.

Once the quality of a review has been appraised, it is then possible to consider its relevance to the local population and the decision that has to be made.

5.3.3.2   Systematic reviews including meta-analysis

If meta-analysis comprises part of any review, the process of appraisal must be more stringent. Meta-analysis is a powerful tool; performed correctly, it produces helpful evidence consistent with, but having narrower confidence intervals than, that from single trials (see Section 6.1.3). However, it is important to be aware that meta-analysis can produce a different conclusion to that generated by the performance of a large RCT. LeLorier et al. found that the outcomes of 12 large RCTs were not predicted accurately 35% of the time by the meta-analyses that had been published previously on the same topic.[10] Moreover, in a review including meta-analysis of magnesium treatment for myocardial infarction, Teo et al. concluded that this therapy was 'effective, safe and simple',[11] whereas in a large RCT known as ISIS-4 (the fourth International Study of Infarct Survival) it was found that magnesium was ineffective.[12] These examples illustrate two main points:

- that the findings from single large RCTs are a superior source of evidence to those from systematic reviews of small trials *if* the large RCT was conducted in the context of a systematic review of previous trials;[1]

- the limitations of meta-analysis.[13]

In an editorial accompanying the paper of LeLorier et al., Bailar concluded that meta-analysis may still be improved.[14] One of the ways in which it is possible to improve the quality of both systematic reviews and meta-analyses was investigated by Moher et al., who found that the quality of the individual trials subjected to meta-analysis had an influence on the interpretation of benefit of the intervention under investigation.[15] The features used to assess the quality of the trial reports are shown in Box 5.4.

There are two further reasons why the results of meta-analyses should be treated with caution.

1. Meta-analyses can be based solely on data from trials found by electronic searches of MEDLINE, which:
   - does not cover all of the world's biomedical journals (see p. 105);
   - finds only those trials that are electronically indexed, about half of the total (see Section 4.1.3.2);
   - finds only those trials that are published, which are usually biased towards the positive.[16]
2. The data from the trials included in a meta-analysis are often heterogeneous, that is, there are important differences among them. Although there are statistical techniques that can be used to minimise the effects of heterogeneity, it still presents a problem.[17]

In the light of these potential sources of bias and error in meta-analyses, as for all other research methodologies, the quality of any meta-analysis should be appraised critically. A checklist of questions for the appraisal of reviews that include a meta-analysis is shown in Box 5.5; these questions should be used in conjunction with those shown in Box 5.3.

5.3.4 Uses and abuses

The systematic review is the best source of evidence for decision-makers. An editorial by Mulrow et al.[19] in the *Annals of Internal Medicine* introduced a series of articles on systematic reviews, which together provide a useful overview of this research methodology and its application. One article of particular interest to those who make decisions about groups of patients and populations is by Bero and Jadad,[20] in which the authors describe how policy-makers and consumers can use the evidence from systematic reviews in decision-making (see Box 5.6). They conclude that as systematic reviews provide an objective

Box 5.4 Features used to assess quality of trial reports (Source: Moher et al.[15])

Randomisation

- Was the study described as randomised (this includes the use of words such as randomly, random, and randomisation)?

An additional point was given if the method to generate the sequence of randomisation was described and it was appropriate (e.g. table of random numbers, computer generated). However, a point was deducted if the method to generate the sequence of randomisation was described and it was inappropriate (e.g. date of birth).

Double blinding

- Was the study described as double blind?

An additional point was given if the method of masking was described and it was appropriate (e.g. identical placebo). However, a point was deducted if the method of masking was described and it was inappropriate (e.g. comparison of tablet versus injection with no double dummy).

Dropouts and withdrawals

- Defined, on the scale, as trial participants who were included in the study but did not complete the observation period or who were not included in the analysis (but should have been described).

The numbers and reasons for withdrawal in each group had to be stated for a point to be awarded. If there were no withdrawals, the report should have said so. If there was no statement on withdrawals, this item was given no point.

Generation of random numbers

- Clinical trials that reported the following methods for generation of their allocation sequence were considered adequate: computer, random numbers table, shuffled cards or tossed coins, and minimisation. Inadequate methods included alternate assignment and assignment by odd/even birth date or hospital number.

Allocation concealment

- Adequate concealment was that up to the point of treatment (e.g. central randomisation). The other category consisted of trials in which allocation concealment was not reported or was inadequate (e.g. alternation).

Box 5.5   Checklist for the appraisal of review articles that include meta-analysis

- Was the searching technique limited to an electronic search of MEDLINE?
- Are the results of the individual trials widely divergent?

It is not appropriate to pool trials in a meta-analysis if the level of heterogeneity is too great.

- Are all the individual trials in the meta-analysis small?

If so, be very cautious.[18]

Box 5.6   Stages in the use of systematic reviews by consumers and policy-makers (Source: Bero and Jadad[20])

- Awareness of the existence of systematic reviews.
- Perception of the advantages and disadvantages of using them.
- Identification of individual reviews.
- Critical evaluation.
- Incorporation into decisions.
- Participation in the design, evaluation, and dissemination of findings.

---

summary of large amounts of information they can be a useful decision-making tool for policy-makers to help them decide what healthcare to provide, and for consumers to help them make decisions about healthcare. Bero and Jadad highlight the scarcity of evidence about the impact of the use of systematic reviews on decision-making by policy-makers and consumers, and recommend that strategies to increase the use of systematic reviews should be evaluated for their usefulness.

One of the first examples of the extensive use of the findings from systematic reviews in a textbook is that written by McQuay and Moore on pain relief.[21] Two other notable texts cover the subjects of cardiology[22] and stroke[23] in an evidence-based way.

References

1. CLARKE, M. and CHALMERS, I. (1998) *Discussion sections in reports of controlled trials published in general medical journals. Islands in Ssarch of continents?* JAMA 280: 280–2.
2. DRASSMAN, D.A., TALLEY, N.J., ALDEN, K.W. and BARRIERO, M.A. (1995) *Sexual and physical abuse and gastrointestinal illness.* Ann. Intern. Med. 123: 782–94.
3. MULROW, C.W. (1987) *The medical review article: state of the science.* Ann. Intern. Med. 106: 485–8.
4. IOANNIDIS, J.P.A. and LAU, J. (1998) *Can quality of clinical trials and meta-analyses be quantified?* Lancet 352: 590.

5. STEWART, L.A. and CLARKE, M.J. (1995) *Practical methodology of meta-analyses (overviews) using updated individual patient data.* Stat. Med. 14: 2057–79.

6. HUNT, D.L. and McKIBBON, K.A. (1997) *Locating and appraising systematic reviews.* Ann. Intern. Med. 126: 532–8.

7. JADAD, A.R., MOHER, M., BROWMAN, G.P., BOOKER, L., SIGOUIN, C., FUENTES, M. and STEVENS, R. (2000) *Systematic reviews and meta-analysis on treatment of asthma: critical evaluation.* Br. Med. J. 320: 537–40.

8. McALISTER, F.A., CLARK, H.D., van WALRAVEN, C., STRAUS, S.E., LAWSON, F.M., MOHER, D. and MULROW, C. (1999) *The medical review article revisited: has the science improved?* Ann. Intern. Med. 131: 947–51.

9. MISAKIAN, A.L. and BERO, L.A. (1998) *Publication bias and research on passive smoking. Comparison of published and unpublished studies.* JAMA 280: 250–3.

10. LeLORIER, J., GREGOIRE, G., BENHADDAD, A. et al. (1997) *Discrepancies between meta-analyses and subsequent large randomised controlled trials.* N. Engl. J. Med. 337: 536–42.

11. TEO, K.K., YUSUF, S., COLLINS, R. et al. (1991) *Effects of intravenous magnesium in suspected acute myocardial infarction: overview of randomised trials.* Br. Med. J. 303: 1499–503.

12. ISIS-4 COLLABORATIVE GROUP (1995) *ISIS-4: a randomised factorial trial assessing early oral captopril, oral mononitrate, and intravenous magnesium sulphate in 58,050 patients with suspected acute myocardial infarction.* Lancet 345: 669–85.

13. YUSUF, S. and FLATHER, M. (1995) *Magnesium in acute myocardial infarction. ISIS4 provides no grounds for its routine use [Editorial].* Br. Med. J. 310: 751–2.

14. BAILAR, J.C. III (1997) *The promise and problems of meta-analysis.* N. Engl. J. Med. 337: 559–60.

15. MOHER, D., PHAM, B., JONES, A., COOK, D.J., JADAD, A.R., MOHER, M. and TUGWELL, P. (1998) *Does quality of reports of randomised trials affect estimates of intervention efficacy reported in meta-analyses?* Lancet 352: 609–13.

16. EASTERBROOK, P.J., BERLIN, J.A., GOPALAN, R. and MATTHEWS, D.R. (1991) *Publication bias in clinical research.* Lancet 337: 867–72.

17. THOMPSON, S.G. and POCOCK, S.J. (1991) *Can meta-analyses be trusted?* Lancet 338: 1127–30.

18. EGGER, M. and SMITH, G.D. (1995) *Misleading meta-analysis: lessons from an 'effective, safe, simple' intervention that wasn't [Editorial].* Br. Med. J. 310: 752–4.

19. MULROW, C.D., COOK, D.J. and DAVIDOFF, F. (1997) *Systematic reviews: critical links in the great chain of evidence.* Ann. Intern. Med. 126: 389–391

20. BERO, L.A. and JADAD, A.R. (1997) *How consumers and policymakers can use systematic reviews for decision making.* Ann. Intern. Med. 127: 37–42.

21. McQUAY, H.J. and MOORE, A. (1998) *An Evidence-Based Resource for Pain.* Oxford University Press, Oxford.

22. YUSUF, F., CAIRNS, J.A., CAMM, J.A., FALLEN, E.L. and GERSH, B.J. (1998) *Evidence-Based Cardiology.* BMJ Publishing, London.

23. WARLOW, C.P, DENNIS, M.S., van GIJN, J., HANKEY, G.J., SANDERCOCK, P.A.G., BAMFORD, J.M. and WARDLAW, J. (1996) *Stroke: A Practical Guide to Management.* Blackwell Science, Oxford.

The interested reader should also consult the Cochrane Database of Systematic Reviews (CDSR), the Cochrane Review Methodology Database, and The Reviewers' Handbook, which are all part of The Cochrane Library (see Appendix I, I.2.1).

5.4 RANDOMISED CONTROLLED TRIALS

The RCT is a very beautiful technique, of wide applicability, but as with everything else there are snags.

Archie Cochrane, Effectiveness and Efficiency, *1989*

5.4.1 Dimensions and definitions

The primary use for an RCT is to evaluate the effectiveness of an intervention, usually a treatment regimen, but it is also possible to apply it to diagnostic interventions, screening programmes or managerial innovations. The defining features of an RCT are shown in Box 5.7.

Box 5.7 The defining features of an RCT

- There must be equipoise, that is, genuine doubt prior to the trial about whether one option is better than another.
- The individuals who might benefit from the intervention are randomly allocated to receive that intervention or not; the latter form the control group, and receive a placebo or the 'standard' treatment.
- All entrants to the trial are followed up in treatment and control groups.
- Individuals in the treatment group remain in that group irrespective of whether they actually receive the intervention; for example, in a trial of breast cancer screening those randomly allocated to receive screening remain in that group even if they do not attend for treatment – this is called randomisation on an 'intention-to-treat' basis.
- The assessment of outcome is made by an assessor who is unaware of the patient's status; this is know as 'blind' assessment.
- All patients are included in the analysis.
- In some types of RCT, such as drug trials, both doctor and patient may be 'blind', i.e. unaware of whether the patient is a member of a treatment group or of the control group – such a trial is known as 'double blind'.

Errors in an RCT may arise as a result of bias or by chance. Bias is manifest as a systematic error that favours either the treatment or the control group. The error is referred to as systematic because if it occurs once it will occur repeatedly due to a flaw in the design or management of the trial. The features of an RCT are designed to minimise bias. Error due to chance is random. Therefore, trials must be carefully designed to ensure that they have sufficient *power* to detect a difference between treatment and control groups, if one exists, or to demonstrate that there is no effect if the treatment is ineffective (Box 5.8).

Box 5.8 Power rules

- The smaller the effect expected in the treatment being tested, the larger the trial necessary to have sufficient power to detect it.
- The larger the trial, the greater its power.

The feature that distinguishes an RCT from a controlled trial is the random allocation of subjects to receive the intervention under investigation.

For an excellent history of the RCT, consult the 'Controlled Trials from History' page at the well-designed website of the Royal College of Physicians of Edinburgh: http://www.rcpe.ac.uk/controlled_trials/index.html

For a book about RCTs that is clear, concise and easy to read, consult Jadad (see Further Reading at the end of this section).

5.4.1.1 Mega trials

To detect a small improvement in health outcome, for example, 5%, a very large trial is needed. Although at first sight it might appear that a 5% improvement is clinically insignificant, for common diseases, such as myocardial infarction, a 5% improvement is of great importance. Large trials, sometimes called 'mega trials', can be designed to demonstrate these small differences in outcome; such trials have made a significant contribution to the management of cardiovascular disease.[1] The main differences between a trial and a mega trial are shown in Table 5.3.

Some of the characteristics of a mega trial can be seen as limitations, for example, the administration of additional treatments may lead to any effect of the experimental therapy being obscured.[2] Any such effects must be borne in mind during the appraisal of mega trial findings. In contrast, some workers feel that certain characteristics that could be regarded as weaknesses, such as simple entry criteria, actually reflect the situation in clinical practice.

Table 5.3   The distinguishing features between trials and mega trials

Characteristics	RCT	Mega trial
Number of subjects	Tens or hundreds	As many as 20 000 each in the treatment and control groups
Number of professionals	Less than ten	Many investigators, sometimes hundreds
Location	Single centre	Multiple centres in several countries
Entry criteria	Restrictive	Simple – wide variety of different types of patient included
Treatment regimen	Only that under investigation	Other treatments in addition to that under investigation may be administered

5.4.1.2   Patient preference in trials

A methodological development of particular importance is the incorporation of patient preference into trials in which the patient's participation in the process of treatment, and therefore his/her motivation, is essential for the intervention to be effective. In drug trials, patient preference is not a significant factor (all the patient has to do is swallow the pills), but in other types of treatment, for example, a study of subcutaneous continuous infusion pumps in the management of diabetes, patient preference needs to be built into the design of the trial.[3]

5.4.1.3   'N of 1' trials

The 'N of 1' trial is a single-patient controlled trial used in the specific circumstances of the care of a patient whose condition, depression for instance, fluctuates widely and is affected by a multiplicity of factors such that the effect of treatment is difficult to assess.[4] In such a situation, after consultation with the doctor, the patient might agree to an 'N of 1' trial. During the trial, personnel in the pharmacy will switch the patient's therapy between active and placebo treatments several times; to be conclusive, the therapy may need to be switched as many as 10 times; neither doctor nor patient is aware of the switches, i.e. they are 'blind'. The doctor and patient will meet at review consultations, but the assessment of treatment outcome is made by a third party, who is also 'blind', i.e. not aware of when the patient was receiving the active drug or the placebo.

5.4.2 Searching

In addition to using the search term for the particular treatment or test that is the focus of the decision, specify the retrieval of RCTs.

The problems usually experienced when searching for trials, because of the limited coverage of MEDLINE and imprecise indexing, are diminishing as the work of The Cochrane Collaboration progresses. Hand-searching of journals, including those covered by MEDLINE and other databases, has revealed many more trials such that about 100 000 are now easily available via The Cochrane Library (see Appendix I, I.2.1). Previously, only about 20 000 RCTs were findable on MEDLINE.

For search strategies to identify RCTs, consult:

LeFEBVRE, C. (1994) *The Cochrane Collaboration: the role of the UK Cochrane Centre in identifying evidence.* Health Libraries Review 11: 235–42.

5.4.3 Appraisal

During the 1970s, although the RCT was regarded as the 'gold standard' for demonstrating the effectiveness of a therapy, there was a growing awareness that this research method also had limitations.

- A survey of 71 negative RCTs showed that the majority of these trials were too small, that is, had insufficient power, to detect important clinical differences, a fact of which the authors seemed unaware.[5]
- A study of 206 RCTs showed that randomisation, one of the main design features of an RCT necessary to prevent bias, was poorly reported. Moreover, in those trials for which randomisation was not described, the effect of treatment was exaggerated by an amount greater than the true effect of the treatment (Table 5.4).[6]

Table 5.4 Methodological quality and estimates of treatment effects in controlled trials (trials with poor evidence of randomisation were compared with trials with adequate randomisation) (Source: Schulz et al.[6])

Methodological issue	Exaggeration of odds ratio (%)
Inadequate method of treatment allocation	Larger by 41%
Unclear method of treatment allocation	Larger by 30%
Trials not double blind	Larger by 17%

- In one review of 196 double-blind trials, it was stated that: 'Doubtful or invalid statements were found in 76% of the conclusions or abstracts'.[7] Bias consistently favoured the new drug in 81 trials and the control in only one trial.[7]
- In a critical appraisal of the relationship between the methodological quality, and other characteristics, of 51 reviews of spinal manipulation as a treatment for low back pain and the conclusions about the effectiveness of this intervention,[8] it was found that one of the factors associated with a positive conclusion (the outcome in 34 reviews) was the presence of a spinal manipulator on the review team.

From these examples, it can be seen that the results of RCTs, like any other research findings, need careful appraisal using explicit criteria.

There are many factors that have been shown to bias a trial, and various checklists of quality criteria have been produced,[9] but these are usually of most use to research workers. Chalmers[10] has identified the three most important factors as follows:

1. inadequate randomisation;
2. failure to blind the assessor of outcome;
3. failure to follow up all the patients in the trial.

These criteria are epidemiological and can be used to assess the quality of a trial; other criteria can be used to assess the size of the effect found in a trial (Box 5.9).

5.4.3.1 Subgroup analysis

It is tempting for the investigators involved in any trial or meta-analysis to analyse data from subgroups of patients to look for treatment effects, particularly if the overall result of the trial is negative. This technique is known as subgroup analysis or data 'dredging'. Any effects of treatment demonstrated by subgroup analysis should be viewed with caution and the analysis appraised carefully using the checklist developed by Oxman and Guyatt[11] (see Box 5.10).

Box 5.9   Checklist for appraising randomised controlled trials (©CASP)

The 11 questions are adapted from: Guyatt GH, Sackett DL, Cook DJ. Users' guides to the medical literature. II. How to use an article about therapy or prevention. JAMA 1993; 270: 2598–601 and 271: 59–63.

A. Are the results of the trial valid?

Screening questions

1. Did the trial address a clearly focused issue?
   An issue can be 'focused' in terms of:
   - the population studied;
   - the intervention given;
   - the outcomes considered.

2. Was the assignment of patients to treatments randomised?
3. Were all of the patients who entered the trial properly accounted for at its conclusion?
   - Was follow up complete?
   - Were patients analysed in the groups to which they were randomised?

Detailed questions

4. Were patients, health workers and study personnel 'blind' to treatment?
5. Were the groups similar at the start of the study? In terms of other factors that might affect the outcome such as age, sex, social class.
6. Aside from the experimental intervention, were the groups treated equally?

B. What are the results?

7. How large was the treatment effect? What outcomes were measured?
8. How precise was the estimate of the treatment effect? What are its confidence limits?

C. Will the results help locally?

9. Can the results be applied to the local population? *Do you think that the patients covered by the trial are similar enough to your population?*
10. Were all clinically important outcomes considered? *If not, does this affect the decision?*
11. Are the benefits worth the harms and costs? *This is unlikely to be addressed by the trial. But what do you think?*

> **Box 5.10** Guidelines for deciding whether apparent differences in subgroup response are real (Source: Oxman and Guyatt[11])
>
> - Is the magnitude of the difference clinically important?
> - Was the difference statistically significant?
> - Did the hypothesis precede rather than follow the analysis?
> - Was the subgroup analysis one of a small number of hypotheses tested?
> - Was the difference suggested by comparisons within rather than between studies?
> - Was the difference consistent across studies?
> - Is there indirect evidence that supports the hypothesised difference?

5.4.4 Uses and abuses

An RCT is the best way of evaluating the effectiveness of an intervention.

5.4.4.1 Interpretation and presentation

A research-based fact is like an uncut diamond, valuable but of little use. The decision-maker has to be able to apply that fact. A checklist of questions that can be used to determine the applicability of research findings is shown in Box 5.11.

> **Box 5.11** Checklist for assessing the applicability of research findings
>
> - How wide are the confidence intervals?
> - What were the exclusion and inclusion criteria?
> - How similar were the patients in the trial to the 'local' patient group?
> - Could the quality of service provided in the trial be reproduced locally?

However, the application of any research information is beset with difficulties because the results of an RCT done on a sample of the whole population must be extrapolated to the local population for which the decision-maker is responsible. This involves judgement, and there are two pervasive but subtle influences that bear upon a decision-maker's judgement and the way in which s/he might apply research findings to the local population.

1. Cultural effects – interpretation
Cultural factors influence the interpretation of research information. In general, physicians in the USA have been quicker to adopt innovations in high technology than their counterparts in the UK. This difference can be illustrated by the differing attitudes towards clotbusting agents.[12] In the USA, tissue plasminogen activator (tPA) is the drug of choice; in the UK, it is streptokinase. However, it can be seen from Fig. 5.2 that tPA is no more effective than streptokinase, which is 10 times cheaper; moreover, streptokinase has fewer adverse effects (see Fig. 5.3). American culture fosters the attitude that a novel intervention should be tried if there is no evidence against its use, whereas the attitude in the UK is that a new intervention should not be introduced until there is strong evidence in favour of its use: New World vs Old; Gung-ho vs Stick-in-the-Mud.

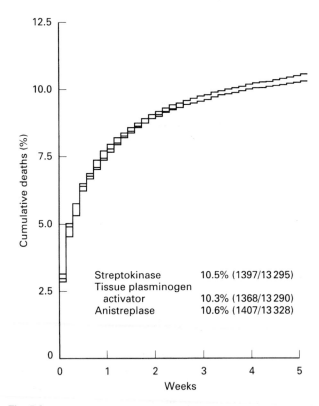

Fig. 5.2
Mortality of three agents compared in ISIS-3 (Source: O'Donnell,[12] with permission, BMJ Publishing Group)

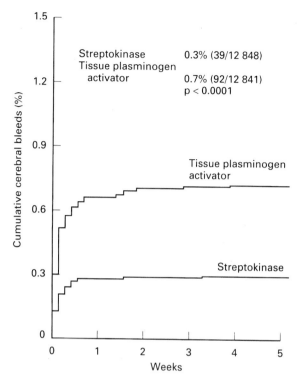

Fig. 5.3
Rates of cerebral bleeds with streptokinase and tissue plasminogen activator in ISIS-3 (Source: O'Donnell,[12] with permission, BMJ Publishing Group)

2. The framing effect – presentation
If a picture is set off by a good frame, it will sell more easily – an experience-based aphorism from the antiques trade. The same applies to research findings: decision-makers are influenced not only by the data but also by the way in which those data are presented. This phenomenon, known as the framing effect, has been recognised by psychologists for years. Indeed, the way in which the pharmaceutical industry presents data to clinicians increases the probability of positive interpretation and therefore of prescribing.

Evidence of the existence of the framing effect is growing. The results of studies in Canada[13] and Italy[14] have shown the degree to which clinicians are influenced by data presented in terms of relative risk reduction. The framing effect has also been shown to influence purchasers. Fahey et al.[15] provided 182 executive and non-executive members of 13 health authorities, family health services authorities, or health commissions with the results from a randomised trial on breast cancer screening, and those from a systematic review on cardiac rehabilitation. However, both sets of results were presented in four different ways, as shown in Table 5.5.

Table 5.5   The framing effect – presentation of the same information in four different ways for two programmes (Source: adapted from Fahey et al.[15])

Method of data presentation	Mammography	Cardiac rehabilitation
Relative risk reduction	34%	20%
Absolute risk reduction	0.06%	3%
Percentage of event-free patients	99.82% vs 99.8%	84% vs 87%
Number needed to treat (NNT)	1592	31

From the 140 questionnaires returned, it was found that the willingness to fund either programme was influenced significantly by the way in which the data were presented. Relative risk reduction stimulated a significantly higher inclination to purchase, followed by the number needed to treat (NNT). It is intriguing to note that only three respondents, 'all non-executive members claiming no training in epidemiology', recognised that the four different modes of presentation of the two sets of data summarised the same results in both cases.

5.4.4.2   Aphoristic warnings

➤ For those who want to influence others, use relative risk reduction as the means of presenting data.
➤ For those who are likely to be influenced by data presentation, never, ever, accept information on the basis of relative risk reduction alone.

Further reading
JADAD, A. R. (1998) *Randomised controlled trials. A User's Guide.* BMJ Books, London.

References

1. YUSUF, S., COLLINS, R. and PETO, T.R. (1984) *Why do we need some large sample randomised trials?* Stat. Med. 3: 409–20.
2. WOODS, K.L. (1995) *Mega-trials and the management of myocardial infarction.* Lancet 346: 611–14.
3. BREWIN, C.R. and BRADLEY, C. (1989) *Patient preferences and randomised controlled trials.* Br. Med. J. 299: 313–15.
4. GUYATT, G., SACKETT, D., TAYLER, W., CHANG, J., ROBERTS, R. and PUGSLEY, S. (1986) *Determining optimal therapy – randomised trials in individual patients.* N. Engl. J. Med. 314: 889–92.

5. FREIMAN, J.A., CHALMERS, T.C., SMITH, H. and KUEBLER, R.R. (1978) *The importance of Beta, the type II error, and sample size in the design and interpretation of the randomised controlled trial.* N. Engl. J. Med. 299: 690–4.
6. SCHULZ, K.F., CHALMERS, I., HAYES, R.J. and ALTMAN, D.G. (1995) *Empirical evidence of bias: dimensions of methodological quality associated with estimates of treatment effects in controlled trials.* JAMA 273: 408–12.
7. GØTZSCHE, P.C. (1989) *Methodology and overt and hidden bias in reports of 196 double blind trials of non-steroidal anti-inflammatory drugs in rheumatoid arthritis.* Control. Clin. Trials 10: 31–56. *Erratum* Control. Clin. Trials 10: 356.
8. ASSENFELDT, W.J.J., KOES, B.W., KNIPSCHILD, P.G. and BOUTER, L.M. (1995) ,*The relationship between methodological quality and conclusions in reviews of spinal manipulation.* JAMA 264: 1942–8.
9. STANDARDS OF REPORTING TRIALS GROUP (1994) *A proposal for structured reporting of randomised controlled trials.* JAMA 272: 1926–31.
10. CHALMERS, I. (1995) '*Applying overviews and meta-analyses at the bedside': discussion.* J. Clin. Epidemiol. 48: 67–70.
11. OXMAN, A.D. and GUYATT, G.H. (1992) *A consumer's guide to subgroup analyses.* Ann. Intern. Med. 116: 78–84.
12. O'DONNELL, M. (1991) *The battle of the clotbusters.* Br. Med. J. 302: 1259–61.
13. NAYLOR, C.D., CHEN, E. and STRAUSS, B. (1992) *Measured enthusiasm: does the method of reporting trial results alter perceptions of therapeutic effectiveness?* Ann. Intern. Med. 117: 916–21.
14. BOBBIO, M., DEMICHELIS, B. and GIUSTETTO, G. (1994) *Completeness of reporting trial results: effect on physicians' willingness to prescribe.* Lancet 343: 1209–11.
15. FAHEY, T., GRIFFITHS, S. and PETERS, T.J. (1995) *Evidence-based purchasing: understanding results of clinical trials and systematic reviews.* Br. Med. J. 311: 1056–60

5.5   CASE-CONTROL STUDIES

For two decades, the case-control study was eclipsed by the RCT as the 'gold standard' in the evaluation of effectiveness, but during the 1990s its distinct and essential contribution regained recognition.

5.5.1 Dimensions and definitions

A case-control study is one in which the individuals selected for the control group have the same characteristics as the individuals in the study group except for the characteristic that is the subject of the hypothesis. In a case-control study of a cancer, for example, the study group comprises those who have the cancer; the characteristics of these individuals, e.g. age, gender, and smoking status, are matched with those of the controls, with the exception that the individuals in the control group do not have cancer.

However, a study in which the outcomes for men who received an intervention, such as prostate cancer screening, simply by virtue of being eligible for a private service are compared with those of men of the same age who have not had the intervention simply because they were not eligible is *not* a case-control study; it is a badly designed and invalid trial.

Case-control studies have several advantageous features:

- they can be less expensive than trials (although some case-control studies are expensive because they involve a large number of subjects);
- they can sometimes be completed relatively quickly.

A case-control study can be used to investigate the following problems:

- the causation of disease;
- the adverse effects of treatment.

5.5.1.1 *Study of the causation of disease*

In a case-control study of people who had lung cancer, it was found that smoking was the main cause of lung cancer: a large proportion of those who had lung cancer smoked whereas only a very small proportion of the control group, none of whom smoked, developed lung cancer.[1]

5.5.1.2 *Study of the adverse effects of treatment*

As the beneficial effects of treatment are usually more common than the adverse effects, a trial with sufficient power to detect the beneficial effects will probably not be powerful enough to detect adverse effects. Adverse effects can be detected either by following patients over many years in a cohort study (Section 5.6) or within a case-control study (current section). In a study of the adverse effects of treatment for high blood pressure,[2] 623 hypertensive patients who were members of a group health co-operative and who had had a first fatal or first non-fatal myocardial infarction were compared with 2032 hypertensive patients, matched for age, sex and calendar year, who had not had a myocardial infarction. The following patients were excluded: those who had been members of the co-operative for less than 1 year; those who did not have a diagnosis of hypertension; those who had had a prior myocardial infarction; those whose infarction had been a complication of a procedure or surgery. Patients entered into the study had to have been taking antihypertensive medicines for at least 30 days – preliminary analysis had shown that the recent starting of beta-blockers and calcium-channel blockers was strongly associated with a risk of myocardial infarction. Initial analysis included only those patients who were free of clinical cardiovascular disease. A strong association between acute myocardial infarction and dose of calcium-channel blocker, administered either alone or in combination with a diuretic, was found. The risk at the highest doses of calcium-channel blockers was three times that at the lowest doses. It is interesting that the authors of this case-control study then performed a systematic review of RCTs,[3] which underlines the need to evaluate a therapy using several different research methods.

5.5.2 Searching

Usually, the first step in any search strategy is to search for RCTs (Section 5.4.2). However, as the results of RCTs alone will not necessarily give all the outcomes of an intervention, it is always useful to search for case-control studies. The most specific way of searching for case-control studies on MEDLINE is to 'explode' (i.e. include this term together with all subordinate terms) the Medical Subject Heading (MeSH) 'case control studies'. It is important to be aware that, as with all study design MeSH terms, its use will generate methodological articles on how to conduct or evaluate a case-control study as well as examples of case-control studies. As most optimal strategies contain both MeSH terms and natural occurring text terms, it is also advisable to use the term 'case control' as a phrase (i.e. in title or abstract). Do not include the word 'studies' in a phrase search because terms such as 'case control design' or even 'case control study' will be missed.

5.5.3 Appraisal

Case-control studies are prone to bias: in a major review of case-control studies, 35 different sources of bias were identified.[4] For the user of research information or a decision-maker, these 35 sources of bias can be distilled into two questions, as follows.

1. Was the selection of control subjects based on a set of criteria that matched the controls with the case subjects

on every criterion except the presence of the disease or risk factor being studied?

2. Were measurements on the control subjects free from bias, e.g. was the observer performing the assessment aware of the patient's status as a case or as a control subject?

5.5.4 Uses and abuses

The main uses of case-control studies are:

- the identification of the causes of disease;
- the identification of rare effects of treatment, usually side-effects.

The main abuse of a case-control study is the evaluation of the effectiveness of an intervention. The appropriate methodology to use for this research question is an RCT.

References

1. DOLL, R. and HILL, A.B. (1952) *The study of the aetiology of carcinoma of the lung.* Br. Med. J. ii: 1271–86.
2. PSATY, B.M., HECKBERT, S.R., KOEPSELL, T.D. et al. (1995) *The risk of myocardial infarction associated with antihypertensive drug therapies.* JAMA 274: 620–5.
3. FURBERG, C.D. PSATY, B.M. and MEYER, J.V. (1995) *Nifedipine. Dose-related increase in mortality in patients with coronary heart disease.* Circulation 92: 1326–31.
4. SACKETT, D.L. (1979) *Bias in analytic research.* J. Chron. Dis. 32: 51–63.

5.6 COHORT STUDIES

Cohort 1489 [a. F. cohorte, ad. L. cohortem (cohors), f. co- + hort-, …] 1. Rom. Antiq. A body of from 300 to 600 infantry; the tenth part of a legion. 2. transf. A band of warriors 1500. 3. fig. A company, band 1719.

Shorter Oxford English Dictionary

5.6.1 Dimensions and definitions

In a cohort study, a group of people is investigated over a particular period of time; any changes that occur during that period are recorded. A cohort study can be either retrospective, for example, a review of all cases of breast, colorectal or prostate cancer treated in seven Californian hospitals between 1980 and 1982,[1] or prospective, that is, the identification of a group of healthy people or patients in order to follow them from one point in time to another.

In a cohort study, subject data can be those collected routinely or those collected specifically for the purpose of the study, or a combination of both.

A cohort study can be used to investigate the following situations.

- The outcome of treatment when it is not possible to perform an RCT for ethical reasons; for example, a study to determine the outcome of prostatectomy.[2] The findings from a cohort study enable quality standards such as the readmission rate[3] to be based on evidence.
- Different approaches to health service delivery and management that cannot be evaluated in an RCT, either because the number of units is too small to confer adequate power upon the trial or because health service policy-makers or managers will not allow their service to be included in such a trial.
- 'Natural experiments', that is, either when changes are made in the organisation or delivery of healthcare for political or managerial reasons, or where different patterns of care exist in similar settings by reason of history and tradition.

Cohort studies have been used to investigate:

- staffing changes: for example, in a study of the effect of introducing on-site physician staffing to intensive care units in hospitals other than teaching centres, it was found that survival improved among patients who had an intermediate likelihood of death;[4]
- the relationship between volume and quality – for some types of intervention an association has been found, particularly for those that are more complex; [5,6]
- the relationship between status and organisation of a hospital, such as teaching vs non-teaching or public vs private, and clinical outcome; although these relationships are complicated, important results can be obtained: for example, in one study, a 'positive correlation between higher mortality rates and hospitals located in States with strict prospective reimbursement programs' was found;[7]
- the relationship between the organisation of a clinical service and clinical outcome: for example, better co-ordination was shown to be associated with lower mortality in intensive care,[8] and the admission of

severely injured patients directly to an operating theatre was shown to reduce 'mortality, morbidity and suffering' in a cohort of patients followed for 9 years after a change in hospital organisation;[9]

- the relationship between professional qualification and clinical outcome – in one study, higher levels of qualification were associated with better outcome,[5] but this finding may reflect a failure to train less highly qualified staff adequately.

It is possible to organise RCTs to assess the benefits of different types of service, such as a geriatric assessment service,[10] or of different methods of healthcare financing (for example, in one RCT the clinical outcomes of a health maintenance organisation and of a fee-for-service organisation were compared[11]). However, for many questions about the relationship between the funding and organisation of healthcare and patient outcomes, a well-conducted cohort study is the most appropriate form of research design.

In the funding or commissioning of research, the balance between promoting direct experimentation, through RCTs, and supporting observational studies, such as a survey of 'high cost patients in 17 acute-care hospitals',[12] must be reviewed continually.

5.6.1.1 *The role of clinical databases*

In a leader in the *British Medical Journal*, Black[13] called for the development of 'high quality clinical databases' which could provide a basis for either observational studies, such as cohort studies, or for RCTs. Databases in which all the cases of a particular type are collected, for example, patients who have leukaemia or all those who have been through intensive care, allow the entire population that has had a particular disorder, or experienced a particular level of care, to be identified and followed up.

Some workers would also argue that such databases provide a better framework for research than RCTs, in which the focus is often on selected subsets of the population.

5.6.2 Searching

It is not necessary to search specifically for cohort studies. A search undertaken in the subject of interest will uncover them.

5.6.3 Appraisal

There are three study design features that are pivotal in the appraisal of any cohort study.

1. The recruitment of individuals
The most important aspect of recruitment is completeness: all of the subjects in a defined time-period should be recruited. If any sampling procedure has been applied to recruitment, such as the recruitment of patients admitted either on weekdays or between 0900 and 1700 hours, it should create suspicion that the study results are biased. It can also be useful to ask: 'What happened to the patients who were not recruited?'. It might be that the more severe cases were referred elsewhere, or those undertaking referral may have referred only mild cases to the hospitals in the study.

2. Study criteria
The criteria used to assess the outcomes of care must be valid. For example, in-patient mortality is not a valid criterion of the quality of hospital care because of variations in duration of patient stay; it is better to use a criterion such as 30- or 60-day mortality. If criteria other than mortality are used, the instruments used to measure variables, such as pain or quality of life, should be validated.

3. Analysis of results
In the analysis of results, the severity of illness should always be taken into account and receive explicit mention in the paper. For example, in studies of intensive care, there is a validated system for assessing the severity of a patient's condition, known as APACHE (acute physiology and chronic health evaluation).[8]

It is also important to control for the effects of co-morbidity, that is, the presence of other diseases that might have influenced outcome.[1] Robust techniques have been developed to do this and must have been applied to the clinical outcome if the results are to be accepted as valid.[14–16]

A checklist of questions that can be used in the appraisal of the findings of any cohort study is shown in Box 5.12.

> **Box 5.12**   Checklist for appraising cohort studies
>
> - Is clear information given about the way in which the cohort was recruited?
> - Were any steps or decisions taken that could have included or excluded more severe cases?
> - If mortality is a criterion, what steps were taken to ensure that all deaths were identified?
> - If other criteria were used, have the instruments used for measurement been validated?
> - Was the severity of disease taken into account in the analysis?
> - Was the presence of other diseases (co-morbidity) taken into account in the analysis?

5.6.4 Uses and abuses

It is appropriate to use cohort studies:

- to assess changes in health service management or organisation;
- to identify uncommon or adverse effects of treatment.

The main abuse of a cohort study is to assess the effectiveness of a particular intervention when a more appropriate method would be an RCT.

References

1. GREENFIELD, S., ARONOW, H.U., ELASHOFF, R.M. and WATANABE, D. (1988) *Flaws in mortality data. The hazards of ignoring comorbid disease.* JAMA 260: 2253–5.
2. FOWLER, F.J., WENNBERG, J.E., TIMOTHY, R.P., BARRY, M.J., MULLEY, A.G. Jr. and HANLEY, D. (1988) *Symptom status and quality of life following prostatectomy.* JAMA 259: 3018–22.
3. HENDERSON, J., GOLDACRE, M.J., GRAVENEY, M.J. and SIMMONS, H.M. (1989) *Use of medical record linkage to study readmission rate.* Br. Med. J. 299: 709–13.
4. THEODORE, C.M., PHILLIPS, M.C., SHAW, L., COOK, E.F., NATANSON, C. and GOLDMAN, L. (1984) *On-site physician staffing in a community hospital intensive care unit.* JAMA 252: 2023–7.
5. KELLY, J.V., and HELLINGER, F.J. (1986) *Physician and hospital factors associated with mortality of surgical patients.* Medical Care 24: 785–800.
6. KELLY, J.V. and HELLINGER, F.J. (1987) *Heart disease and hospital deaths: an empirical study.* Health Serv. Res. J. 22: 369–95.
7. SHORTELL, S.M. and HUGHES, E.F.X. (1988) *The effects of regulation, competition and ownership on mortality rates among hospital inpatients.* N. Engl. J. Med. 318: 1100–7.
8. KNAUS, W.A., DRAPER, E.A., DOUGLAS, M.S. and ZIMMERMAN, J.E. (1986) *An evaluation of outcome from intensive care in major medical centers.* Ann. Intern. Med. 104: 410–18.
9. FISCHER, R.P., JELENSE, S. and PERRY, J.F. Jr. (1978) *Direct transfer to operating room improves care of trauma patients.* JAMA 240: 1731–2.

10. STUCK, A.E., SIU, A.L., WIELAND, G.D., ADAMS, J. and RUBENSTEIN, L.Z. (1993) *Comprehensive geriatric assessment: a meta-analysis of controlled trials.* Lancet 342: 1032–6.
11. WARE, J.E., RODGERS, W.H., DAVIES, A.R. et al. (1986) *Comparison of health outcomes at a health maintenance organisation with those of fee-for-service care.* Lancet i: 1017–22.
12. SCHROEDER, S.A., SHOWSTACK, J.A. and ROBERTS, H.E. (1979) *Frequency and clinical description of high-cost patients in 17 acute-care hospitals.* N. Engl. J. Med. 300: 1306–9.
13. BLACK, N. (1997) *Developing high quality clinical databases.* Br. Med. J. 315: 381–2.
14. KNAUS, W.A. and NASH, D.B. (1988) *Predicting and evaluating patient outcomes.* Ann. Intern. Med. 109: 521–2.
15. SEAGROATT, V. and GOLDACRE, M.J. (1994) *Measures of early postoperative mortality beyond hospital fatality rates.* Br. Med. J. 309: 361–5.
16. JENCKS, S.F. and DOBSON, A. (1987) *Refining case-mix adjustment. The research evidence.* [Special article] N. Engl. J. Med. 317: 679–86.

5.7 SURVEYS

5.7.1 Dimensions and definitions

A survey is an investigation of what is happening at a point in, or during a period of, time. For example, in a survey of 61 US hospitals in which the approaches to quality improvement were investigated in relation to an objective measure of clinical efficiency (length of stay), it was found that the most important determinant of quality was the management culture within a hospital rather than the specific quality improvement techniques utilised.[1]

To increase the power of a survey, it can be combined with statistical analysis. For example, in a study of the factors that promoted or hindered physician satisfaction with the hospital in which they worked, regression analysis was conducted on the survey results.[2]

However, the best way to increase the validity of a survey is to repeat it either after a period of time has elapsed or after some intervention has been undertaken: this type of study in which a group of people, patients or service providers is followed over a period of time is called a cohort study (see Section 5.6). Surveys, however, give the fastest return on investment.

5.7.2 Searching

The appropriate technique for searching for surveys will depend on the subject of the survey that you require. It is common practice to use the Medical Subject Heading

(MeSH) 'Health surveys' but it usually needs to be supplemented by an additional MeSH modifier (e.g. Mortality, Birth Rate, Vital Statistics, Demography, Morbidity, Incidence, Prevalence). It is also possible to use the subject of the survey such as disease – 'coronary disease' – with a subheading such as epidemiology or mortality, or an intervention – 'coronary angiography' – with a subheading such as stastistics and numerical data, trends or utilisation. The MeSH term 'Health care surveys' can be used to search for statistical measures of utilisation and other aspects of the provision of healthcare services including hospitalisation and ambulatory care.

5.7.3 Appraisal

Gentle Reader,

Visualise Great Tew, a village that lies on the side of an Oxfordshire hill, where the cottages are thatched and the pub serves real ale.

In 1066, it was owned by the Bishop of Bayeux, who was landlord to 42 souls. Fascinating detail about the mills, meadows and pasturage of Great Tew can be found in the Domesday Book, the first great survey of England, when King William I 'sent men all over England to find out ... what or how much each landowner held ... in land and livestock and what it was worth ...'.

The survey commissioners were required to take evidence on oath, and four Frenchmen and four Englishmen from each hundred were sworn to verify the detail. In addition, a second set of commissioners was sent out 'to shires they did not know, or they were themselves unknown, to check their predecessors' survey and report culprits to the King'.

Commentary

Not only was the survey of 1085 thorough, but King William also recognised that the quality of a survey, even the most comprehensive conducted by the highest authority, needed to be appraised.

> **Box 5.13** Checklist for the appraisal of a survey
>
> - How was the population to be surveyed chosen? Was it the whole population or a sample?
> - If a sample, how was the sample chosen? Was it a random sample or was it stratified to ensure that all sectors of the population were represented?
> - Was a validated questionnaire used? Did the authors of the survey mention the possibility of different results being obtained by different interviewers, if interviewers were used?
> - What procedures were used to verify the data?
> - Were the conclusions drawn from the survey all based on the data or did those carrying out the survey infer conclusions? *Inference is acceptable, but it must be clearly distinguished from results derived solely from the data.*

5.7.4 Uses and abuses

The appropriate uses of a survey are:

- to obtain a snapshot of a service at a specific point in time;
- to study complicated situations;
- to determine the acceptability of an intervention to patients.

Although it is possible to identify the existence of problems during a survey, it is difficult to determine the cause(s) of those problems; additional research is often required in such a situation.

It is not possible to use a survey to measure any changes over time.

References

1. SHORTELL, S.M., O'BRIEN, J.L., CARMAN, J.M. et al. (1995) *Assessing the impact of continuous quality improvement/total quality management: concept versus implementation.* Health Serv. Res. J. 30: 377–401.
2. BURNS, L.R., ANDERSEN, R.M. and SHORTELL, S.M. (1990) *The effect of hospital control strategies on physician satisfaction and physician hospital conflict.* Health Serv. Res. J. 25: 527–60.

5.8 DECISION ANALYSIS

In evidence-based healthcare, although decisions are based on a careful appraisal of the best evidence available, how is that evidence incorporated into the decision-making process? One approach is to discuss any evidence together with information on the resources available and on the needs or values of the population under consideration. A more systematic approach is to describe the evidence that must be taken into account in addition to estimating the impact of any of the various options available – this approach is known as decision analysis.

5.8.1 Dimensions and definitions

Lilford and Royston[1] have described decision analysis as:

> ... the bridge from knowledge to action. To inform action, empirical or theory-based knowledge about the effects of actions must be set into a 'real-world' context where some facts are uncertain, where information must be brought together from disparate sources and where decisions must be based not only on professional expertise but also on patient preferences. Decision Analysis provides a framework for doing this and can thus help bridge the gap between knowledge and action. The Decision Analysis bridge can be traversed in both directions: one way to help translate existing knowledge into action; the other to indicate what new knowledge is needed to inform action.

Decision analysis is a technique that enables a quantification to be made of the effects or impacts of the different options involved in any decision. However, most decisions are not a simple choice between option A or option B because option A and option B may have different consequences. Decision analysis usually involves:

- establishing a set of objectives and settling upon the relative importance of each, that is, their utility or value;
- identifying alternative courses of action;
- establishing the likely outcomes of these actions, together with the probability of each of them occurring.

The analysis of a decision can be expressed as a 'decision tree' in which the consequences of various decisions are displayed together with the probability of each event occurring. To construct a decision tree, the correct computer software is necessary; elegant software is available for designing decision trees.[2] It is also important to base any decision tree on robust information about the natural history of the condition under discussion, and on good evidence about the effects of different interventions.

Once a decision tree has been constructed, it is possible to incorporate values. Patients or members of the public can be asked to assign values to the good and bad outcomes of a decision, otherwise known as utilities and disutilities, respectively. A decision tree for screening for Down's syndrome for a population of 100 000 pregnancies is shown in Fig. 5.4.[3] Values were assigned to the outcomes by women who participated in the study. A value of 0 was given to a healthy live-birth, and that of 1 to a Down's syndrome live-birth; miscarriage as a result of amniocentesis and a termination because of Down's syndrome were each given a weighting of 0.3.

To calculate the course of minimum expected disutility for any branch of a decision tree, the probabilities are multiplied by the disutilities. To use the example shown in Fig. 5.4: without screening, 100 Down's syndrome babies would be born. On the basis of various assumptions (shown in Fig. 5.4), screening would detect 40 Down's syndrome babies (terminations) and 30 women would miscarry healthy babies as a result of amniocentesis. Therefore the expected disutility of a screening programme is:

> 40 terminations because of Down's syndrome + 30 miscarriages because of amniocentesis × 0.3 = 21

The expected disutility of not screening for Down's syndrome is:

> 40 Down's syndrome births × 1.0 = 40

Thus, screening results in a net gain of 19 'utility units'.

The same technique can also be used to compare different screening policies. The decision tree in Fig. 5.5 shows the impacts of five different screening policies for detecting Down's syndrome before birth,[4] the decision

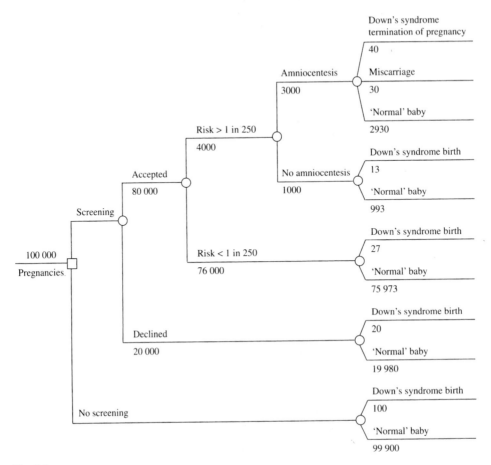

Fig. 5.4
Decision tree for Down's syndrome screening for a population of 100 000 pregnancies (Source: Thornton and Lilford,[3] with permission, BMJ Publishing Group)

analysis of which included financial cost but not disutilities. It also included sensitivity analysis, which enables the effect of variations in one or more of the variables, such as the cost of ultrasound or the specificity of the serum test, to be examined.

5.8.2 Searching

Search for decision analysis articles using the term 'decision support techniques'.

5.8.3 Appraisal

A checklist of questions useful in the appraisal of the quality of a decision analysis is shown in Box 5.14.

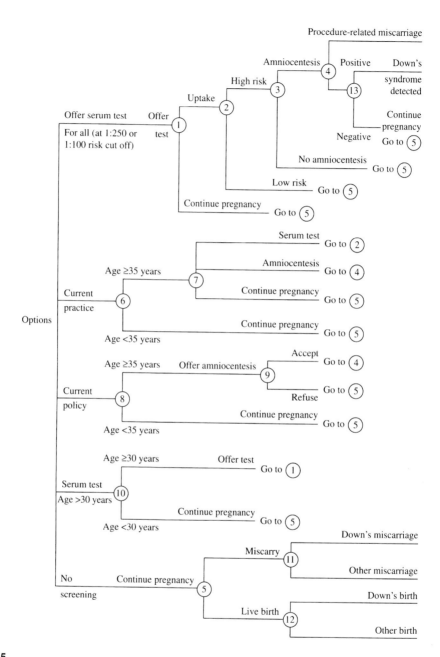

Fig. 5.5
Decision tree for five screening policies for detecting Down's syndrome before birth (Source: Fletcher et al.,[4] with permission, BMJ Publishing Group)

> **Box 5.14** Checklist for the appraisal of a decision analysis
>
> - What proportion of the branches in the decision tree represent good data based on good-quality research?
> - If utilities or disutilities have been used, were they based on surveys of people with the health problem, surveys of a sample of the general population or estimates of the author's personal values?
> - Has sensitivity analysis been performed to determine whether the estimate of effectiveness used in the decision analysis is higher or lower than the true level of effectiveness?
> - Has sensitivity analysis been performed to determine whether the estimate of the incidence of side-effects is higher or lower than the true incidence of side-effects?
> - Has sensitivity analysis been performed to test the analysis at estimates of financial cost higher or lower than the cost estimates used in the decision analysis?
> - Has sensitivity analysis been used to test the effect of higher or lower utilities being assigned to different options?
> - Have all the costs that should be taken into account been included?

Critical appraisal of a decision analysis will necessitate an assessment of the original parameters used to perform the analysis. For example, the decision analysis in which the impacts of various screening policies for detecting Down's syndrome were compared[4] was subject to the following criticisms:

- the assumption of an uptake of 75% for amniocentesis was overoptimistic;[5]
- age-specific values for sensitivity and specificity were not used;[6]
- the costs were overestimated;[7]
- the detection rates and the false-positive rates were too low.[8]

Although Fletcher et al dealt with these criticisms,[9] they pointed out that:

One of the advantages of using decision analysis as a tool for considering the consequences of different screening policies is that the assumptions and numerical values on which the model's predictions are based are explicit. If there is debate about the assumptions or the numbers that should be used in the calculations it is easy to recalculate the model with the new numbers.

A critical approach to decision analysis therefore does not necessarily reveal flaws in the technique, but instead helps to clarify any assumptions that may have been implicit or 'fudged' (Fig. 5.6), and can be used to improve the decision analysis through an iterative process.

5.8.4 Uses and abuses

The main use of decision analysis is to provide a decision-maker with an estimate of the impact an intervention may have on the population or group of patients for whom it is intended.

It should *not* be used to evaluate the effectiveness of an intervention

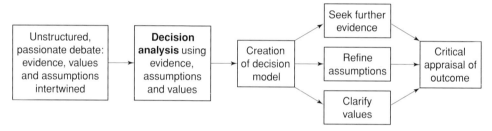

Fig. 5.6
The iterative process of decision analysis

References

1. LILFORD, R. and ROYSTON, G. (1998) *Decision Analysis in the selection, design and application of clinical and health services research.* J. Health Services Research & Policy 3: 159–66.
2. Smltree decision analysis software. J. Hollonberg, 16B Pine North, Roslyn, NY 11576, USA.
3. THORNTON, J.G. and LILFORD, R.J. (1995) *Decision analysis for medical managers.* Br. Med. J. 310: 791–4.
4. FLETCHER, J., HICKS, N.R., KAY, J.D.S. and BOYD, P.A. (1995) *Using decision analysis to compare policies for antenatal screening for Down's syndrome.* Br. Med. J. 311: 351–6.
5. MURRAY, D. and TENNISON, B. (1995) *'Decision analysis and screening for Down's syndrome.' Estimate of uptake of amniocentesis is overoptimistic [Letter].* Lancet 311: 1371.
6. SPENCER, K. (1995) *'Decision analysis and screening for Down's syndrome.' Not using age specific values invalidates study [Letter].* Lancet 311: 1371–2.
7. REYNOLDS, T.M. (1995) *'Decision analysis and screening for Down's syndrome.' Costs were overestimated [Letter].* Lancet 311: 1372.
8. WALD, N.J., KENNARD, A., WATT, H. et al. (1995) *'Decision analysis and screening for Down's syndrome.' Testing should be in all women [Letter].* Lancet 311: 1372.
9. FLETCHER, J., HICKS, N.R., KAY, J.D.S. and BOYD, P.A. (1995) *'Decision analysis and screening for Down's syndrome.' Authors' reply [Letter].* Lancet 311: 1372–3.

5.9.1 Dimensions and definitions

Qualitative research can be used to gain an understanding of health and health services, and as such has a role to play in a science-based health service. The basic disciplines of qualitative research are social anthropology and sociology.

The other types of research methodologies described in this chapter (Sections 5.4–5.8) are examples of quantitative research, the basic disciplines of which are epidemiology, biostatistics, psychology and economics. Although each of these two types of research is fiercely defended by its proponents, there is much common ground for agreement and increasingly health service professionals are beginning to understand that both qualitative and quantitative research are necessary.

Qualitative research has two main functions.

1. To comprise part of a research programme that has a qualitative and a quantitative component. Sometimes quantitative research is preceded by qualitative work; for example, in the design of a study to identify the reasons why different services have different rates of intervention – in this case, it is appropriate to conduct structured or semistructured interviews with lead consultants and managers to help design the quantitative research protocol. Similarly, in the preparation of patient questionnaires, it is often useful to discuss with focus groups of patients what they perceive to be the useful outcomes of treatment, otherwise outcomes chosen by clinicians and research workers might bear little relation to what is important to patients.
2. To complement quantitative research; for example, to capture information that complements data obtained from patient questionnaires, and which can increase the validity of the information obtained using quantitative methods.

However, qualitative research should not be regarded as merely a complement and supplement to quantitative research. It can often be used to generate hypotheses for the solution of a problem, which can then be tested using either quantitative methods, by building on the findings of the qualitative research, or a combination of qualitative and quantitative methods. The relationship between qualitative and quantitative research methods is shown in Fig. 5.7.

The defining features of a qualitative research study are shown in Box 5.15. The types of question best answered by qualitative research are shown in Box 5.16, most of which are related to people's behaviour, beliefs and attitudes.

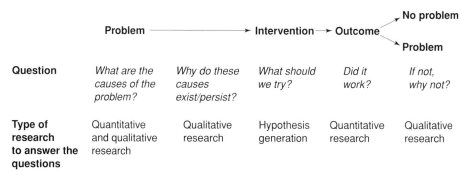

Question	What are the causes of the problem?	Why do these causes exist/persist?	What should we try?	Did it work?	If not, why not?
Type of research to answer the questions	Quantitative and qualitative research	Qualitative research	Hypothesis generation	Quantitative research	Qualitative research

Fig. 5.7
The relationship between qualitative and quantitative research

---

Box 5.15 The defining features of a qualitative research study

- An explicit peer-reviewed protocol.
- Ethics committee approval.
- A theoretical framework.
- A clear project management protocol.
- A means of identifying whether there are biases in the collection of information or drawing of conclusions.

Box 5.16 Examples of questions it is appropriate to address using qualitative research methods

- Why is it that people continue to smoke when the evidence about the harmful effects of smoking is incontrovertible and known to a proportion of those who smoke?
- Why do people not take the medicine prescribed for them?
- Why do clinicians adopt innovations of unproven effectiveness and of unknown effect while failing to adopt innovations of proven effectiveness?
- Why are nurses and doctors not able to work with one another with ease?
- What difference has the involvement of doctors in management made to the management of health services?

5.9.2 Searching

There are no Medical Subject Headings (MeSH) that adequately encompass the concept of qualitative research. A search for a specific subject will usually yield articles that include those which take a quantitative approach and those which take a qualitative approach; it is possible to differentiate between them only by reading the abstract. It is probable that a higher yield of qualitative research articles will be obtained when searching nursing and allied health databases, such as CINAHL or the British Nursing Index.

5.9.3 Appraisal

The first step in appraisal is to determine whether the use of qualitative research in a study was appropriate.[1] The second step is to judge the quality of the qualitative research. As there are now good sources of information about qualitative research methods, it is possible to draw up criteria that can be used to judge quality. A checklist for the appraisal of qualitative research is shown in Box 5.17.

Box 5.17   Checklist for the appraisal of qualitative research

- Was the research question clearly identified?
- Was the setting in which the research took place clearly described?
- If sampling was undertaken, were the sampling methods described?
- Did the research workers address the issues of subjectivity and data collection?
- Were methods to test the validity of the results of the research used?
- Were any steps taken to increase the reliability of the information collected, for example, by repeating the information collection with another research worker?
- Were the results of the research kept separate from the conclusions drawn by the research workers?
- If quantitative methods were appropriate as a supplement to the qualitative methods, were they used?

5.9.4 Uses and abuses

The main use of qualitative research is to gain an understanding of the working of any health service, which is particularly important to those who must make decisions about groups of patients or populations.

The main abuse of qualitative research methods is to evaluate the effectiveness or safety of an intervention; in this situation, it is necessary to use quantitative methods.

Reference

1. MAYS, N. and POPE, C. (1996) *Qualitative Research in Health Care*. BMJ Publishing Group, London.

5.10 HALLMARKS FOR KNOWLEDGE

A *hallmark* is a mark used at Goldsmiths' Hall and Government Assay Offices for marking the standard of gold and silver. The *carat* is a measure of the purity of gold; the word is derived from the Arabic 'quarat' meaning carob bean, chosen as a measure because the seeds of that plant show little variation one from the other. Pure gold.is 24 carats. (See Margin Fig. 5.1 for the hallmark for 18 carat gold assayed in Glasgow from 1914.)

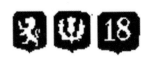

Margin Fig. 5.1

Since its foundation in 1327, The Goldsmiths' Company in London has been hallmarking gold such that any purchaser is fully aware of the quality of the gold they are buying. In the development of the National electronic Library for Health (NeLH) in the UK, early thought was given to setting up a knowledge hallmarking system.

5.10.1 The need for hallmarking

Those who use information about health and healthcare need to appraise, or be assured of, the quality of that information before it can be applied to a local problem or decision. An assurance of a certain level of quality, as measured against a standard, of health information as indicated by a knowledge hallmark would be useful for all those who do not necessarily have time to appraise everything.

5.10.2 The pitfalls of hallmarking

There are several problems associated with hallmarking knowledge.

- Knowledge is more difficult to assay than gold – beyond the particular quality standard, quality may not be uniform.
- Hallmarking could be perceived as an instrument of censorship – the assay of knowledge is value-laden unlike the assay of gold, an inert metal.

5.10.3 Examples of knowledge hallmarks in the healthcare sector

Examples of knowledge hallmarks in the healthcare sector include:

- the titles of certain journals, e.g. *The Lancet* or the *New England Journal of Medicine (NEJM)*;
- the Cochrane Collaboration logo (see Margin Fig. 5.2), which is used to signify that a systematic review conforms to the standards set out in *The Cochrane Collaboration: the reviewers' handbook* – these standards delineate the methods that should be used to search for evidence, appraise its quality and combine data if a systematic review is to be included in The Cochrane Library;
- DISCERN – the output of a national project to establish quality thresholds for information on treatment choices, aimed at users in the NHS, charities, the pharmaceutical industry and other health service suppliers. All the potential user groups mentioned were involved in developing the quality criteria used to set the quality threshold. The *DISCERN Handbook: Quality criteria for health information – user guide and training resource* has been published, and a Quick Reference Guide to the DISCERN Criteria, and the DISCERN Instrument are available at: http://www.discern.org.uk/

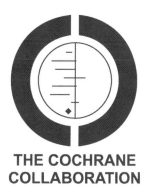

THE COCHRANE COLLABORATION

Margin Fig. 5.2

5.10.4 The unreliability of some knowledge hallmarks

5.10.4.1 The use of declarative titles – a Christmas cracker from the New England Journal of Medicine

The *New England Journal of Medicine* is one of the world's most prominent medical journals and health service professionals tend to regard it as a source of clear and definitive advice.

On 24 December 1998, the *New England Journal of Medicine* published as its lead article a paper entitled 'Symptomatic benefit from eradicating *Helicobacter pylori* infection in patients with nonulcer dyspepsia'.[1] In itself, the style of the title is significant. Hitherto, the Editor of the *New England Journal of Medicine* had not been keen to use what are known as declarative titles, i.e. titles that announce or declare the findings of a study. Previously, titles that described the study method had been used; for instance, a traditional descriptive title for this paper would have been, 'A randomised controlled trial of the eradication of *Helicobacter pylori* in patients with dyspepsia but with no evidence of an ulcer'.

Readers who had then tunnelled their way through five pages of dense text would have felt a sense of relief as they reached page 1874 believing that they had unearthed the foundation for an evidence-based policy. The bombshell hit them on page 1875 where the six pages of the issue's second article, entitled 'Lack of effect of treating *Helicobacter pylori* infection in patients with nonulcer dyspepsia',[2] stated the opposite. However, an editorial was published in which these two contradictory studies were reconciled[3] so the editors were not as mischievous as one might at first suppose.

This example of the unreliability of hallmark journals highlights the benefits of the systematic review as a scientific method (see Section 5.3).

5.10.4.2 Peer-review – the death of another sacred cow

Mantra: Indian 1808. [Sanskrit mantra lit. 'instrument of thought', f. man to think.] A sacred text or passage, esp. one from the Vedas used as a prayer or incantation.

Shorter Oxford English Dictionary

The only thing that will stop you publishing an article is a shortage of postage stamps.

Traditional research proverb

For a research article to be published in one of the hallmark journals, it must undergo the process of peer-review, in which the paper is sent to one or more experts in the field for comment before it is accepted for publication. Indeed, in recent years, 'peer review' has reached the status of a mantra. In the past, publication of an article in a peer-reviewed journal was taken as a guarantee about the quality of research. However, it is now becoming clear that there are flaws in the process of peer-review, and it is necessary to be much more critical of it. At the time of writing, the deliberations of participants at three international congresses on peer-review have been published in biomedical publications. The third congress, held in September 1997 in Prague, was attended by people from 46 countries. An entire issue of the *Journal of the American Medical Association* (JAMA) (15 July 1998) was devoted to the conference presentations which highlighted the variability and unreliability of peer-review.

One attempt to resolve some of the problems is to make the peer-review process open, for example, by identifying the peer-reviewers and any conflicts of interest they might have. However, it would appear from the study by van Rooyen et al.[4] that open peer-review has no effect, either beneficial or adverse, on:

- the quality of peer-reviews;
- the peer-reviewers' recommendations.

Despite this finding, the Editor of the *British Medical Journal* decided to introduce a system of open peer-review in 1999 'for largely ethical reasons',[5] emphasising that, although evidence-based decision-making means making a decision based on evidence, values and resources must also be taken into account. Peer-review as a process will continue to be used, but in future it must be more rigorous, evidence-based and open.[6]

5.10.5 Caveat lector

It may be that the only approach which is workable, honest and open is:

- to provide as much information as possible about the methods used to arrive at the conclusion in the written document;
- to provide the reader with the skills to appraise research information such that it is possible for each individual to decide if that information is fit for their purpose, and the decision that must be made.

References

1. McCOLL, K., MURRAY, L., EL-OMAR, E. et al. (1998) *Symptomatic benefit from eradicating* Helicobacter pylori *infection in patients with nonulcer dyspepsia.* N. Engl. J. Med. 339: 1869–74.
2. BLUM, A.L., TALLEY, N.J., O'MORAIN, C. et al. (1998) *Lack of effect of treating* Helicobacter pylori *infection in patients with nonulcer dyspepsia.* N. Engl. J. Med. 339: 1875–81.
3. FRIEDMAN, L.S. (1998) Helicobacter pylori *and nonulcer dyspepsia.* N. Engl. J. Med. 339: 1928–30.
4. Van ROOYEN, S., GODLEE, F., EVANS, S., BLACK, N. and SMITH, R. (1998) *Effect of open peer review on quality of reviews and on reviewers' recommendations: a randomised trial.* Br. Med. J. 318: 23–7.
5. SMITH, R. (1998) *Opening up BMJ peer review.* Br. Med. J. 318: 4–5.
6. GODLEE, F. and JEFFERSON, R. (eds). (1999) *Peer review in health sciences.* BMJ Publishing Group, London.

Gentle Reader,

Empathise with the doctor. He had turned his head to respond to the greeting, and was shocked to find himself looking at what appeared to be a statue carved in Carrara marble: white sheets, white cover, white pillowslip, white hair and white face. 'How are you, doctor?', the occupant of the bed asked cheerily. The doctor struggled to recall the face, one of so many seen in a hectic year during the course of two busy surgical jobs. 'How are you?', said the doctor, dissembling well and still trying to recollect where he had seen the face before. 'I'm fine, doctor,' said the patient, 'but it doesn't seem like 5 months since I was last admitted. I've had such good care throughout.' Five months, last March, vascular surgery: the face came back, but not the name. 'That's a long time', said the doctor. 'Yes, but it's been wonderful whatever he's done, although I'm still trying to get used to this', replied the patient, waving his hand at the unnaturally narrow mound in the bed where two legs should have lain but now there was only one.

Back in the ward office the doctor reviewed the case notes. The man had come in for a routine aortic graft. Although he had had symptoms of claudication, they were not very severe. No-one had recommended the effective and safe therapy of exercise, which should be standard practice before the knife is considered. The patient's first operation had been
uneventful, but 7 days later he had thrown off a clot that had blocked the artery to his left leg; after two more operations, the leg had been amputated. During his recovery from the amputation, he had developed a venous thrombosis in the remaining leg and suffered a severe pulmonary embolus. Whilst he was seriously ill from the pulmonary embolus, another clot had formed, this time in the artery leading to his intestine, and part of his intestine had been removed, giving him malabsorption.

He was now medically stable, waiting for a rehabilitation bed, and a place in the unit where amputees are helped to adjust to, and cope with, the loss of a limb.

Commentary

Perhaps it is unwise to speak of the outcome of care as if there is only one; there are frequently many outcomes, even though each clinician may see only one. The patient described in this prologue had thought that his initial operation was absolutely necessary, and he was tremendously grateful for what he considered to be a life-saving act. The various clinicians who had seen him during his progress through the healthcare system had each formed their own opinion about the effectiveness, appropriateness and cost-effectiveness of the care he had received, and the outcomes of that care, at each stage of his perilous journey.

CHAPTER 6

ASSESSING THE OUTCOMES FOUND

6.1 FIVE KEY QUESTIONS ABOUT OUTCOMES

Once it has been established that the research is of sufficiently good quality for the outcomes of that research to be included within the framework of the decision, those outcomes must be assessed. There are five key questions about outcomes.

- How many outcomes were studied?
- How large were the effects found?
- With what degree of confidence can the results of the research be applied to the whole population?
- Does the intervention do more good than harm?
- How relevant are the results to the local population or service about which the decision is being made?

For the clinician, there is also a sixth question:

- 'How relevant is the research to this particular patient?'

6.1.1 How many outcomes were studied?

The proposition that an intervention 'is effective' implies that there is only one outcome of care and only one objective in the design of that intervention. This is rarely the case. There are various outcomes of disease, and, if effective care is given, these outcomes may be ameliorated or improved (see Table 6.1).

Table 6.1 The outcomes of disease

Outcomes of untreated disease	Outcomes of effective care of disease
Death	Lower morbidity
Disability	Functional ability improved
Disease status deteriorates and risk of complications increases	Disease status improves and risk of complications decreases
Distress about effects of disease	Feeling better

Although in Table 6.1 the beneficial outcomes of care have been presented, the possibility that adverse effects may also occur must always be considered. The balance between good and harmful effects of treatment should be weighed very carefully.

6.1.2 How large were the effects found?

The beneficial effect of a treatment for either an individual patient or a group of patients can range from 0.1% to 100%.

- For individual patients, benefit is measured by the magnitude of the effect, which ranges from no effect to complete cure.
- For a group of patients, magnitude of effect must also include the proportion of patients who will benefit, which is usually expressed as the odds ratio.

The odds ratio is the ratio of the frequency of the key event, such as mortality, in the group receiving treatment to the frequency of the key event in the control group.

6.1.2.1 Which yardstick?

In a situation where a condition was previously untreatable, any new treatment must be compared with a placebo in trials.

If there is a treatment for the condition already available, it is important to compare the new treatment with that already in use to identify any differences in the effectiveness, safety, acceptability and cost between the two. This may seem self-evident, but sometimes a difference in any of these criteria does not exist.

Some trials, particularly those funded by the pharmaceutical industry, are designed to compare a new treatment with placebo irrespective of whether other therapies for that condition are already available; using this strategy, it is possible to give the impression that the new treatment may be more effective than it actually is.

6.1.3 With what degree of confidence can the results of the research be applied to the whole population?

Research studies produce results, but these results are not necessarily the answer to the decision faced by the decision-maker. Research is always conducted on a sample of the population of interest; for example, even in a mega-trial of myocardial infarction in which 46 000 patients are enrolled, those 46 000 comprise only a sample of the millions of people who will have a heart attack. Thus, a well-designed research study generates information about what happens only when the group of patients in that study are given a treatment; it must not be assumed that the results of the study can be applied automatically to the whole population.

The degree to which the results of any study are generalisable can be expressed as a probability, both numerically and diagrammatically, using confidence intervals. The results of individual research studies are shown as single points in Fig. 6.1. However, each of the results plotted is only an estimate of the true effect as each study was done on a sample of the population. Although each sample could represent the whole population perfectly, the method of sampling always introduces errors. It is possible, however, to estimate the range of values within which the true result actually lies; this range is known as the confidence interval.

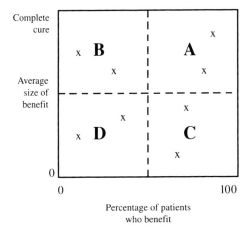

Fig. 6.1
Results of research studies. **x** represents the result for a single therapy; **A** represents good value, **D** poor value. If the effect is in either **B** or **C**, the judgement is more difficult

It is usual practice to calculate the 95% confidence intervals, which indicate there is a 95% probability that the effect of treatment in the whole population would lie within the range of values. The larger the sample of the population studied, the narrower will be the range of values within the confidence intervals (see Box 6.1).

Box 6.1   Confidence intervals

- The larger the sample of patients, the narrower will be the confidence intervals.
- The narrower the range of the confidence intervals, the greater will be the degree of confidence about the general applicability of the results.
- If both ends of the range of confidence intervals lie on the side of the line which indicates that treatment does more good than harm, then it will be effective in all circumstances.

An alternative way to express this is that there is a 1 in 20 chance that the effect in the whole population will lie outside this range. Although it is possible to calculate narrower confidence intervals, for example, 99%, these often produce such a wide range of results that the preferred convention is to use 95% confidence intervals.

It can be seen from Fig. 6.2 that, for high-risk patients, even if the result of the research is, by chance, more optimistic than the true effect in the whole population, the intervention is effective because there is a clear benefit at the lowest end of the confidence intervals – point B. For individuals at low risk, even if the result of

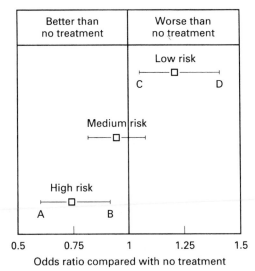

Fig. 6.2
Rate of coronary events in individuals receiving cholesterol-lowering treatments divided by rate of coronary events in individuals not receiving treatment, shown with 95% confidence intervals (Source: adapted from *Bandolier* 1995; 5: 4)

the research is, by chance, more pessimistic than the true effect, the intervention is ineffective because there is no benefit at the highest end of the confidence intervals – point C. For those at medium risk, it would be unwise to generalise from these results because the range in which the true effect lies includes both ends of the confidence interval, indicating that the intervention might be either beneficial or harmful.

A cumulative meta-analysis, that is, an analysis of the data from all the trials as reported year on year, is shown in Fig. 6.3. It can be seen that the confidence intervals narrow as the numbers of patients included in the meta-analysis increase.

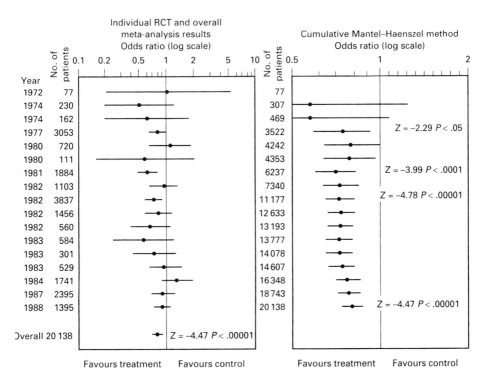

Fig. 6.3
Results of 17 RCTs of the effects of oral beta-blockers for secondary prevention of mortality in patients surviving a myocardial infarction presented as two types of meta-analyses. On the left is the traditional one, revealing many trials with non-significant results but a highly significant estimate of the pooled results on the bottom of the panel. On the right, the same data are presented as cumulative meta-analyses, illustrating that the updated pooled estimate became statistically significant in 1977 and has remained so up to the present. Note that the scale is changed on the right-hand graph to improve clarity of the confidence intervals (Source: Antman et al., *JAMA*, 8 July 1992, vol 268, p. 242. Copyright 1992, American Medical Association)

Although the increasing size of any trial narrows the confidence intervals, it is not necessary to design a mega-trial for every intervention to be tested because it is the size of the effect being forecast that determines the size of a trial, as follows.

- If a treatment is expected to cure someone who has a disease that was hitherto 100% fatal, only one patient is needed, as was the case with penicillin in the treatment of osteomyelitis.
- If a treatment might reduce mortality by 5%, thousands of subjects will have to be entered into the trial to demonstrate this effect (see Section 5.4.1.1).
- If the effect of treatment might be greater than 5%, fewer patients will be necessary.

It is possible to estimate the number of patients required to ensure that a trial will be of sufficient size to produce a definite result. This is known as estimating the power of a trial (see Box 6.2 for the power rules).

Box 6.2 Power rules

- The smaller the effect predicted, the larger the trial required to produce a result.
- The larger the trial, the greater the power.
- The greater the power, the narrower the confidence intervals.
- If the power calculations are correct and the size of the beneficial effect is as predicted, both ends of the confidence interval will lie on the same side of the line as the result.

6.1.4 Does the intervention do more good than harm?

When an intervention has beneficial effects, it is important not only to record their existence but also to indicate the probability of both good and harm occurring. Few treatments benefit every patient and the balance of good and harm should always be estimated (see Fig. 6.4).

One of the many ways in which Scottish law is better fitted for purpose than English is the possibility of a verdict in addition to 'guilty' and 'not guilty', that of 'not proven' – a judgement of the strength of evidence. Similarly, in evidence-based healthcare, rather than classifying interventions as either 'effective' or 'ineffective', it is more accurate to classify them as:

- proven to do more good than harm – 'not guilty';
- proven to do more harm than good – 'guilty';
- of unproven effect – 'not proven'.

It must always be borne in mind that because an intervention has not been shown to be effective does not mean that it is ineffective, but neither can it be assumed to do more good than harm. Such an intervention should be evaluated in a well-designed research study.

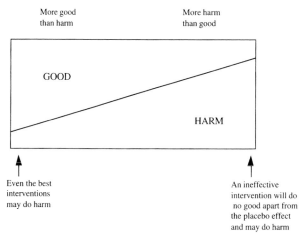

Fig. 6.4
The balance of good and harm

6.1.4.1 L'Abbé plots

The L'Abbé plot, developed by Kristen L'Abbé and colleagues, provides a simple graphical way of representing the results of individual trials in a systematic review. Each point on the L'Abbé scatter plot is one trial in the review. The proportion of patients achieving the outcome with the intervention under study is plotted against the event rate in controls. For trials of a treatment regimen, if the intervention is better than the control the points will be in the upper left of the plot between the y axis and the line of equality; if the intervention is no better than the control, the points will be on the line of equality; if the control is better than the intervention, the points will be in the lower right of the plot between the x axis and the line of equality (see Fig. 6.5). For trials of prophylaxis, the pattern will be reversed: because the intervention reduces the number of adverse events, it is to be expected that a smaller

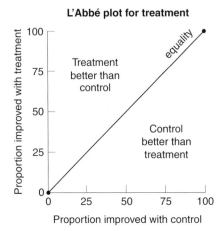

Fig. 6.5
L'Abbé plot for treatment

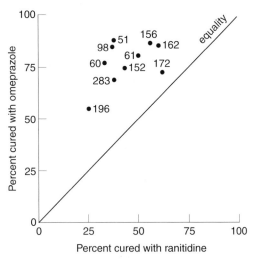

Fig. 6.6
L'Abbé plot showing the overall effects of omeprazole versus ranitidine treatment on short-term endoscopic healing of erosive oesophagitis after 8 weeks. It can be seen from this plot that for all trials ($n = 23$) omeprazole was more effective than ranitidine, and that about 80% of patients are healed on omeprazole, whereas only 45% are healed on ranitidine (Source: *Bandolier, the second annual; issues 21–34, S-4–7.*)

proportion of patients receiving the intervention will be harmed when compared with the controls. Thus, if the intervention is better than the control, the points will be between the x axis and the line of equality. An illustration of the L'Abbé technique is shown in Fig. 6.6.

The use of L'Abbé plots gives an indication of the level of agreement among trials. If the points fall within a consistent 'cloud', then it is likely that there is a homogeneous effect. If the points scatter, especially if they cross the line of equality, the effect is heterogeneous and gives cause for concern about the intervention, or the patients being treated and their condition.

6.1.5 How relevant are the results to the local population or service?

In protocols for research studies, especially trials, the criteria for the inclusion and exclusion of patients are stipulated. The use of these criteria ensures that a homogeneous group of patients is selected from which the intervention and control groups are randomised. However, this selection of a study population raises problems; for instance, how applicable are the results of a study of the treatment of heart failure in patients under the age of 75 years to patients who are over the age of 75 years? One way to increase the applicability of the findings would be to use less stringent inclusion criteria, thereby decreasing the proportion of patients excluded from the trial, but this strategy may also reduce the validity of the trial.

If certain results are considered to be applicable to the whole population, are they also relevant to any local population that is the subject of a decision? Is a study of primary care in the Netherlands relevant to Northampton? Is the treatment given in a teaching hospital in Canada relevant to a district general hospital in Kent? A checklist of questions that can be used to assess the relevance of research findings to the local population is shown in Box 6.3.

> **Box 6.3**   Checklist for assessing the relevance of research findings to the local population
>
> 1. Does the population studied differ from the local population in ways that are likely to be important with respect to:
> * genetic composition?
> * health status, e.g. is there a higher or lower prevalence of risk factors of disease in the local population?
> * beliefs and attitudes, e.g. is the local population likely to be more or less compliant with invitations to attend for screening?
> 2. Does the local healthcare service have the potential to reproduce the service provided in the trial?
> 3. Could a similar level of resources as that available to the research workers be channelled into the local service?
> 4. Are the skills to deliver a service of adequate quality available locally? If not, is it possible to develop those skills at an affordable cost?

6.1.6 The clinician's dilemma

Gentle Reader,

Empathise with Mr B. 'What do you think, doctor?' asked Mr B, who had been found to have narrowing of the arteries to his brain after investigation for a transient ischaemic attack. His GP had put him on aspirin and referred him to hospital. Mr B knew the aspirin was safe and effective, and he had no trouble taking it. However, after numerous tests, the hospital doctor had advised him to have an operation on his carotid arteries – an endarterectomy – not unlike, he was cheerily told, rodding out pipes that had become furred up. So here he was, back in the surgery of his GP, whom he trusted, asking, 'What do you think, doctor?'.

Gentle Reader,

Empathise with the GP. On being asked what she thought by Mr B, she was assailed by so many different thoughts. Why didn't consultants make the decisions? Isn't it just great to be a GP, trusted by both the patient and the consultant to whom the referral had been made! She thought of Mrs B, who had Alzheimer's disease: if Mr B has a stroke, she's had it. But there again, he might not: not everyone with carotid artery stenosis does. What if he dies on the table? Some people do. What are the risks and benefits for Mr B? Where do I find the evidence? Why are these bloody difficult decisions always booked into a routine slot in morning surgery?

Commentary

Carotid endarterectomy is effective: it does more good than harm, but some people are harmed by the operation.[1] In fact, some of those who suffer harm would not have had a stroke even if they had not had the operation. It is essential for any clinician to know how to target treatment to individual patients who are at high risk of a poor outcome without treatment but who are also at a low risk of a poor outcome with treatment. In making this particular decision, the GP and Mr B were fortunate because an epidemiologist had actually completed and published the necessary research.[2]

Only 20% of people at risk of carotid stenosis becoming stroke will have a stroke on medical treatment alone. Thus, 80% will not. If everyone at risk of stroke had a carotid endarterectomy, some of the 80% would be harmed. Fortunately, a risk factor can be calculated that indicates which of those with carotid stenosis are most likely to benefit from an operation, and would therefore have a higher than average probability of being helped rather than harmed.[3]

As outlined earlier, the additional question for clinicians in relation to outcomes is:

'How relevant is this research to this particular patient?'

The key issue a clinician must consider is the 'baseline risk of the patient', that is, the degree of risk of a particular individual who shares the same characteristics as the patients in the trial.[4] Although this issue does not have to be addressed by health service decision-makers directly, they should be cognisant of the dilemma faced by the clinician and the patient, both of whom have to weigh up not only the probability of good and harmful outcomes occurring but also the magnitude of any beneficial and of any adverse effects (see Fig. 6.7).

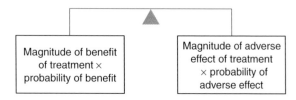

Fig. 6.7
The balance between the magnitude of beneficial effects and
that of adverse effects

One approach that can be taken to help clinicians and
patients resolve this dilemma is the use of a decision
support system. A computer-based decision support
system (CDSS) has been defined as any software designed
to aid the clinician directly in clinical decision-making, in
which the characteristics of individual patients are matched
to a computerised knowledge base for the purpose of
generating patient-specific assessment or recommendations
that are then presented to the clinician for consideration.[5]
For advice on how to use an article evaluating the clinical
impact of a computer-based clinical decision support
system see Randolph et al.[6]

References

1. EUROPEAN CAROTID SURGERY TRIALISTS COLLABORATIVE
   GROUP (1991) *MRC European Carotid Surgery Trial: interim results for
   symptomatic patients with severe (70–99%) or with mild (0–29%) carotid
   stenosis.* Lancet 337: 1235–43.
2. ROTHWELL, P.M. (1995) *Can overall results of clinical trials be applied to
   all patients?* Lancet 345: 1616–19.
3. ROTHWELL, P.M. and WARLOW, C.P. (1999) *Prediction of benefit from
   carotid endarterectomy in individual patients: a risk modelling study.
   European Carotid Surgery Trialists' Collaborative Group.* Lancet 353:
   2105–10.
4. GUYATT, G.H., JAESCHKE, R.Z. and COOK, D.J. (1995) *Applying the
   findings of clinical trials to individual patients.* ACP Journal Club Mar–Apr;
   122: A12–13.
5. HUNT, D.L., HAYNES, R.B., HANNA, S.G. and SMITH, K. (1998)
   *Effects of computer-based clinical decision support systems on physician
   performance and patient outcome: a systematic review.* JAMA 280: 1339–46.
6. RANDOLPH, A.G., WAYNES, R.B., WYATT, J.C., COOK, D.J. and
   GUYATT, G.H. (1999) *Users' guides to the medical literature: XVIII. How to
   use an article evaluating the clinical impact of a computer-based clinical
   support system.* JAMA 282: 67–74.

6.2 MEASURING OUTCOMES

6.2.1 Problems and pitfalls of performance measurement

During the last decade of the 20th century, there was great enthusiasm for outcome measurement. However, there are many difficulties associated with the use of outcome measures (see Section 6.8.1.2). In an important article, David Eddy has identified the reasons why it is difficult to measure healthcare quality and outcome.[1] He divides the problems into two types: natural problems and man-made problems. It is possible to rectify the latter, whereas it is possible only to work around the former.

6.2.1.1 Natural problems

- *Probability factor*: almost all health outcomes are probabilistic, that is, it is not possible to guarantee a good outcome for every patient, therefore measures of quality need to give some indication that probabilistic factors are being monitored, e.g. using probability or P values when expressing the difference between two services.
- *Low frequency*: many important health problems occur at a low frequency at the level of service management; for example, cervical cancer is rare at the level of the individual screening programme, although it is a major problem nationally.
- *Long delays*: it may take 5–10 years to detect and therefore measure a clinical outcome, this affects not only the feasibility of measurement but also its usefulness to the manager or clinician. For example, there will be a lapse of time before potential changes in the incidence of stroke become manifest following the introduction of a hypertension control programme.
- *Control over outcomes*: other factors may influence the outcome. For example, the prevalence of smoking is determined not only by the effectiveness of a health education programme but also by taxation policy.
- *Level of clinical detail*: this relates to the imprecision of clinical concepts; in order to derive an appropriate measure, it is necessary to have an operational definition of the disease under investigation, but this will differ among the various clinicians involved in any one service.

- *Comprehensibility*: some biological outcomes and process measures are not comprehensible in terms of the outcomes about which patients are concerned.

6.2.1.2 Man-made problems

Man-made problems are consequent upon the way in which a healthcare system has evolved.

- *Inadequate information systems*: systems that do not have the capacity to measure what they are intended to measure.
- *Too many measurers and measures*: for example, different sectors within the performance management system may request different measures of performance.

The two other man-made problems that Eddy identifies are *health plan complexity* and *funding*, both of which are specific to the US healthcare system.

It is also possible to add *inconsistency* or *lack of continuity* to Eddy's list of man-made problems, i.e. those responsible for measuring performance may change the measures to be used from year to year.

Process
 | ⟋Chance
 |⟋
 ↓
Outcome

Good process ≠ Good outcome
 (but it helps)

Margin Fig. 6.1

6.2.2 In praise of process

As the use of outcome measures for managing services is beset with many difficulties, many people prefer to use evidence-based process measures (see Margin Fig. 6.1), i.e. measures of processes for which there is good evidence that if such processes were applied consistently the required outcome would be achieved. For a discussion of the use of process measures in the assessment of quality, see Section 6.8.1.1.

Reference

1. EDDY, D.M. (1998) Performance measurement problems and solutions. Health Aff. 17: 7–26.

Equity: 1. The quality of being equal or fair; impartiality; even-handed dealing. 2. That which is fair and right …

Shorter Oxford English Dictionary

To do equyte and justice.

William Caxton

Equity was my crowne.

Job, xxix.14

6.3.1 Dimensions and definitions

The definition of equity has occupied philosophers for many years; indeed, there is no simple definition. However, one of the objectives of the NHS, explicit at the time of its institution and still implicit in many of the decisions made, is to provide equity of care in relation to assessed need. Equity, therefore, is different to equality; no-one would argue that different patient groups should have equal shares of NHS resources. Equity implies social justice, and fairness is one of the values on which NHS commissioning decisions are based.

6.3.1.1 Measuring equity

Although social justice, or fairness, is felt keenly by everyone, can it be measured? Cost-utility analysis is a form of economic appraisal in which the quality-adjusted life year (QALY) is used as an outcome measure. It is theoretically possible to calculate the total number of QALYs provided for each patient group by a purchaser: *if* the QALY were a perfect measure of health benefit and *if* the purchaser had achieved perfect equity, the total number of QALYs for each patient group would be the same. Such an exercise might be impossible to undertake due to the amount of effort it would require, and it may be spurious given the imperfections inherent in the QALY as a measure.

6.3.1.2 *Assessing equity: evidence-based cuts at the margin*

There is one way in which evidence could be used to assess the equity of a purchaser's decisions: by analysis of the effects of marginal changes. If it were possible to identify the total amount of money spent on different disease categories (for example, eye disease, diseases of the ear, nose and throat, and diseases of the mouth), it would then be possible to determine the effects of either removing £500 000 from, or adding £500 000 to, each programme budget. The effects of reducing spending on diseases of the ear, nose and throat by £500 000 could then be compared with the effect of increasing expenditure on eye disease by the same amount. This approach might prove useful in that it would narrow the debate about cuts to a relatively limited set of service changes; it would encourage decision-makers to seek evidence useful in the quantification of the effects of such marginal changes on the population served.

6.3.2 Searching

When searching for articles on equity, it is probably most useful to search using the word 'fairness'.

6.3.3 Appraisal

When appraising articles on equity, the key issue is the definition of equity used by the authors. If the term is not clearly defined, it will be difficult to appraise the article. A checklist of questions for the appraisal of research information on equity is given in Box 6.4.

Box 6.4   Checklist for the appraisal of research information on equity

- Is the definition of equity clearly set out in the article?
- Is the definition of equity original or do the authors cite another source from which it was derived?
- Do the authors identify or discuss how their own values could influence the interpretation of the findings?
- Are there any data describing the opinions of individuals other than the authors about the equity of a particular decision or resource allocation?

6.3.4 Applicability and relevance

Equity is an issue that inhabits the moral high ground; those who claim to argue in favour of equity put themselves in a strong moral position. Those who argue from this position should be treated with a high index of suspicion because they could be arguing, either consciously or unconsciously, for a change that will confer benefit on them rather than on society as a whole.

6.4 EFFECTIVENESS

London has seen the birth of many revolutionary ideas, one of the greatest of which is the National Health Service. This idea, first current in the 1930s,[1] was developed in many a draughty hall and lecture theatre. At one of these rallies, the young Archie Cochrane bore a banner carrying the slogan: 'All effective treatment must be free'.

The only reaction then, he reported,[2] was from someone who damned it for having Trotskyite tendencies. From this small beginning, the concept of effectiveness has become a major driving force for change in modern healthcare.

6.4.1 Dimensions and definitions

The effectiveness of an intervention, from single treatments through to services including the professionals within them, is the degree to which the desired health outcomes are achieved in clinical practice.

The quality of a service is the degree to which it conforms to pre-set standards of care (see Section 6.8.1).

Earlier definitions of effectiveness were broader and included efficiency;[3] today efficiency, or cost-effectiveness, is almost always used as a distinct criterion (Section 6.7), although it is not uncommon for the media to use the term 'efficient' when epidemiologists would use the term 'effective' (see Margin Fig. 6.2).

The efficacy of an intervention is the degree to which the desired health outcomes are achieved *in the best possible circumstances.*

This distinction between efficacy and effectiveness is important and has implications for decision-makers who must apply the results of research. Research may be performed in an environment in which the level of

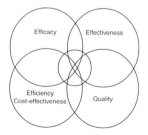

Margin Fig. 6.2

resourcing and/or the number of skilled staff are greater than those available to the local service. For this reason, it is vital to consider not only the results of research but also the relevance of those results to the particular population or group of patients about which the decision is being made: an intervention may be efficacious in an RCT at Massachusetts General Hospital, but will it be effective on a wet Thursday in Barchester District General Hospital?

6.4.1.1 Assessing effectiveness from the patient's perspective

It is essential to assess effectiveness not only from a clinical perspective, the focus of which is death, disease status and the functional ability of a patient, but also from the perspective of an individual patient.

The delivery of effective and safe healthcare by professionals who are sensitive to the needs of a patient can engender the following emotional responses in the patient:

- the patient feels better because intervention has brought about an improvement in his/her health;
- the patient feels happy because s/he has been treated as an individual by a sensitive professional during the process of care.

The various combinations of the relationship between a patient's state of health and their degree of happiness with the process of care are presented in Matrix 6.1.

	Happiness with process of care	
	Low	High
State of health after care — No improvement – still feeling poorly — or feeling worse	A	B
Feeling better	C	D

Matrix 6.1

As can be seen, it is possible for a patient not to improve, or indeed to deteriorate, during the process of care but still to be happy with the way in which care was given (outcome B). It is also possible for a patient to feel better because the disease causing the problem has been dealt with effectively while feeling unhappy about the process of care (outcome C). The ideal outcome is D. The worst outcome is A, in which a patient's health does not improve and the patient is unhappy about the process of care. Such patients are difficult to assess because their view about the process of care may be influenced by the poor outcome for health status. Outcome A is the least satisfactory for both patients and clinicians.

6.4.1.2 Improving outcomes by providing emotional support

Not only may health outcome influence the patient's perception of the process of care, but the converse can also occur: the effectiveness of care may be increased if the patient's emotional needs are met by giving the patient support (see Margin Fig. 6.3). This has been clearly demonstrated in an RCT of women in labour.[4] In comparison with the control group, the provision of emotional support by a professional or voluntary carer was found:

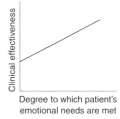

Margin Fig. 6.3

- to shorten the duration of labour;
- to reduce the rate of Caesarean section;
- to lessen the use of forceps;
- to decrease the length of stay of infant hospitalisation.

6.4.1.3 Improving outcomes through patient participation

The other important factor determining clinical outcome is the extent of participation the professional allows the patient in the process of care (see Margin Fig. 6.4). In a controlled study, known as the 'friendly' dentists trial,[5] dental patients were assigned alternately to one of two 'treatment' groups: one group received care from dentists who were instructed to say things like 'Your opinion is more important than mine'; the other group comprised the control subjects and received care from dentists who behaved in the 'usual' manner. It was found that outcome improved with patient participation.

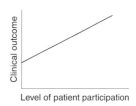

Margin Fig. 6.4

6.4.1.4 Improving outcomes through process: in the absence of an effective technical intervention

The process of care is of greater importance when treating patients in whom there is no apparent structural disease but who have distressing symptoms, such as headache.[6] In this type of health problem, the nature of the process of care is the main factor determining outcome.

6.4.2 Searching

To search for evidence of effectiveness, consult the various databases in the sequence of steps shown below.

Step 1: The Cochrane Database of Systematic Reviews (CDSR; see Appendix I, I.2.1.1)

Step 2: The Database of Abstracts of Reviews of Effectiveness (DARE; see Appendix I, I.2.1.2)

Step 3: EMBASE (see Appendix I, I.2.7) and MEDLINE (see Appendix I, I.2.6), for:
- systematic reviews;
- RCTs;
- other types of study.

Step 4: Specialist databases (see Appendix I, I.2.8)

Use 'effectiveness' as a search term.

6.4.3 Appraisal

Evidence of effectiveness can be generated by several different types of research study. In Box 6.5, the different research methods have been ranked in order of validity for obtaining evidence of effectiveness; for this ranking to hold, all the research must be of high quality.

Box 6.5 Research methods ranked in order of validity for obtaining evidence of effectiveness

1. Large RCTs (Section 5.4).
2. Systematic reviews of RCTs (Section 5.3).
3. Individual RCTs of inadequate size to detect adverse effects of treatment.
4. Controlled trials without randomisation.
5. Observational studies, such as cohort (Section 5.6) or case-control studies (Section 5.5), preferably from more than one research group.
6. Reports of expert committees, the writing of which has been based upon the sources of evidence cited and not simply the opinion of eminent committee members.

A checklist of questions for the appraisal of research evidence on effectiveness is shown in Box 6.6.

Box 6.6   Checklist for the appraisal of research evidence of effectiveness

1. Does the research provide evidence about adverse effects (Section 6.5) and the patients' perspectives of outcome (Section 6.6)?
2. What is the magnitude of the beneficial effect?
3. With what degree of confidence can the findings in a research setting be reproduced in ordinary clinical settings?

Once evidence has been found and its quality appraised, it is necessary to address the implications of the research findings (see Box 6.7 and Table 6.2).

Box 6.7   The possible implications of evidence of effectiveness for the provision of healthcare in a local service

- If the trial results are negative, that is, no effect is shown, and this treatment is being delivered within the 'local' service, search for other evidence because the treatment may not be effective.
- If the trial results are positive and this treatment is being delivered within the local service, ascertain how large the effect is at what risk and at what cost. (The NNT is of use in this assessment.)
- If the trial results are positive and this treatment is not being delivered within the local service, consider implementing the research findings but beware of the five positive biases (Table 6.2).

Table 6.2   Five positive biases

Bias	Cause
Submission bias	Research workers are more strongly motivated to complete, and submit for publication, positive results
Publication bias	Editors are more likely to publish positive studies[7]
Methodological bias	Methodological errors such as flawed randomisation produce positive biases[8]
Abstracting bias	Abstracts emphasise positive results[9]
Framing bias	Relative risk data produce a positive bias[10]

6.4.3.1 *Experimental studies of effectiveness*

1. The odds ratio: the relative benefit

The magnitude of any beneficial effect is often expressed in relative terms as the odds ratio.

- In a controlled trial, if the odds ratio is equal to 1, the treatment probably has no effect.
- If the odds ratio is less than 1, the treatment probably has a beneficial effect when compared with the intervention applied to the control group.
- If the odds ratio is greater than 1, the treatment is probably less effective than the intervention applied to the control group.

For a lucid explanation of the odds ratio, follow the example given in The Cochrane Collaboration: The Reviewers' Handbook in The Cochrane Library (see Appendix I, I.2.1)

The presentation of trial data in terms of relative risk introduces a bias: readers interpret the results as being more positive than they actually are – known as the framing effect (Section 5.4.4.1). It is therefore important to consider the absolute reduction in risk that a treatment will produce.

2. NNT: the absolute benefit

The number needed to treat (NNT) is a comprehensible measure of the absolute effects of treatment.[11] McQuay and Moore describe it as a clinically useful measure of the effort required to obtain a beneficial outcome with an intervention, and suggest it is particularly useful for expressing the relative effectiveness of several different interventions.[12] The NNTs for various interventions-to-outcomes are set out in Table 6.3. The clarity gained by presenting data in this way is striking: for example, only 15 people with severe high blood pressure have to be given treatment to prevent one stroke, but among people with mild hypertension 700 have to be treated to prevent one stroke. The same concept can be applied to adverse outcomes, in which case the measure is referred to as the number needed to harm (NNH).

Table 6.3   NNTs for various interventions (Source: extracts from *Bandolier* 1995; 17: 7, and McQuay and Moore[12])

Intervention	Outcome	NNT
CABG in left main stenosis	Prevent 1 death at 2 years	6
Carotid endarterectomy in high-grade symptomatic stenosis	Prevent 1 stroke or death in 2 years	9
Simple antihypertensive therapy for severe hypertension	Prevent 1 stroke, MI or death in 1 year	15
Simple antihypertensive therapy for mild hypertension	Prevent 1 stroke, MI or death in 1 year	700
Treating hypertension in the over-60s	Prevent 1 coronary event	18
Aspirin in severe unstable angina	Prevent MI or death in 1 year	25
Aspirin in healthy US physician	Prevent MI or death in 1 year	500
Graduated compression stockings for venous thromboembolism	Episodes of venous thrombo-embolism	9
Triple therapy for peptic ulcer	Eradication of *H. pylori*	1.1
Triple therapy for peptic ulcer	Ulcers remaining cured at 1 year	1.8
Permethrin for headlice	Cure	1.1
Antibiotics for dogbite	Infection	16

6.4.3.2   *Observational studies of effectiveness*

It had been hoped that health service data collected routinely on computer systems would enable the effectiveness of new technology to be evaluated within observational studies. Unfortunately experience thus far has not fulfilled early expectations. The principal reason for this is the absence of a 'control' group in this methodology. Consequently, it is impossible to know if the effects of treatment are generalisable or if they are due to factors such as the preferential selection of patients for one particular intervention as opposed to another. Large databases of outcomes cannot be used to provide definitive answers about effectiveness: as one authority states, 'while databases can suggest problems and offer answers, they cannot prove them; database analysis must be followed by trials.'[13]

The potential of and pitfalls associated with observational studies are exemplified by the investigations of the safety of prostatic surgery. Transurethral resection of the prostate gland (TURP) for the condition benign prostatic hypertrophy became fashionable in the 1970s; by the mid 1980s, it was in common use. In 1989, the results of an observational study indicated that TURP was associated with a higher long-term mortality rate than the traditional operation of open prostatectomy (OP) – an increase of 45%.[14] Other evidence against the use of TURP was also published.[15,16] However, all the possible reasons for this difference in mortality had not been taken into account. In particular, during analysis of the results, no allowance had been made for the differences in selection criteria between those used for men undergoing OP and those used for men undergoing TURP. These differences pertain because there is an increase in short-term morbidity and mortality associated with OP. In an excellent study, Seagroatt[17] adjusted the data for differences in selection criteria and came to the opposite conclusion, as follows:

> The apparent excess in long-term mortality after TURP is unlikely to be caused by the operation itself. It is more likely to reflect relatively low long-term mortality in OP patients as a consequence of the OP patients having been relatively fitter than those having TURP.[17]

Thus, it is not possible to convict TURP of causing excess mortality; any previous convictions were made on the basis of flawed evidence. Seagroatt also concluded that any differences in long-term mortality can be 'answered only in a randomised clinical trial', but emphasised that such a trial may be impossible to organise.[17]

6.4.4 Applicability and relevance

Confidence intervals provide the best guide to the applicability of research results. The narrower the confidence intervals, the more confident a decision-maker can be that the research evidence represents the effect it is possible to obtain in the whole population.

A checklist of questions for the assessment of the applicability and relevance of research evidence on effectiveness is shown in Box 6.8.

> **Box 6.8** Checklist for assessing the applicability of research evidence of effectiveness to the local population and service
>
> - Is the study population similar to the local population:
>   - genetically?
>   - socially?
>   - medically?
> - Is the service or treatment under investigation similar to that available locally in terms of:
>   - skills?
>   - resources?

References

1. WEBSTER, C. (1988) *The health services since the war: volume 1*. HMSO, London.
2. COCHRANE, A. (1972) *Effectiveness and efficiency*. Nuffield Provincial Hospitals Trust, London.
3. DOLL, R. (1974) *Surveillance and monitoring*. Int J. Epidemiol. 3: 305–14.
4. KENNELL, J., KLAUS, M., MCGRATH, S., ROBERTSON, S. and HUNTLY, C. (1991) *Continuous emotional support during labor in a US hospital*. JAMA 265: 2197–201.
5. LEFER, L., PLEASURE, M.A. and RESENTHAL, L. (1962) *A psychiatric approach to the denture patient*. J. Psychosom. Res. 6: 199–207.
6. FITZPATRICK, R. and HOPKINS, A. (1981) *Referrals to neurologists for headaches not due to structural disease*. J. Neurol. Neurosurg. Psychiat. 44: 1061–7.
7. EASTERBROOK, P.J., BERLIN, J.A., GOPALAN, R. and MATTHEWS, D.R. (1991) *Publication bias in clinical research*. Lancet 337: 867–72.
8. SCHULZ, K.F., CHALMERS, I., GRIMES, D.A. and ALTMAN, D. (1994) *Assessing the quality of randomization from reports of controlled trials published in obstetrics and gynecology journals*. JAMA 272: 125–8.
9. GØTZSCHE, P.C. (1989) *Methodology and overt and hidden bias in reports of 196 double-blind trials of nonsteroidal anti-inflammatory drugs in rheumatoid arthritis*. Control. Clin. Trials 10: 31–56. [Published erratum: GØTZSCHE, P.C. (1989) Control. Clin. Trials 10: 356.]
10. FAHEY, T., GRIFFITHS, S. and PETERS, T.J. (1995) *Evidence-based purchasing: understanding results of clinical trials and systematic reviews*. Br. Med. J. 311: 1056–60.
11. COOK, R.J. and SACKETT, D.L. (1995) *The number needed to treat: a clinically useful measure of treatment effect*. Br. Med. J. 310: 452–4.
12. McQUAY, H.J. and MOORE, A. (1997) *Using numerical results from systematic reviews in clinical practice*. Ann. Intern. Med. 126: 712–20.
13. TEMPLE, R. (1990) *Problems in the use of large data sets to assess effectiveness*. Int. J. Technol. Assess. Health Care 6: 211–19.
14. ROOS, N.P., WENNBERG. J.E., MALENKA, D.J. et al. (1989) *Mortality and reoperation after open and transurethral resection of the prostate for benign prostatic hyperplasia*. N. Engl. J. Med. 320: 1120–4.
15. ANDERSEN, T.F., BRONNUM-HANSEN, H., SEJR, T. and ROEPSTORFF, C. (1990) *Elevated mortality following transurethral resection of the prostate for benign hyperplasia! But why?* Med. Care 28: 870–81.
16. SIDNEY, S., QUESENBERRY, C.P., SADLER, M.C. et al. (1992) *Reoperation and mortality after surgical treatment of benign prostatic hypertrophy in a large prepaid medical care program*. Med. Care 30: 117–25.
17. SEAGROATT, V. (1995) *Mortality after prostatectomy: selection and surgical approach*. Lancet 346: 1521–4.

6.5   SAFETY

Arthur Dent	*If I asked you where the hell we were, would I regret it?*
Ford Prefect:	*We're safe.*
Arthur Dent:	*Oh good.*
Ford Prefect:	*We're in a small galley cabin in one of the space ships of the Vogon Constructor Fleet.*
Arthur Dent:	*Ah, this is obviously some strange usage of the word safe that I wasn't previously aware of.*

Douglas Adams,
The Hitch Hiker's Guide to the Galaxy, *1979*

6.5.1   Dimensions and definitions

Safety and risk are inversely related to one another, as follows:

> Safety = 1 – risk of adverse effects

The risk associated with an intervention is the 'probability' that an adverse effect will occur.

The use of the word 'probability' is interesting: perhaps not surprisingly, most people use the 1576 definition, given in the *Shorter Oxford English Dictionary* as 'something which, judged by present evidence, is likely to happen', rather than the 1718 mathematical definition which is 'the amount of antecedent likelihood of a particular event as measured by the relative frequency of occurrence of events of the same kind in the whole course of experience'. Words used to describe frequency, such as 'likely', 'often', 'sometimes', 'possible' and 'frequently', can be interpreted by different individuals differently. This difference in interpretation is also evident in expressions of 'subjective possibility' (*SOED*); for example, 'Side-effects may occur'. In an interesting study by Lichtenstein and Newman,[1] a questionnaire was sent to a random selection of 225 male employees at the System Development Corporation to determine the correspondence between numerical probabilities and a range of associated verbal phrases.

Subjects were asked to give the probability number (from 0.01 to 0.99) that reflected the degree of probability implied by each phrase; 188 scorable replies were received. The results are shown in Table 6.4.

Table 6.4 Ranking of probability phrases (Source: Lichtenstein and Newman[1])

Most likely	1	Highly probable
↑	2	Very likely
	3	Very probable
	4	Quite likely
	5	Usually
	6	Good chance
	7	Predictable
	8	Likely
	9	Probable
	10	Rather likely
	11	Pretty good chance
	12	Fairly likely
	13	Somewhat likely
	14	Better than even
	15	Rather
	16	Slightly more than half the time
	17	Slight odds in favour
	18	Fair chance
	19	Toss-up
	20	Fighting chance
	21	Slightly less than half the time
	22	Slight odds against
	23	Not quite even
	24	Inconclusive
	25	Uncertain
	26	Possible
	27	Somewhat likely
	28	Fairly unlikely
	29	Rather unlikely*
	30	Rather unlikely*
	31	Not very probable
	32	Unlikely
	33	Not much chance
	34	Seldom
	35	Barely possible
	36	Faintly possible
	37	Improbable
	38	Quite unlikely
	39	Very unlikely
	40	Rare
Least likely	41	Highly improbable

* This probability phrase was scored differently in terms of the mean, median, σ, and range.

Despite a few generally held distinctions, for instance, that 'probable' implies a higher frequency than 'possible', the variation in the weighting given to different words is so great that numbers have to be used, but which numbers?

Risk can be expressed in two ways:

1. relative risk;
2. absolute risk.

Relative risk can be expressed using a numerical scale: for example, the relative risk of impotence in men who remain on the thiazide treatment for high blood pressure is 2.3, with 23% of men on thiazides being impotent after two years' treatment in comparison with only 10% of those receiving placebo.[2]

Absolute risk is used to express probability either as a simple percentage, for example, 'About 60% of patients will experience adverse effects', or as the number needed to harm (the NNH – see Section 6.4.3.1). Some patients may find the NNH more comprehensible than a percentage, i.e. the number of patients treated with thiazide diuretics that would result in one person being harmed over and above the risk in the general population is 8. To continue with the example, the number needed to cause an extra case of impotence (NNI), is calculated by converting the relative risk to an absolute figure using the following formula:

$$\frac{\text{NNH}}{(\text{risk in treated population} - \text{risk in untreated population})} = 1$$

As for all other outcome estimates, confidence intervals should be given.

A new measure, which has been derived from the NNT and the NNH, is the likelihood of being helped to being harmed (LHH).[3] It was developed by Sharon Straus at the Centre for Evidence-Based Medicine in Oxford to give an indication of the potential adverse effects of new treatments; in the past, emphasis has been given to the potential benefits. The LHH is the balance of the NNT and the NNH.

6.5.2 Searching

Step 1:   Specify the intervention in question: the drug, test or operation.
Step 2:   Specify adverse effects or risk of adverse effects.

It is not normally useful to stipulate a publication type. Although the best evidence is provided by a systematic review of RCTs, other methods of research can be helpful, therefore, it is important not to limit the boundaries of the search in this way.

6.5.3 Appraisal

The two main questions in the critical appraisal of research information about safety are:

1. Which is the best research method to give information about the risks of treatment?
2. How good is the quality of the research?

6.5.3.1   Which method?

The research methods that can generate information about safety, and the risk of adverse effects of treatment are:

- systematic review of RCTs (Section 5.3), which is generally better than an RCT for this purpose;
- RCT (Section 5.4);
- survey (Section 5.7) and cohort study (Section 5.6);
- case-control study (Section 5.5).

Systematic reviews of any of these methods of research (Section 5.3) are better than single studies provided the quality of the primary research is good.
   It is relatively rare for the results of RCTs to generate useful evidence about the harmful effects of treatment, principally because adverse effects usually occur less frequently than beneficial effects. A trial designed with sufficient power to demonstrate the beneficial effects of treatment (Section 5.5.1.2) will probably not have sufficient power to detect any adverse effects, and it is often necessary to perform a cohort study.
   A cohort study is a research design in which one or more groups of patients are followed over time. For example, in the UK, thousands of women who were and were not taking oral contraceptives have been followed for years. However, those women not taking oral contraceptives

cannot be compared directly with those who are; for instance, even though deep vein thrombosis may have been detected more often in pill users, it is possible that non-users may not have been prescribed the pill because they were considered to be at high risk of thrombosis.

Prospective cohort studies are less prone to bias and can be used when it is not possible to conduct an RCT. For example, most anaesthetists might refuse to participate in an RCT in which the hypothesis that epidural anaesthesia causes backache is tested. However, it did prove possible to follow 329 women for six weeks after delivery, 164 of whom had had epidural anaesthesia and 165 of whom had not. The results of this prospective study of these two cohorts did not show that backache was an adverse effect of epidural anaesthesia.[4]

The most appropriate study design to identify the adverse effects of drugs may be the case-control study despite the fact that this research methodology may introduce a greater degree of bias than that introduced by cohort studies.

A major source of bias is introduced if data that were collected previously are reviewed. In an elegant experiment, 112 anaesthetists were asked to review 21 cases for which there had been adverse anaesthetic outcomes classified as either permanent or temporary. In addition, the authors generated 21 matching alternate cases identical to the original except that in each case a plausible outcome of opposite severity was substituted. The original and the alternate cases were randomly assigned to two sets and presented to the anaesthetists. The results were startling:

- the proportion of cases in which care was deemed 'appropriate' *decreased* by 31% when the outcome was changed from temporary to permanent;
- the proportion of cases in which care was deemed 'appropriate' *increased* by 28% when the outcome was changed from permanent to temporary.

From this study, it can be seen that foreknowledge of the outcome of care can alter the reviewer's perception of the appropriateness of that care, and therefore his/her perception of the safety of the procedure.[5]

6.5.3.2 Appraising the quality of studies on safety

Although the quality of each type of research study needs to be appraised against the criteria set out in the relevant sections of this book, there are also some general questions that should be used in the appraisal of any study designed to investigate adverse effects (see Box 6.9).

Box 6.9   Checklist for appraising the quality of a study designed to investigate adverse effects

1. Was the assessment of outcomes free from bias?
2. Was there an adverse effect greater than would be expected by chance, taking into account the confidence intervals?
3. How important is the adverse effect clinically?
4. If more than one study is available, are the results consistent among them?

6.5.4 Applicability and relevance

Evidence revealing risks associated with drug treatment can usually be applied to the whole population: the results will be relevant to all patients of the same type as those described in the original trial. In contrast, the risks associated with particular surgical operations or interventions, in which the skill of the professional is an important determining factor, may vary according to the professionals involved; therefore, the risk could be smaller or greater than that reported in the literature.

   A checklist of questions for the assessment of the applicability and relevance of research findings on safety is shown in Box 6.10.

Box 6.10   Checklist for assessing the applicability and relevance of research evidence of safety

1. Were the professionals participating in the study more highly specialised or more experienced in this intervention than those who will be treating the local population?
2. Would the quality of training be important in determining the frequency of adverse effects?
3. Were the patients in the research study different from those in the local population, either by being fitter or by having more advanced disease?

References

1. LICHTENSTEIN, S. and NEWMAN, R.J. (1967) *Empirical scaling of common verbal phrases associated with numerical probabilities.* Psychon. Sci. 9: 563–4.
2. MEDICAL RESEARCH COUNCIL WORKING PARTY (1981) *Adverse reactions to bendrofluazide and propanolol for the treatment of mild hypertension.* Lancet ii: 539–43.
3. SACKETT, D.L., STRAUSS, S.E., RICHARDSON, W.S., ROSENBERG, W. and HAYNES, R.B. (2000) *Evidence-based medicine: how to practice and teach EBM.* 2nd Edition. Churchill Livingstone, Edinburgh.
4. MACARTHUR, A., MACARTHUR, C. and WEEKS, S. (1995) *Epidural anaesthesia and low back pain after delivery: a prospective cohort study.* Br. Med. J. 311: 1336–9.
5. CAPLAN, R.A., POSNER, K.L. and CHENEY, F.W. (1991) *Effect of outcome on physician judgements of appropriateness of care.* JAMA 265: 1957–60.

6.6   PATIENT SATISFACTION AND PATIENTS' EXPERIENCE OF CARE

Gentle Reader,

Empathise with Mr R. He spat accurately into the bucket that served as both spittoon and urinal. Disabled by a stroke and a gas lung sustained in an afternoon during the First World War when the gas came 'rolling towards us', he was unable to climb the stairs to get to the bathroom of his damp council house. The room in which he lived was heated by only a small electric fire; mould had formed an opulent brocade on the walls. Although the young doctor and social worker were apologising for their inability to improve his health and environment, his views were clear. 'I'm grateful for all you're doing, but don't worry about me; I'm all right. Sixty years ago today I was up to my waist in mud and water.'

Commentary

Satisfied with his lot, satisfied with his services, this Old Contemptible would never have dreamed of complaining, even when the quality of care was manifestly poor. However, times have changed and patient satisfaction can no longer be taken for granted.

6.6.1 Dimensions and definitions

6.6.1.1 Acceptability of care

Finally, I will admit one thing: there is no way in which I would ever have a colonoscopy as a screening procedure.

Lecture given by a doctor about a pilot screening programme using colonoscopy to detect colorectal cancer

Acceptability is a theoretical construct used in service planning and technology assessment. It is applied to interventions before they have been introduced into a service to test patients', or members' of the public, willingness to be treated in a particular way. Once an intervention has been introduced, acceptability as a concept becomes subsumed within the measurement of patient satisfaction and patients' experience of care.

6.6.1.2 Patient satisfaction

The level of a patient's satisfaction with care is directly related to the degree to which his/her expectations have been met (see Margin Fig. 6.5).

However, the assessment of patient satisfaction, although necessary, is not sufficient: satisfaction is determined not only by patient expectations but also by the quality of the service. Despite this, patient satisfaction is an imperfect measure with which to assess the quality of any service: it is possible for patients to be delighted with healthcare in which the quality of clinical practice was poor if their expectations were low.

Prior
expectations

Dissatisfaction

Satisfaction

Delight

Experience of care

Margin Fig. 6.5

6.6.1.3 Patients' experience of care

As patient satisfaction is an imperfect measure for the assessment of quality, it is necessary to investigate the patient's *experience* of care and make a judgement about the quality of that experience irrespective of whether the patient is satisfied (Margin Fig. 6.6). For instance, it is possible for a patient to be satisfied with the amount of information provided and the way in which it was provided, despite the fact that the information is wrong and misleading. It is essential, therefore, to complement the question 'Were you satisfied with the information you were given?' with the question 'What information were you given?'.

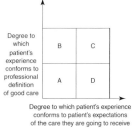

Degree to which patient's experience conforms to professional definition of good care

B   C

A   D

Degree to which patient's experience
conforms to patient's expectations
of the care they are going to receive
(= Patient Satisfaction)

Margin Fig. 6.6

This novel approach of gathering patients' experiences was developed in the USA, where it has been used to improve medical care in hospitals.[1] Indeed, increasing use is being made of systems designed to assess patient experience, and The Picker Institute Europe, which was established in 1997 as a sister organisation to the Picker Institute in the USA, is now extending the use of this approach throughout Europe (see http://www.picker.org/Europe/Default.htm).

In the UK, in a survey of 5150 randomly chosen NHS patients recently discharged from 36 NHS acute hospitals, patients were interviewed 2–4 weeks after discharge by means of a structured questionnaire.[2] They were asked direct questions about their experience during treatment in hospital, including aspects such as communication with staff, pain management, and discharge planning. They were also asked general questions about their degree of satisfaction with care. The authors' conclusion was that asking patients direct questions about what had happened rather than how satisfied they were with treatment gave a better understanding of what might be wrong with a service and provided a stronger base upon which healthcare professionals and managers could make improvements to care.

A patient's experience is determined by three inter-related aspects of care (see Margin Fig. 6.7):

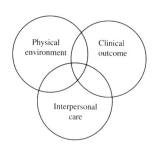

Margin Fig. 6.7

1. the clinical outcome;
2. the physical environment in which care is received;
3. the interpersonal relationships of care, namely, how patients are treated by the professionals giving care.

1. Clinical outcome: expectations and experience
Although a patient's expectations may be determined by many factors, the single most important factor is what the patient remembers the clinician said about clinical outcomes, such as:

- the magnitude of health improvement that could be expected, e.g. complete cure or alleviation of symptoms;
- the probability that there would be a benefit;
- the nature of side-effects that occur most commonly;
- the probability that any of those side-effects would be suffered personally.

The optimal information exchange in a consultation is when the patient remembers all that the clinician said; however, this does not always occur (see Margin Fig. 6.8). Thus, the most important factor is the quality of the clinician's communication.

The various reactions a patient might have are shown in Matrix 6.2.

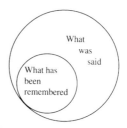

Margin Fig. 6.8

	Beneficial effect as predicted or expected	Beneficial effect absent or not as great as predicted or expected
No side-effects	Delighted	Disappointed
Side-effects as expected or predicted	Modified delight	Very disappointed
Side-effects worse than expected or predicted	Response dependent upon personality and other factors, e.g. satisfaction with interpersonal care	Desolate

Matrix 6.2

Patients' reactions may also vary depending upon:

- factors over which the health service has no influence, e.g.
  - the patient's personality;
  - the advice of ambulance-chasing lawyers;
- factors over which the health service has influence, e.g.
  - the physical environment in which care is received;
  - the quality of interpersonal care.

2. The physical environment: expectations and experience
Certain aspects of the physical environment in which care is delivered are of particular importance to patients:

- quality of food;
- availability of parking;
- the standard of cleanliness;
- the comfort of the bed;
- the 'external' environment (is it possible to see trees from the bed?);
- ease of access by public transport.

If the clinical outcome is satisfactory and the interpersonal care is good, satisfaction with the physical environment will be a bonus. If the patient is pleased with clinical outcome and interpersonal care, deficiencies in the physical environment are unlikely to lead to overall dissatisfaction and the registration of a complaint.

If there is dissatisfaction with the clinical outcome or interpersonal care, a high-quality physical environment is unlikely to compensate for deficiencies in these more important aspects of care. Furthermore, a low-quality environment may provide a focus for the discontent of a patient or their relatives if there is dissatisfaction with other aspects of care that are difficult to articulate.

3. *Interpersonal care: expectations and experience*

> Asking why his daughter needed further tests, a father was told: 'Your last child died of cancer. Draw your own conclusions.'

> During a delivery, a junior doctor was told: 'Go slow, man, or you'll tear the baby's head off.'

> A woman complaining of a 'congested' nose was told: 'Don't use long words. Use your own language, woman.'

> *Extracts from an article by William Evington entitled* 'Physician, heal thyself' *in the Thursday Review of* The Independent, *8 July 1999*

Frank rudeness in healthcare professionals is an obvious cause of dissatisfaction and distress for both patients and their relatives. However, it is more common for failures in a professional's behaviour to be of a subtle non-verbal nature. It is important that any patient receives the impression that s/he:

- is an individual and not just a number;
- has a problem that the professional is taking seriously;
- is the sole focus of that professional's attention during any interaction.

A healthcare professional may subscribe to this approach, but if it is not translated into appropriate behaviour the patient is unable to appreciate it: patients are not mind-readers.

6.6.1.4 Is the measurement of patient satisfaction of any use?

The measurement of patient satisfaction is not completely pointless. One of the objectives of any manager should be to satisfy a patient's desire for safe and effective treatment, delivered by professionals who care about that patient, in pleasant surroundings.

6.6.1.5 Does patient satisfaction bring physician satisfaction?

In the 'friendly' dentists trial,[3] two approaches to dental practice for people who required dentures were investigated: in the treatment group, the dentists discussed care options with patients, involved them in decision-making and shared both the responsibility and pleasure of a satisfactory outcome; the control group received treatment in the usual manner. The outcome of the trial demonstrated clearly that the 'friendly' dentists achieved better clinical outcomes than the conventional dentists.

Evidence of the effectiveness of patient participation in the process of care was also produced by a cross-sectional survey of 7730 patients from the practices of 300 physicians, which was part of the Medical Outcomes Study.[4] It was found that:

- the greater the level of patient participation, the greater the degree of patient satisfaction;
- physicians who had primary care training or training in interviewing scored higher than those who lacked such training;
- physicians in higher volume practices were rated as less participatory than those in lower volume practices;
- physicians who were satisfied with the level of professional autonomy were rated as more participatory than those who were dissatisfied.

The authors raise the fascinating possibility that:

> Because participatory decision-making style is related to patient satisfaction and loyalty to the physician, cost-containment strategies that reduce time with patients and decrease physician autonomy may result in suboptimal patient outcomes.

As this survey was conducted within the US healthcare system, and the questionnaire developed in the USA, the results cannot be taken at face value by healthcare professionals working in other countries. However, there appears to be strong evidence that a participatory, 'friendly' style of practice is better for patient care and, if patients can vote with their feet, for business. Longer, 'friendlier' consultations in which the patient participates seem to be cost-effective in the long term, although the investment may be greater in the short term.

In an editorial, entitled 'The physician interviewer in the era of corporatization of care',[5] Lipkin opened with a challenging metaphor:

> With the increasing corporatization of medicine, are physicians becoming Sisyphean drudges toiling futilely, forced to roll the stone uphill faster and faster, losing patients, pride in quality care, autonomy, and their own health? This increasingly prevalent self-image – correlated with high rates of burnout and fundamental dissatisfaction with the profession – contrasts with the happier, Pegasus-like myth of the physician soaring on the wings of science and professionalism, experiencing the joys of effectiveness, altruism, moral probity, and wealth that attracted so many of us to medicine. Implicit in much Sisyphean negativism is victimization – by the nature of things, in Camus' existentialist version, and by the medical-industrial complex, in others. The extent to which we have perpetuated our own victimization and the extent to which it is remediable through our own actions are empiric questions.

Lipkin argues that improving interviewing skills improves both a physician's and a patient's satisfaction with care. As each physician will undertake 200 000–300 000 consultations during his/her professional life, such a strategy would improve physician performance and make them feel better. Thus, the development of better interviewing skills should not be seen simply as an altruistic device to improve patient satisfaction, but as part of a self-interested campaign for physician survival.

6.6.2 Searching

As patient satisfaction is determined to a great extent by the local characteristics of a particular service, as opposed to its effectiveness, studies of patient satisfaction may not be considered to be research and, as such, may not be indexed in MEDLINE or EMBASE. However, it is still worth searching both databases using 'satisfaction' and 'patient's perception of outcome' as keywords.

6.6.3 Appraisal

Critical skills are needed for two tasks.

1. The appraisal of an instrument for measuring satisfaction. There are many such instruments, usually a combination of a questionnaire and an interview, either face to face or by telephone. A checklist of questions for the appraisal of any instrument used to assess patient satisfaction is shown in Box 6.11.
2. The appraisal of the study of patient satisfaction. Although the main focus of the appraisal is on the instrument used to measure satisfaction, it is also important to assess the overall study design (see Box 6.12).

Box 6.11 Checklist for the appraisal of instruments used to assess patient satisfaction

1. How has the instrument been tested?
2. What is the interobserver variability, i.e. how different are the answers if different people use the questionnaire on the same person?
3. How good is the instrument at measuring the three aspects of care that determine satisfaction: interpersonal care, the physical environment and clinical outcome?
4. How comprehensible are the questions to people of different reading abilities or different ethnic backgrounds?

Box 6.12 Checklist for the appraisal of study designs used to assess patient satisfaction

1. How well did the survey assess the experience of the patients as opposed to their reaction to that experience?
2. Was the sample interviewed a representative sample of the population served by the service or was it biased?
3. Are the results applicable to the population in general?
4. Are the results relevant to the local population?

6.6.4 Applicability and relevance

Surveys of patient satisfaction are primarily of use to the service about which they have been conducted. The degree to which any of the results are a function of patient expectations, which vary from one population to another, and the quality of the service those patients received make it difficult to apply findings about one service to others elsewhere. However, the reasons for complaint revealed by such surveys (e.g. noise), as opposed to the degree of patient dissatisfaction found, may be useful because they can indicate causes of dissatisfaction that could be relevant to any population.

References

1. CLEARY, P.D., EDGMAN-LEVITAN, S., WALKER, J.D. et al. (1993) *Using patient reports to improve medical care: a preliminary report from 10 hospitals*. Qual. Manage. Health Care 2: 31–8.
2. BRUSTER, S., JARMAN, B., BOSANQUET, N. et al. (1994) *National survey of hospital patients*. Br. Med. J. 309: 1542–6.
3. LEFER, L., PLEASURE, M.A. and RESENTHAL, L. (1962) *A psychiatric approach to the denture patient*. J. Psychosom. Res. 6: 199–207.
4. KAPLAN, S.H., GREENFIELD, S., GANDEK, B. et al. (1996) *Characteristics of physicians with participatory decision-making styles*. Ann. Intern. Med. 124: 497–504.
5. LIPKIN, M. Jr. (1996) *Sisyphus or Pegasus? The physician interviewer in the era of corporatization of care*. Ann. Intern. Med. 124: 511–12.

> **Oxymoron:** a rhetorical figure by which
> contradictory terms are conjoined so as to give point
> to the statement or expression (now often loosely = a
> contradiction in terms)
>
> *Shorter Oxford English Dictionary*

In recent years, the arguments used by the pharmaceutical companies have changed; no longer do they claim that a new drug is more effective, they emphasise that the drug is much more *cost*-effective for the health service, the implication being that even though the cost of prescribed medication may be more expensive, savings are made elsewhere in the healthcare system.

Robert Evans, one of the world's leading health economists, wrote a leader for the *Annals of Internal Medicine*[1] which should be read by anyone who receives information about the cost-effectiveness of new drugs. It is a commentary on, and critique of, a report entitled *Economic Analysis of Health Care Technology*.[2] Evans points out that the work of the Taskforce described in the report was funded entirely by the pharmaceutical industry, and asserts that the industry was giving a verisimilitude of objectivity to a technique that should be assumed to be biased. His criticisms are typically forthright; for example, he states that:

> A pseudodiscipline, 'pharmaco-economics', has been
> conjured into existence by the magic of money, with
> its own practitioners, conferences, and journals. There
> are a lot of drugs and there is a lot of money, so the
> 'field' is booming.

In response to two letters in which the original leader was criticised, he concludes:

> In the end, drug buyers and reimbursers will have to
> do their own evaluations and make their own
> purchasing decisions. Offers of participation and
> scientific cooperation from sellers always spring from
> the same underlying motive, to move the product.
> What else can they do?[3]

This may seem a cynical line to take but this issue must be faced, especially as studies of cost-effectiveness have an increasingly important role to play in the appraisal of new interventions.

A similar line of argument was taken in a leader published in the *British Medical Journal* entitled 'Promoting cost-effective prescribing'.[4] Freemantle et al. pointed out that drug companies have been criticised for using economic analyses as marketing devices, and those working for funders of health services have been criticised for favouring the containment of costs at the expense of benefits for patients. Freemantle et al. emphasise the need for the development of scientifically rigorous guidelines for the conduct of economic analyses to be linked either to a regulatory mechanism or positive incentives. They highlight the fact that the guidelines in the UK, drawn up by the Department of Health and the Association of British Pharmaceutical Industries (ABPI), were prepared with minimal consultation of those working in the field, and there is no evidence of scientific rigour having been applied in contrast with the guidelines developed for use in Canada or Australia (see Fig. 7.3).

6.7.1   Dimensions and definitions

The concept of cost-effectiveness has evolved from earlier conceptions of efficiency.

6.7.1.1   Productivity and efficiency

Wittgenstein proposed that when a word caused more confusion than clarification its use should be discontinued; this is now the case for the word 'efficiency'. The term is often used as if it were synonymous with productivity, and it is common in the NHS for efficiency to be calculated by relating the outputs of a service (i.e. episodes of care) to the inputs (i.e. costs), which is actually the method of calculating what is more accurately termed productivity (see Box 6.13 for examples of measures of productivity).

6.7.1.2   Cochrane's definition of efficiency

In his excellent work *Effectiveness and Efficiency*,[5] Cochrane's definition of the term 'efficiency', although it is similar to that of productivity (he cites, for example, 'length of stay' as one measure), encompasses one important difference: he focused on *effective* interventions, and in doing so brought the numerator closer to that of an outcome. For Cochrane,

---

Box 6.13 Examples of productivity measures (usually referred to as efficiency measures)

$$\text{Productivity} = \frac{\text{Output}}{\text{Input}}$$

1. $\dfrac{\text{Episodes of care}}{\text{Cost}}$

2. $\dfrac{\text{No. episodes of care}^6}{\text{No. professionals}}$

3. $\dfrac{\text{No. operations}}{\text{No. surgeons}}$

4. $\dfrac{\text{No. operations}}{\text{No. bed-days}}$

---

the provision of a service of proven ineffectiveness, or of unproven efficacy, was inefficient *ipso facto* no matter how cheaply that intervention was delivered. Thus, his use of the term 'efficiency' is closer to a definition of 'cost-effectiveness'.

6.7.1.3 The advent of the concept of cost-effectiveness

There are two main ways in which linguistic inexactitude can be clarified:

- reaching a consensus about a definition or set of definitions at a national or international conference and disseminating the outcomes;
- introducing a new word that will express the meaning more clearly.

In the case of 'efficiency', the second strategy has been followed, and the term cost-effectiveness has been introduced.

Cost-effectiveness is calculated by relating the outcomes of a service (e.g. number of lives saved) to the inputs (i.e. costs):

$$\text{Cost-effectiveness} = \frac{\text{Outcomes}}{\text{Cost}}$$

However, when measuring cost-effectiveness, it is essential to remember that the outcomes of care may be adverse as well as beneficial:

$$\text{Cost-effectiveness} = \frac{\text{Beneficial outcomes} - \text{adverse outcomes}}{\text{Cost}}$$

6.7.1.4 Assessing cost-effectiveness: the use of outcome measures

Initially, the beneficial outcome of an intervention designed to prevent mortality was expressed only in terms of the number of extra years of life resulting from that intervention.

$$\text{Beneficial outcome} = \frac{\text{Extra years of life}}{\text{No. bed days}}$$

Subsequently, it was recognised that the quality of life during those extra years is an important consideration. In order to determine the quality of life during those extra years, various studies were undertaken to ascertain the value people attach to different states of health and illness. It was found that a consensus could be reached about the values people attach to certain states, ranging from a factor of 1, which represents excellent health, to 0, which represents the worst state of health. A method was then developed that enabled a combination of a patient's levels of disability and of distress, such as pain, to be assessed.[7] It was then possible to estimate the quality of life during the extra years as well as the quantity, and these two measures were combined to produce the quality-adjusted life year (QALY).

> The number of extra years of life obtained
> ×
> the value of the quality of life during those extra years
> =
> quality-adjusted life years (QALYs)

The concept of QALYs is now in fairly widespread use.

However, decisions are rarely based solely on the calculation of QALYs. Many decision-makers use this measure as an initial screen for classifying interventions into one of three groups, as follows:

1. those that are very expensive and are not to be considered further;
2. those that are very cheap and should be provided – a 'no-brainer' decision;
3. those that require further investigation.

For the busy decision-maker, it is unfortunate that the majority of interventions fall into the third group.

Another approach is described in *The Global Burden of Disease*, a text of tremendous importance. In it, Murray and Lopez[8] introduce the concept of the disability-adjusted life year (DALY), the focus of which is 'non-fatal health outcomes'. This type of approach emphasises the importance of neuropsychiatric conditions, principally depression. They describe a programme of work being undertaken by the World Health Organization to estimate the global burden of disease. To complete such an estimation, it was necessary to develop techniques to estimate the causes of death in the absence of robust data, and then to summarise the 'descriptive epidemiology of disability', namely:

- incidence, i.e. the number of new cases per year;
- prevalence, i.e. the number of people living at any one time with a disability;
- health expectancy, and the years of life lived with each type of disability.

It is also possible to use this technique to calculate variations in disease burden, such as:

- that in different regions of the world;
- that which could be attributed to 10 major risk factors;
- projections to the year 2020 (Fig. 6.8).

Using this approach, it is possible to predict the changing pattern of disease, thereby facilitating the identification of opportunities for disease prevention and health improvement. From Fig. 6.8, it can be seen that as some of the traditional diseases of poor countries drop down the list, in which the rank order of DALYs for the 15 leading causes in the world are shown for the year 1990 against the projection for the year 2020, other diseases that appear to

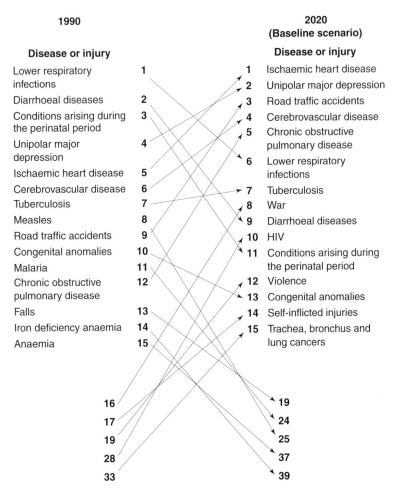

Fig. 6.8
Change in the rank order of DALYs for the leading causes (world) 1990–2020
(Source: Murray and Lopez[8])

be consequent upon development, notably ischaemic heart disease and depression, move up.

6.7.1.5 Marginal and opportunity costs

To determine the cost of an operation, the cost of a unit, including all fixed costs, is divided by the number of operations performed by that unit.

$$\frac{\textit{Total cost of the unit, including salaries and capital charges (£10\,000\,000)}}{\text{Number of operations (1000)}} = £10\,000 \text{ per op.}$$

A marginal cost is the cost of any *additional* interventions performed by a unit for which the cost of working at a particular rate has already been calculated. For instance, in a unit in which 1000 operations are undertaken at a cost of £10 000 each, the fixed costs will be £9000 per operation whereas the cost of the consumables per operation will be £1000. Thus, the marginal cost of 100 extra operations will be £100 000, i.e. the cost of the consumables at £1000 for each extra operation.

Opportunity costs are defined as those uses, other than the one being resourced, on which the same amount of money could be spent. For example, the opportunity costs of the £100 000 that might be spent on 100 more cardiac operations could be expressed as the number of chiropody treatments or cataract operations that it is possible to purchase with the same amount of money.

6.7.1.6 Economic evaluations

There are many different approaches to the evaluation of cost-effectiveness:

- cost-benefit analysis – an assessment of the return on investment in terms of money
- cost-utility analysis – an assessment of the return on investment in terms of QALYs which is a more sophisticated form of cost-benifit analysis;
- cost-effectiveness – an assessment of the relative merits of different methods of achieving the same objective.

Cost-benefit and cost-utility analyses enable decision-makers to assess the benefit that will be gained from investing resources in a particular type of health service, and then to compare the benefits of investing resources in services designed to treat different health problems. As an example, the results would allow the return on investment in an immunisation programme to be compared with the return that might be obtained from investment in another child health programme, or a different preventive programme for adults, or any other form of healthcare.

Studies of cost-effectiveness enable decision-makers to compare the costs of different ways of tackling the same health problem.

- The results of a cost-benefit or cost-utility analysis would help a decision-maker to assess the returns on investing £100 000 additional resources in either a renal transplantation programme or a cardiac surgery programme; the decision-maker might then wish to carry out a cost-effectiveness study of the alternatives to renal transplantation.
- The results of a cost-effectiveness analysis would help the decision-maker assess the relative cost-effectiveness of dialysis and of transplantation as methods of treating end-stage renal failure.

6.7.2 Searching

Step 1: Specify the search term for the health problem and the intervention.

Step 2: Search for terms that will identify papers in which the focus is on the costs of the particular health problem and the cost-effectiveness of the intervention.

6.7.3 Appraisal

In 1996, the Panel on Cost-Effectiveness in Health and Medicine published recommendations for reporting cost-effectiveness analyses[9] in order:

- to enhance the transparency of study methods;
- to assist researchers in providing complete information;
- to facilitate the presentation of comparable results across studies.

Neumann et al.[10] investigated the quality of reporting in 228 cost-utility analyses (i.e. measured in terms of QALYs) published in English from 1976 to 1997. Analyses were audited against the following categories:

- disclosure of funding;
- framing;
- reporting of costs;
- reporting of preference weights;
- reporting of results;
- discussion.

They found that in most studies modelling assumptions (82%), comparator intervention (83%), sensitivity analysis (89%), and study limitations (84%) were reported. However, in 34%, the source of funding was not disclosed, a finding that gives credence to Robert Evans' misgivings discussed earlier in this section (see page 209). It is interesting to note that the quality of published analyses was found to be higher in general clinical journals and journals that published a greater number of these analyses.

A checklist of questions for the appraisal of economic evaluations is shown in Box 6.14.

Box 6.14   Checklist for the appraisal of economic evaluations of healthcare (Source: Adapted from Drummond et al.[6])

1. Was a well-defined question posed in an answerable form?
2. Was a comprehensive description of the competing alternatives given (i.e. can you tell who did what to whom, where, and how often)?
3. Was there evidence that the programme's effectiveness had been established? [How strong was the evidence of effectiveness?]
4. Were all the important and relevant costs and consequences for each alternative identified?
5. Were costs and consequences measured accurately in appropriate physical units (e.g. hours of nursing time, number of physician visits, lost work-days, life-years gained)?
6. Were costs and consequences valued credibly?
7. Were costs and consequences adjusted for differential timing?
8. Was an incremental analysis of the costs and consequences of alternatives performed? [Were the additional (incremental) costs generated by one alternative over another compared to the additional effects, benefits, or utilities generated?]
9. Was allowance made for uncertainty in the estimates of costs and consequences?
10. Did the presentation and discussion of study results include all issues of concern to users?

6.7.4 Applicability and relevance

Cost-benefit and cost-effectiveness analyses are of most use to decision-makers; however, the results of research studies are of limited relevance to decision-makers who are responsible for populations other than those in which the study was performed. Therefore, the findings of any research study must be carefully appraised for applicability and relevance to the local situation. This is because, although the effectiveness of a service is universal, a service's cost-effectiveness is influenced by local factors such as the incidence and prevalence of disease, and resource constraints. A cost-benefit study of a coronary revascularisation programme is a function of the incidence and prevalence of coronary artery disease in the population served, and the prevailing resource constraints such as the availability of skilled cardiac surgeons. Similarly, if the opportunity costs are expressed in terms of tuberculosis control, they are influenced not only by the incidence and prevalence of tuberculosis in that population but also by the relevant resource constraints such as the availability of trained nursing staff.

In assessing whether an economic appraisal is relevant and can be applied to the local service, it is necessary to ask two questions, as follows:

- how similar is the study population to the local population?
- how similar are the healthcare costs and level of available resources in the research study to healthcare costs and resources available locally?

Although data showing the relative costs and benefits of different programmes are more useful than absolute data about a single programme, the results of all economic studies must be used with caution.

References

1. EVANS, R.G. (1995) *Manufacturing consensus, marketing truth: guidelines for economic evaluation.* Ann. Intern. Med. 123: 59–60.
2. TASK FORCE ON PRINCIPLES FOR ECONOMIC ANALYSIS OF HEALTH CARE TECHNOLOGY (1995) *Economic analysis of health care technology. A report on principles.* Ann. Intern. Med. 123: 61–70.
3. EVANS, R.G. (1996) *Principles of economic analysis of health care technology. [Response to letters]* Ann. Intern. Med. 124: 536.
4. FREEMANTLE, N., HENRY, D., MAYNARD, A. and TORRANCE, G. (1995) *Promoting cost-effective prescribing.* Br. Med. J. 310: 955–6.
5. COCHRANE, A. (1972) *Effectiveness and efficiency.* Nuffield Provincial Hospitals Trust, London.
6. DRUMMOND, M.F., O'BRIEN, B., STODDART, G.L. and TORRANCE, G.A. (1997) *Methods for the economic evaluation of health care programmes.* 2nd Edition. Oxford University Press, New York.
7. ROSSER, R. and KIND, P. (1978) *A scale of valuations of states of illness: is there a social consensus?* Int. J. Epidemiol. 7: 347–58.
8. MURRAY, C.J.L. and LOPEZ, A.D. (Eds) (1996) *The Global burden of Disease.* World Health Organization, Geneva.
9. SIEGEL, J.E., WEINSTEIN, M.C., RUSSELL, L.B., and GOLD, M.R. for the Panel on Cost-Effectiveness in Health and Medicine (1996) *Recommendations for reporting cost-effectiveness analyses.* JAMA 276 1339–41.
10. NEUMANN, P.J., STONE, P.W., CHAPMAN, R.H., SANDBERG, E.A. and BELL, C.M. (2000) *The quality of reporting in published cost-utility analyses, 1976–1997.* Ann. Intern. Med. 132 964–72.

6.8   QUALITY

Quality, in the context of treating patients in the UK, can be defined as doing the right things right to the right people at the right time.

This definition integrates three concepts that have been widely used in the last few years.

> *quality* (new definition) = *clinical effectiveness* (doing the right thing)
> +
> *appropriateness* (right people, right time)
> +
> *quality* (doing things right – old definition of quality)

This approach to quality is at the heart of the UK Government's paper *A First Class Service: quality in the new NHS.*[1] In this consultation paper, the elements necessary to ensure the delivery of a good-quality health service were outlined, together with the mechanisms that will be used to implement them (see Box 6.15).

6.8.1   Dimensions and definitions

The definition of quality based on doing the right things to the right people at the right time and getting it right first time is inspiring but difficult for a health service manager to use on a daily basis. The older definition by Avedis Donabedian is more useful in these circumstances: the quality of a service is the degree to which it conforms to pre-set standards of care.

Standards are usually developed as part of a system of care, and each system of care comprises a set of activities that have common objectives. Whenever possible, the objectives for any service should be expressed in terms of the population served (see, for example, the original objectives for the NHS Breast Screening Programme in Box 6.16).

The effectiveness of a professional or a service is the degree to which the objectives of care are achieved.

Box 6.15   Elements important in the delivery of a good-quality health service, and the mechanisms that will be used to implement them in the NHS (Source: Department of Health[1]).

Setting quality standards
- The National Institute for Clinical Excellence (NICE)
- The National Service Frameworks

Delivering quality standards
- Clinical governance
- Lifelong learning
- Professional self-regulation

Monitoring quality standards
- The Commission for Health Improvement
- A National Framework for Assessing Performance
- National Survey of Patient and User Experience

Action for quality

Box 6.16   Original objectives of the NHS Breast Screening Programme

The aim of the programme is to reduce mortality from breast cancer in the population screened.
- To identify and invite eligible women for mammographic screening.
- To carry out mammography in a high proportion of those who were invited.
- To provide services that are acceptable to those who receive them.
- To follow up all women referred for further investigations.
- To minimise the adverse effects of screening – anxiety, radiation and unnecessary investigations.
- To diagnose cancers accurately.
- To support and carry out research.
- To make effective and efficient use of resources for the benefit of the whole population.
- To enable those working in the programme to develop their skills and find fulfilment in their work.
- To encourage the provision of effective acceptable treatment which has minimal psychological or functional side-effects.
- To evaluate the service regularly and provide feedback to the population served.

6.8.1.1 Quality assessment by measuring the process of care

The process of care is the sequence of healthcare activities undertaken from the initial consultation of a healthcare professional by a patient to the completion of the course of treatment.

For each of the objectives set for a service, relevant healthcare activities need to be defined, the rates of delivery for which can be used to measure progress towards the objective. The healthcare activities chosen to indicate the rate of progress towards an objective were termed process measures by Donabedian.[2]

The processes of care measured should be those for which there is good evidence of effectiveness. For example, for an assessment of the quality of a maternity service, the proportion of women going into labour prematurely who were given antenatal steroids[3] is an evidence-based process measure; in the assessment of the quality of care received by those suffering an acute myocardial infarction, the proportion of patients who receive streptokinase treatment within an hour of arriving at hospital is also an evidence-based process measure. By using such evidence-based process measures, the performance of an individual or service can be defined. This represents an objective assessment of what is being achieved.

A standard is a subjective judgement of a level of performance that *could* be achieved. Different levels of quality standard can be set (see Fig. 6.9).

- The *minimal* acceptable standard below which no service should fall without urgent remedial action being taken.
- The *excellent* or *optimal* standard: the best level of service that can be achieved. Although this is a worthy standard, it is often achieved only by exceptional people and/or people working in exceptional circumstances. The excellent or optimal standard may be regarded by colleagues in other services as atypical and therefore it is of little use for motivating the majority of service providers.
- The *achievable* standard: the level of performance achieved by the top quartile of services; if one quartile of services can achieve a certain level of performance, almost all services have the potential to do so.

A comparison of actual performance with the standard enables a target for quality improvement to be set. These

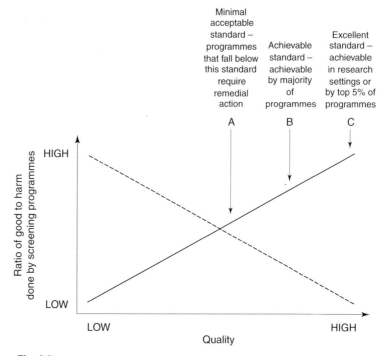

Fig. 6.9
Levels of quality standard set in the context of the ratio of the amount of good (—) and harm (- - - -) done by screening programmes of different levels of quality

elements can be combined into a system of care as shown in Fig. 6.10.

Process measures are better suited to the management of local services than outcome measures. For example, in a cervical screening programme, although mortality rates from cervical cancer are the only measures those responsible for evaluating national policy should use, for local decision-makers this outcome measure is not a good indicator of service quality for two reasons.

1. Changes in mortality rates are influenced by factors other than service quality, for example, changes in the incidence of cervical cancer.
2. Changes in mortality rate reflect the quality of the service pertaining several years ago, whereas the manager or purchaser needs information about the current state of quality.

Objectives	Criteria	Standards		Present position	Targets
		Minimal	Achievable		
To cover the population who would benefit from cervical screening	Percentage of women who have **not** had a hysterectomy who have had a readable smear in the last 5 years	50%	80%	70 general practices under 50% 17 practices more than 80%	By the end of year: 1 out of 70 general practices less than 50% 35 general practices over 80%

Fig. 6.10
Standards incorporated into a system of care for cervical screening

6.8.1.2 Quality assessment by measuring the outcome of care

The outcome of care is the result of undertaking healthcare activities.

When outcome measures were first proposed they were hailed as the ultimate measures that would enable the patient and purchaser to distinguish between a service of good quality and one of poor quality. Further experience with outcome-based measures of quality has stemmed this initial enthusiasm for two main reasons.[4]

1. The health status of an individual, a group of patients or a population receiving a service is determined by several factors other than the quality of that service, notably, severity of illness and state of health before treatment.
2. The collection of valid information about outcomes in ordinary service settings is difficult due to the problems of obtaining accurate data on what are known as confounding variables, namely, factors other than quality of care that could explain the variation in outcome.

Outcomes are rarely of use in measuring quality because it has not proved feasible to collect information on outcomes in large databases of sufficiently good quality to allow the adequate evaluation of existing services. However, there is still hope that such databases could be used to provide useful information on the quality of services delivered by individual institutions or clinicians.

Despite the numerous practical problems that must be resolved to ensure that databases contain accurate data on each and every case treated within a service, outcome measures, e.g. mortality rates for patients with specific conditions such as myocardial infarction, are being used to construct 'league tables' of hospital quality. Unless there is complete data coverage in a database, any conclusions drawn from database analysis may be misleading. However, completeness of data (in terms of quantity and quality) does not resolve all of the problems in using outcome measures because, in any comparison, factors such as co-morbidity and disease severity must be taken into account.

'Co-morbidity' is the presence of other conditions that may be relevant to a patient's outcome; 'severity' describes the stage of disease a patient has reached. Those hospitals at which there are selective admission procedures, i.e. certain patients who have significant co-morbidity or a severe form of a disease are excluded, may appear to achieve better outcomes than those hospitals at which either all patients are admitted or more difficult cases are treated. Indeed, the standard of care at hospitals with selective admission procedures may be no better than that in a hospital to which all cases are admitted; it may even be worse. Failure to correct for co-morbidity and/or disease severity is the most common reason why false conclusions are drawn from the analysis of such databases. Any league tables generated from databases for which co-morbidity and disease severity data are not routinely collected are of limited credibility, particularly with reference to those hospitals at which performance appears to be poor.

In addition to the need to collect robust data and to correct for co-morbidity and disease severity when assessing quality through outcome measures, it is also important to investigate the method used to calculate the outcome indicator. In an interesting historical study, Iezzoni[5] highlights the fact that even hospital mortality rates can be calculated in such a way as to distort perceptions of performance. During the 19th century, William Farr and Florence Nightingale argued that urban hospitals, particularly those in London, were more dangerous than rural hospitals. They supported this contention with data showing the number of deaths ('mortality per cent. on inmates') at the 106 principal hospitals in England, which were published in the *24th Annual Report of the Registrar-General*. According to this data, mortality at the 24 London hospitals was 90.84% compared with a mortality of 12.78% at the Royal Sea Bathing Infirmary (Margate). However, Farr had calculated the death rates as follows: total number of deaths at the hospital in 1861 divided by the number of patients at the hospital on 8 April 1861. As can be seen, the numerator reflected the figures for an entire year whereas the denominator reflected the figure for a single day in that year. As Iezzoni points out, Farr had actually calculated death rates per occupied hospital bed and not mortality rates per total number of hospitalised patients. Farr's methodology inflated the apparent mortality rates; when calculated as the annual number of deaths divided by the total number of inpatients treated during the year, the mortality rates for the general wards of 14 London hospitals averaged 9.7%.

6.8.1.3 Reporting outcomes in the public domain

The benefits and hazards of reporting medical outcomes in the public domain are set out in an excellent article[6] about the work of the New York (NY) State Department of Health to reduce mortality after coronary artery bypass grafting (CABG). In 1989, the NY State Cardiac Advisory Committee helped the NY Department of Health to set up a Cardiac Surgery Reporting System in order to collect information about demographic variables, risk factors and complications, and mortality after operation. In 1990, the Department published the risk-adjusted mortality rates for each hospital. Using the Freedom of Information Law, a newspaper then sued the Department to obtain the original data from which these rates had been calculated and won. The data were published in December 1991 to a stormy reaction from the participating surgeons. Despite this, the NY Department of Health continued with the programme.

An analysis of the data showed that from the beginning of 1989 through to the end of 1992 there was a 41% decline in risk-adjusted operative mortality. Although no comparable data exist, and many factors could explain the decline in mortality, it is reasonable to assume that the reporting system was responsible for part of the improvement seen, which may have resulted from the ability to identify surgeons who had poor records, usually those performing only a small number of procedures.

Between 1989 and 1992, 27 low-volume surgeons stopped performing CABG in New York State.

Although the Cardiac Surgery Reporting System was bold and scientifically rigorous, it should be possible to use this type of approach elsewhere to improve performance for specific procedures that are relatively few in number but which have dramatic outcomes (e.g. death). It is not unrealistic to pursue an objective of making hospital- and operator-specific information publicly available for a small number of interventions.

6.8.2 Searching for and appraising evidence on standards of care

6.8.2.1 Searching for papers on quality standards

Step 1: Specify the intervention.
Step 2: Select terms to define the parameters that are relevant:
- quality;
- audit;
- standards;
- guidelines.

6.8.2.2 Appraising evidence on quality standards

The most appropriate form of study design is one in which a service is monitored over a period of time, not only to measure performance against agreed quality standards but also to assess the effects of the interventions designed to improve quality by measuring performance on at least two separate occasions. A checklist of questions for the appraisal of evidence on quality is shown in Box 6.17.

Box 6.17   Checklist for the appraisal of evidence on quality

1. Is there good evidence that the intervention used as the indicator of quality is an effective intervention?
2. Are there standards relating to acceptability and safety?
3. Is there clear information about the method used to develop the standards, e.g. are the standards set by taking the cut-off point for the top quartile of several services?
4. Is there only one measure of quality or are there several measures?

6.8.3 Searching for and appraising evidence on variations in healthcare outcome

The search for and appraisal of evidence about standards of care and means of quality improvement is often driven by the healthcare professionals or managers within a service. However, external forces, such as the publication of inter-hospital audit results or hospital mortality league tables, may also raise the issue. Although the identification of poor performance can provoke denial in those working within a service, it is possible to take a scientific approach to quality improvement.

6.8.3.1 Searching for papers on variations in healthcare outcome

Step 1: Take the disease or health problem and explode the term.
Step 2: Combine the search results with the name of the operation and/or with the term 'mortality'. It may be necessary to explode 'mortality'.

6.8.3.2 Appraising evidence on variations in healthcare outcome

Large databases can also be manipulated to compare different types of institution, for example:

• teaching hospitals vs non-teaching hospitals;
• services providing a high volume of care vs those providing a low volume.

For this type of comparison, it is not possible to perform an RCT; however, the 'natural experiment' created by the variety of health services provided presents an opportunity to identify the determinants of quality.
   A checklist of questions for the appraisal of studies designed to investigate a possible managerial problem or to identify the determinants of service quality is shown in Box 6.18.

6.8.4 Applicability and relevance

Is it possible to apply the results of studies on quality of care from one organisation, or population, to another? It has been argued, that because health service provision and methods of payment vary greatly from one population to

---

Box 6.18 Checklist for the appraisal of studies of quality in the provision of healthcare (Source: Adapted from Naylor and Guyatt [7])

1. Are the outcome measures accurate and comprehensive?
   Large databases tend to include only simple outcome measures, such as death, and rarely hold data on measures such as disability or quality of life.
2. Were there clearly identified and appropriate comparison groups?
3. Were the comparison groups similar with respect to important determinants of outcome other than the one of interest?
   For example, when comparing teaching hospitals with non-teaching hospitals, the question must be asked: 'Are the two groups of patients similar from the point of view, for example, of the prognosis?'.
   Useful appraisal questions to ask include:

   • Did the investigators measure all known important prognostic factors?
   • Were measures of patients' prognostic factors reproducible and accurate?
   • Did the investigators show the extent to which patients differ on these factors?
   • Did the researchers use some form of multivariate analysis to adjust for all the important prognostic factors?
   • Did additional analysis (particularly in low-risk subgroups) demonstrate the same results as the primary analysis?

4. Were all possible hypotheses examined?
   Often the report of an observational study has as a focus the most dramatic finding, e.g. a difference between teaching and non-teaching hospitals, but when comparing services in which there are differences in the same outcome measure more than one explanation is possible.

   • Who did the operation, e.g. specialist or generalist?
   • When was it done, e.g. day or night, weekday or weekend?
   • Where was it done, e.g. in a large-volume or small-volume service?
   • How was it done?
   • Which operation was done?

---

another, work on quality is not generalisable but is specific to the population in which the study was done.

Although it is true that the *results* of studies of quality are not generalisable (poor quality of care in a service such as cervical screening in one population does not mean that the quality of cervical screening will be poor in all populations), the identification of criteria that can be used to set standards and measure quality, and the identification of the reasons for quality failure, are generally applicable. For example, in the study of CABG in New York State,[6] the identification of the high risk of mortality associated with low-volume surgeons is a generalisable finding. It is immaterial whether the high mortality rate arose because those surgeons were less practised in the operation or because fewer patients were referred to those surgeons by physicians who were aware of their colleagues' performance (a common quality standard used within the profession), the association was demonstrated and is relevant to all the parties involved – patients, physicians, providers and purchasers.

References

1. DEPARTMENT OF HEALTH (1999) *A First Class Service: consultation document on quality in the new NHS.* Available at: http://www.open.gov.uk/doh/newnhs/quality.htm
2. DONABEDIAN, A. (1980) *The definition of quality: a conceptual exploration. In: Explorations in quality assessment and monitoring. Volume I: The definition of quality and approaches to its assessment?* Health Administration Press, Ann Arbor.
3. CROWLEY, P.A. (1995) *Antenatal corticosteroid therapy: a meta-analysis of the randomized trials, 1972 to 1994.* Am. J. Obstet. Gynecol. 173: 322–5.
4. SCHROEDER, S. A. and KABCENELL, A. I. (1991) *Do bad outcomes mean substandard care?* JAMA 265: 1995.
5. IEZZONI, L.I. (1996) *100 apples divided by 15 red herrings: a cautionary tale from the mid-19th century on comparing hospital mortality rates.* Ann. Intern. Med. 124: 1079–85.
6. CHASSIN, M.R., HANNAN, R.L. and DeBUONO, B.A. (1996) *Benefits and hazards of reporting medical outcomes publicly.* New Eng. J. Med. 334: 294–8.
7. NAYLOR, C.D. and GUYATT, G.H. (1996) *User's Guides to the Medical Literature. X. How to use an article reporting variations in the outcomes of health services.* JAMA 275: 554–8.

6.9 APPROPRIATENESS

6.9.1 Dimensions and definitions

Appropriateness is a measure of the way in which an intervention is used in clinical practice. It is based on a subjective judgement about whether it is right to give a particular intervention to an individual, a group of patients, or a population. It is assessed on a balance of probabilities: the probability of doing good against the probability of doing harm; however, the judgement must also take into account the context in which care is being delivered – what is appropriate at the Mayo Clinic may not be appropriate in Chelyabinsk.

An intervention is considered to be appropriate if the balance of good to harm is sufficiently high to justify the administration of an intervention. Interventions are considered to be inappropriate if the balance of good to harm is too low to justify the administration of an intervention.

The appropriateness of care provided to an individual patient or group of patients can be determined in several different ways:

- by asking an independent clinician or group of clinicians and patients to pass judgement on the intervention given;
- by comparing the intervention given to a patient with clinical guidelines indicating which patients are most likely to benefit, or least likely to be harmed, by that intervention.

As the distinction between appropriateness and inappropriateness is a matter of judgement, there is a spectrum of potential categories. In many studies of appropriateness, three categories are identified (see Fig. 6.11):

- clearly appropriate;
- clearly inappropriate;
- a class in between where clinicians, experts and patients disagree depending upon their values.

Unequivocally appropriate	The grey zone	Unequivocally inappropriate

Fig. 6.11
The spectrum of judgements about appropriateness

The concept of appropriateness is particularly useful when making decisions about what Naylor has called the 'grey zones of clinical practice', namely, aspects of care for which the evidence is scarce or the evidence available is not relevant to the patient or the service under consideration.[1]

6.9.1.1 Appropriateness for individual patients

In clinical practice, any judgement of appropriateness should take into account the needs, values and expressed wishes of the individual patient. Chemotherapy with agents that carry a high probability of side-effects may be appropriate for a patient who has potentially curable cancer but may be inappropriate for a patient who has incurable cancer, depending upon the relative values the patient attaches to a few more months of life on the one hand and to suffering from side-effects on the other. Hitherto, financial cost has not been a factor in clinical decisions about appropriateness relating to individual patients.

6.9.1.2 Appropriateness for groups of patients or populations

For groups of patients and populations, the concept of appropriateness relates not only to the benefits and risks but also to the costs of intervention. Furthermore, the appropriateness of providing an intervention or a service for any population may change with the volume of service provided.

If resources are limited, a service is usually given to those who are most likely to benefit. As resources increase, the threshold for intervention changes and the intervention is offered to people who are at lower risk or less severely affected. The benefit obtained decreases with each unit of increase in resources – known as the law of diminishing returns – with a flattening of the cost-benefit curve (Fig. 6.12).

However, interventions have adverse as well as beneficial effects. Donabedian, who invented the concept of 'structure, process and outcome' in healthcare evaluation, also introduced the benefit-to-harm graph.[2] He argued that when the volume of healthcare offered is increased, the cost–benefit curve flattens but the cost–harm curve does

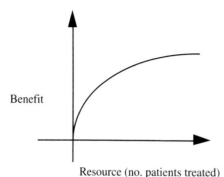

Fig. 6.12
The law of diminishing returns – the decrease in the amount of benefit obtained for each unit of increase in resources (Source: Donabedian; see ref. 2, p. 229)

not; namely, side-effects may be as common in individuals at low risk or who have mild disease as in those at high risk or who have severe disease. For each unit increase in resources or volume of care, there is a concomitant increase in adverse effects (Fig. 6.13).

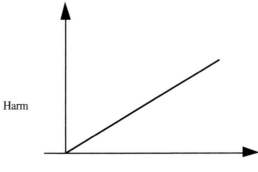

Fig. 6.13
The balance of benefit to harm – for each unit of increase in resources, or volume of healthcare, there is an increase in adverse effects (Source: Donabedian; see ref. 2, p. 229)

Thus, as the proportion of a population covered by a health service increases, the balance of good to harm changes. This can be expressed most simply by subtracting harm from good and showing the net benefit graphically (Fig. 6.14). For an example of this phenomenon in the treatment of gallstone disease, see Fig. 6.15.

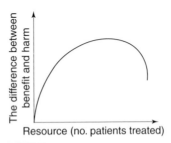

Fig. 6.14
The balance of benefit to harm – the net benefit to the population as the proportion receiving healthcare increases (Source: Donabedian; see ref. 2, p. 229)

**Laparoscopic cholecystectomy is safer
than conventional cholecystectomy.
The consequences of this in Maryland
are of great interest.**

The procedure of cholecystectomy becomes safer

↓

Patients who would not have been
considered for open cholecystectomy,
because of frailty or relatively minor
symptoms, are referred for treatment
by laparoscopic cholecystectomy

↓

The rate at which cholecystectomy
is done increases by 28%

↓

The operative mortality
declines from 0.84% to 0.56%

↓

However, owing to the increase in the
number of operations being done the
total number of people dying as a result
of the procedure does not change

Fig. 6.15
The epidemic of cholecystectomies (Source: Steiner et al.[3])

6.9.1.3 Identifying concerns about appropriateness

There are several ways in which the appropriateness of use
of a particular intervention may be identified as being a
matter of concern, notably:

- as part of an audit project;
- following the publication of an article on
  appropriateness;
- following the publication of a league table showing
  variations in the rate of use of a particular intervention
  by different clinicians or services; in such situations,
  pressure to change will fall on the professional or service
  deemed to be the least appropriate, i.e. at the end of the
  league table that denotes poor performance.

Evidence-based analysis of variations in levels of use may
indicate variations in appropriateness of use (variations in
outcome may indicate variations in quality) (Table 6.5).
Indeed, during the past decade, the results of an increasing
number of studies have demonstrated wide variations in
rates of care provided. Some of the variations observed are

Table 6.5   The underlying problems indicated by variation

Variation	Possible problem
In outcome	Quality
In rates of intervention, i.e. in process	Appropriateness

far greater than can be explained by variations in the incidence and prevalence of disease. In one of the classic studies of this phenomenon, Wennberg et al. compared the provision of hospital services in Boston and in New Haven.[4] The two communities receiving hospital care were similar demographically (in terms of percentages of those who were below the poverty line, black, and aged 65 years or over). In both Boston and New Haven, a large proportion of the resident population was admitted to major teaching hospitals. Excluding any beds occupied by non-residents, it was found that people in Boston occupied 4.5 beds per thousand population, whereas people in New Haven occupied only 2.9. The overall rates of admission in Boston were found to be nearly 50% higher than those in New Haven, with the average length of stay being 7% longer.

Other studies of this phenomenon have disclosed variations in the provision of care for almost every condition in which clinical judgement plays a part. The results of these studies emphasise the need for detailed study of clinicians' behaviour and in particular the ways in which their interpretation of the evidence, influenced by local custom, culture and practice, result in one population receiving a different level of care, and thereby consuming a different amount of resources, to a similar population living elsewhere.

6.9.1.4   *It may be appropriate but is it necessary?*

Once all ineffective interventions and services have been excluded, if resources are limited it may not be possible to provide all of the effective and appropriate services. The team from the RAND Health Sciences Program has developed a new criterion that can be used to evaluate appropriate interventions: necessity.[5] Their definition of appropriateness is that the benefits should sufficiently outweigh the risks to make the procedure worth performing, and they extend this definition by proposing criteria that can be used to decide whether a procedure is necessary (see Box 6.19).

Box 6.19   Criteria for identifying necessary interventions (all four must be met) (Source: Kahan et al.[5])

- The procedure must be *appropriate*, as defined above.
- It would be improper care not to recommend this service.
- There is a reasonable chance that the procedure will benefit the patient. Procedures with a low likelihood of benefit but few risks are not considered necessary.
- The benefit to the patient is not small. Procedures that provide only minor benefits are not necessary.

A high necessity rating indicates that it is improper clinical judgement not to recommend the procedure; a low necessity rating indicates that there are alternative courses of action (including no action) that are equally or almost equally appropriate. This is an important and novel way of thinking about procedures and is already being used by the RAND team.

Necessity can be measured by asking a panel of clinicians to rate a set of cases. Although there is, as would be expected, variation in rating, there is sufficient consistency for the measure of necessity to be useful. One obvious use is to determine which procedures are not necessary to the well-being of patients. However, the RAND team points out that the converse is also possible, namely, that patients do not receive necessary treatment either because of costs or because of the judgement of the clinicians. The RAND team reviewed 243 patients with angina who had positive exercise stress tests. They found that patients who were under the care of a cardiologist were more likely to receive a 'necessary' exercise stress test than those who were under the care of a generalist or primary care physician.[6]

6.9.1.5 Who defines necessity?

Hitherto, the definition of necessity has been made by doctors (see Fig. 6.16).

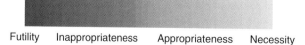

Futility   Inappropriateness   Appropriateness   Necessity

Fig. 6.16
The spectrum of appropriateness for healthcare interventions from futility to necessity

However, dramatic changes to the conception of appropriateness are taking place, and two of the other stakeholders in medical decision-making – patients on the one hand, and payers on the other – are becoming much more influential.

Rosenbaum et al.[7] have identified three issues in the definition of necessity.

1. Who has the power to decide what is meant by necessity?
2. What evidence can and must be used to justify the decision?
3. Who bears the burden of proof: must the insurer demonstrate with acceptable evidence that a recommended treatment is unnecessary, or does the patient bear the burden of demonstrating that the treatment in question is necessary?

It is interesting to note there is no mention of the clinician in this discussion – a portent of things to come?

6.9.1.6 Medical futility

A consideration of what constitutes appropriate care has led to the identification of some interventions as not only inappropriate but also futile.[8]

The definition of futility is problematic, but a useful definition has been developed by the Council on Ethical and Judicial Affairs of the American Medical Association.

> In the course of caring for a critically ill patient it may become apparent that further intervention will only prolong the final stages of the dying process. At this point, further intervention is often described as futile.[9]

The Council recognises there has been controversy in both the literature and clinical practice about what comprises a futile intervention. It has been suggested that futile interventions are those which sustain life for patients in a persistent vegetative state, or continue 'aggressive' therapy, for example, chemotherapy for people with advanced terminal cancer who have no realistic expectation of cure or symptom relief. Owing to the difficult position that many clinicians find themselves in when dealing with patients at the end of life, the Council on Ethical and Judicial Affairs reviewed the problems they had to face and proposed a 'fair process' for managing futility cases.

The process comprises seven steps: four aimed at deliberation and resolution; two aimed at securing alternatives in case of irresolvable differences; and a final step designed to achieve 'closure' when other alternatives have been exhausted.

Step 1: A good attempt should be made to negotiate an understanding of what would constitute futile care for a particular patient *before* the critical illness occurs.

Step 2: Joint decision-making should also be made at the bedside between the patient, or a proxy person, and the clinician; this process of joint decision-making should make use of outcomes data whenever possible, include the clinician's and patient's or proxy's goals for treatment, and comply with established standards of informed consent.

Step 3: The assistance of an individual (consultant and/or patient representative) should be engaged to facilitate the resolution of any conflicts.

Step 4: An institutional committee, such as a Clinical Ethics Committee, should be involved if it is not possible to resolve any conflicts.

Step 5: This occurs if the deliberations of the institutional committee coincide with the wishes of the patient but the clinician remains unhappy. In this situation, care of the patient is transferred to another physician whose views about futility in the case under consideration coincide with those of the patient and the institutional committee.

Step 6: This occurs if the deliberations of the institutional committee support the clinician's position but the patient and/or the person acting for the patient remains unpersuaded. In this situation, it may be necessary to transfer the patient to another institution.

Step 7: This occurs if either Step 5 or Step 6 proves impossible. In this situation, if the request is considered to conflict with medical ethics, the intervention need not be provided. The legal consequences of this course of action are 'uncertain'.

This process is shown in Fig. 6.17.

In making decisions about the futility of further intervention, the model outlined above emphasises the

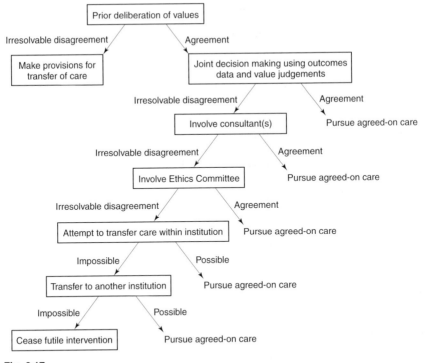

Fig. 6.17
The process for considering futility cases devised by the American Medical Association Council on Ethical and Judicial Affairs[9]

need for a decision-making process and structure within a healthcare organisation, supported by an institutional committee. Such committees are usually called clinical ethics committees, to distinguish them from research ethics committees, which consider the ethical implications of research protocols. The role of clinical ethics committees is evolving, and different types of ethics committees have developed in different kinds of healthcare organisation and in various countries.

Herb and Lazar[10] have identified three main themes of work for ethics committees:

1. education;
2. policy review and evaluation;
3. case review.

However, they emphasise that these functions become interwoven because the consideration of individual cases tends to reveal problems that may require the development of new policies and/or necessitate individual, team or organisational learning.

During the consideration of ethical issues, it is important for ethics committees to base their decisions on evidence. Studies of evidence and ethical-based decision-making in the treatment of patients who have a poor prognosis are now being published. In an important study of the 'aggressive surgical management' of patients with penetrating brain injuries, usually from gunshot wounds, the relatives of patients were given evidence about the probable outcome of surgical management. Levy et al.[11] found that it was possible to make evidence-based decisions about aggressive surgical treatment that were satisfactory to the relatives, but that also limited the number of pointless new surgical procedures while still 'liberally' favouring those patients who had even a small chance of surviving to live independently. The authors emphasised the need to see the role of the physician as being not only a surgical interventionist but also 'a provider of information and co-decision-maker' (see Sections 10.2–10.4).

6.9.2 Searching

Step 1: Specify the intervention for which there are different rates of utilisation. The relevant MeSH term is 'utilization review', an American term similar to 'clinical audit'. It may be necessary to explode 'utilization review'.

Step 2: Search for 'guideline' or 'practice guideline' under publication type.

Step 3: The relevant MeSH term is 'guidelines'; the term should be exploded to include 'practice guidelines'.

Step 4: The keywords 'guideline' and 'appropriateness' can be used. The MeSH term for appropriateness is 'regional health planning', which it may be necessary to explode.

6.9.3 Appraisal

Most of the research published on appropriateness is a review of data about patients that were collected previously. A checklist of three sets of questions useful for the appraisal of evidence of appropriateness is shown in Box 6.20.

> **Box 6.20** Checklist for the appraisal of evidence of appropriateness (Source: Adapted from Naylor and Guyatt[12])
>
> 1. Are the criteria evidence based?
>   - Is there evidence to support the judgements about:
>   – right patient?
>   – right place?
>   – right time?
>   – right intervention?
>   – right professional?
>   - What is the quality of the evidence on which the judgements have been made and the criteria chosen?
>   - How good was the agreement between experts on the panel?
>   - Were patients' views on outcomes taken into account?
> 2. How scientifically was the study done?
>   - Were steps taken to minimise bias, for example, by using more than one auditor or by using explicit criteria to audit notes?
>   - Was the sample of patients representative and large enough to produce valid results?
> 3. Are the criteria relevant to the local service?
>   - How similar is the local population to the population studied?
>   - Were the clinicians on the panel similar to local professionals?
>   - How different from the local facility was the facility studied?

6.9.4 Applicability and relevance

Appropriateness is a subjective measure of whether an intervention, or level of intervention, is right; this judgement of 'rightness' is influenced by the incidence or prevalence of the disease in the population and by the resources available.

Although the results of studies of appropriateness may not be generalisable, they may be of relevance to different populations because they can reveal areas of clinical uncertainty. Thus, a study of appropriateness could indicate an interesting area to investigate in the local health service; if validated, the methods used in the study can probably be transposed to the local service, with modification. However, the levels of intervention judged to be 'right' for the local population must be determined according to local circumstances.

References

1. NAYLOR, C.D. (1995) *The grey zones of clinical practice.* Lancet 345: 840–2.
2. DONABEDIAN, A. (1980) *Explorations in Quality Assessment and Monitoring. Volume 1: The definition of quality and approaches to its assessment.* Health Administration Press, Ann Arbor.
3. STEINER, C.A., BASS, E.B., TALAMINI, M.A., PITT, H.A. and STEINBERG, E.P. (1994) *Surgical rates and operative mortality for open and laparoscopic cholecystectomy in Maryland.* N. Engl. J. Med. 330: 403–8.
4. WENNBERG, J.E., FREEMAN, J.L. and CULP, W.J. (1987) *Are hospital services rationed in New Haven or over-utilised in Boston?* Lancet i: 1185–8.
5. KAHAN, J.P., BERNSTEIN, S.J., LEAPE, L.L. et al. (1994) *Measuring the necessity of medical procedures.* Med. Care 32: 357–65.
6. BOROWSKY, S.J., KRAVITZ, R.L., LAOURI, M. et al. (1995) *Effect of physician specialty on use of necessary coronary angiography.* J. Am. Coll. Cardiol. 26: 1484–91.
7. ROSENBAUM, S., FRANKFORD, D.M., MOORE, B. and BORZI, P. (1999) *Who should determine when health care is medically necessary?* N. Engl. J. Med. 340: 229–32.
8. ZUCKER, M.B. and ZUCKER, H.D. (1997) *Medical Futility and the Evaluation of Life-Sustaining Interventions.* Cambridge University Press.
9. COUNCIL ON ETHICAL AND JUDICIAL AFFAIRS, AMERICAN MEDICAL ASSOCIATION (1999) *Medical futility in end-of-life care. Report of the Council on Ethical and Judicial Affairs.* JAMA 281: 937–41.
10. HERB, A. and LAZAR, E.J. (1997) *Ethics committees and end-of-life decision making.* In: Zucker, M.B. and Zucker, H.D. (eds) *Medical Futility and the Evaluation of Life-Sustaining Interventions.* Cambridge University Press.
11. LEVY, M.L., DAVIS, S.E., McCOMB, G. and APUZZO, M.L.J. (1996) *Economic, ethical, and outcome-based decisions regarding aggressive surgical management in patients with penetrating craniocerebral injury.* J. Health Communication 1: 301–8.
12. NAYLOR, C.D. and GUYATT, G.H. (1996) *User's guides to the medical literature. XI. How to use an article about a clinical utilization review.* JAMA 275: 1435–40.

Gentle Reader,

Empathise with the Secretary of the Faculty of Public Health Screening Committee. He was musing on the particular lightness of green that makes the leaves of early summer stand out sharply against the blue sky of May. The movement of the leaves was a comfort to him. He looked at them for at least three minutes before letting his eyes drop for a second time to the letter, written in all innocence but disturbing in content, that lay on the desk before him.

Dear Colleague,

I would be grateful to know the evidence to support the introduction of screening for abdominal aortic aneurysm which we are currently considering. The proposal is strongly supported. It would have a very beneficial impact on our efficiency index because many more people would be referred to hospital, but I would also be interested to know what health benefits we can describe to the health authority.

Commentary

Organisations take on a life of their own. The culture of an organisation imbues any decision-making with the prevailing preoccupation, in this case a preoccupation with productivity. To counteract this, a different hierarchy within the decision-making process is vital, one in which it is possible to ask the following questions.

- *Will the proposal have a beneficial effect on health?*
- *Is there a harmful effect, and what is the balance between benefit and harm?*
- *What is the cost of the innovation?*
- *How does this proposal compare with other proposals currently under consideration?*
- *Is it possible to deliver the new service at acceptable levels of quality and cost?*

CHAPTER 7

THE EVIDENCE-BASED ORGANISATION

7.1 CREATING THE CONTEXT FOR AN EVIDENCE-BASED ORGANISATION

I am the Master of this College
What I know not is not knowledge
> Benjamin Jowett, Master of Balliol College.

Wife of Oxford Classics Don: *Tell me, Mr Einstein, what is it that you do?*

Einstein: *Physics.*

Wife of Oxford Classics Don: *My husband tells me that anyone who has a First in Greats can get up physics in a fortnight.*

At some point in the past, it may have been true that all there was to know could be known by one individual, but the claims of the Oxford Dons quoted above seem to us now a trifle bold. Organisations, however, particularly those that consist of large numbers of individuals, should have the capacity to manage all the knowledge that they need. Indeed, knowledge management has become one of the dominant management trends of the last decade.

7.1.1 Types of knowledge

Of fundamental importance in thinking about knowledge management is the distinction between two types of knowledge:

- tacit knowledge is practical and subjective, for example, knowing what other people in the organisation are doing;
- explicit knowledge is theoretical and objective, for example, the published results of formal research.

Tacit knowledge can be converted into an explicit form in two ways:

- concepts and models are combined into new forms;
- knowledge is externalised, e.g. the interpretation of a strategy into recommendations.

Explicit knowledge can be absorbed into the tacit knowledge base by a process closely related to learning by doing.

Evidence-based decision-making has largely been based on the use of explicit knowledge, but it is possible to use knowledge that is tacit.

The new electronic journal *Impact* (available at: http://www.jr2.ox.ac.uk:80/Bandolier/ImpAct) publishes tacit knowledge that would never appear in conventional medical or management journals. This tacit knowledge is precisely the type of knowledge that people need to make a difference. It is important to recognise that evidence for decision-making can be derived from experience as well as from formal research.

The characteristics of tacit and explicit knowledge are shown in Table 7.1.

Table 7.1   The characteristics of tacit and explicit knowledge

Tacit knowledge	⟷	Explicit knowledge
Created by clinicians, patients and managers	⟷	Created by researchers
Rarely published; sometimes not even written down	⟷	Published in scientific journals
States how to do it	⟷	States what to do
May be only locally applicable	⟷	Generalisable
Traditionally of low value	⟷	Traditionally highly valued

7.1.1.1   Knowledge from experience

As indicated above, the results of formal research are not the only source of knowledge that is useful to organisations. Experience, particularly in the context of learning from adverse events, can be a valuable form of knowledge if it is used to improve or remedy organisational performance. However, in the past, learning from experience was perceived as ineffective, and potentially harmful in that it might be a way of replicating 'errors'. One of the fields in which learning from adverse events has been successful is aviation, where the primary aim has been to improve safety measures and practices.

In a recent report from the Expert Group on Learning from Adverse Events in the NHS,[1] it was estimated that as many as 850 000 serious adverse healthcare events might occur in the NHS hospital sector each year at a cost of over £2 billion; half of these events are considered to be preventable. The report contains an assessment of how the NHS learns from adverse events. It is concluded that the NHS is a 'passive' rather than an 'active' learning organisation, which has a culture of blame and of the superficial analysis of adverse events, and therefore misses many of the learning points that could have been used to improve both safety and performance, and thereby quality of care. Several recommendations are made for changing this culture in the NHS; there is also a recommendation to establish a national mandatory reporting scheme for adverse health events and specified near misses. This report demonstrates how it is possible for an organisation to learn from itself as well as from the literature.

7.1.2 The learning organisation

The introduction of evidence-based decision-making into an organisation requires cultural change, but in order to integrate an evidence-based approach to decision-making the entire organisation must focus on learning. The characteristics of a learning organisation have been most elegantly described by Peter Senge in his influential book *The Fifth Discipline – the Art and Practice of the Learning Organization.*[2] He has identified five disciplines that are necessary for any organisation to become a learning organisation:

1. personal mastery – the discipline of continually clarifying and deepening one's personal vision and objectivity;
2. making mental models – the discipline of creating with metaphors and language a mental model of what the organisation is, what it stands for, and how it works;
3. building shared visions – the discipline of translating the vision of an organisation's leader or leaders from the objectives shared by a few to a vision for everyone in that organisation;

4. team learning – the discipline of ensuring that the collective intelligence of a team is greater than the sum of the individual intelligence; if a team is dysfunctional, the intelligence of a team will be less than the summed intelligence of the individuals;
5. systems thinking – what Senge calls 'the fifth discipline' – the discipline in which individual elements are linked together into a coherent set of activities with a common set of objectives.

7.1.3 Hypertext organisations

Organisations can be described in many different ways using a variety of images and metaphors. In his book *Images of Organisation*,[3] Morgan discussed the way in which images are used to characterise an organisation. The images employed are often dictated by the predominant management theorists of the time, for example, Taylor created the concept of the organisation as machine.

Organisations have also been likened to:

- families;
- brains;
- neural networks.

However, organisations can also be described in terms of their working methods or *modus operandi*. Knowledge-creating organisations, i.e. organisations that produce new knowledge and new ways of working in addition to managing the knowledge produced by others, have been described as hypertext organisations.

In the hypertext organisation:

- each individual belongs to a team, which is usually composed of people who have similar skills;
- the organisation is in the process of undertaking several projects;
- a leader is assigned to each project, together with various individuals who will be working on it, who are almost always drawn from more than one team;
- each individual usually works on more than one project.

Although it is not possible to represent the structure of a hypertext organisation as a matrix, the use of browsers within such an organisation would enable each project and each team, and even each individual, to have their own Web page.

7.1.4 The knowledge-rich organisation

Once a culture change has occurred and evidence-based management skills have been developed sufficiently for individuals to undertake an evidence-based approach to decision-making, it is vital to have the capacity to provide knowledge when and where it is needed. Although the provision of knowledge alone does not necessarily effect change, without knowledge poor decisions are often made.

Good knowledge management, particularly that of tacit knowledge, enables individuals to find new ways of doing things, e.g. new know-how, new techniques, and new services.

In managing tacit knowledge, organisations have tended to depend on central filing systems, newsletters, notice boards, team briefings and communication strategies, all of which are, at best, only partially successful. However, new opportunities for the management of tacit knowledge are being made available with Web technology, in particular software such as Autonomy (see http://www.autonomy.com). The advantages of using this type of software are demonstrated in the following hypothetical example. Imagine an expert who works for a large computer company in Florida who must visit a healthcare manager in Puerto Rico where, as in the rest of Latin America, managed care is being introduced.[4] The reason for the meeting is to discuss software solutions that link billing to diagnosis. Once back in Florida, the computer expert enters a note of the meeting onto the Intranet of his company using Autonomy, which enables him to identify rapidly two other people, one in Hungary and one in Denmark, who have been involved in discussions to develop a similar package.

7.1.5 The evidence-based knowledge-rich learning organisation

Is it possible to encompass all these theories into a vision for the 21st century organisation? Perhaps the most appropriate metaphor to use is that of the organisation as a human being, an entity that is greater than a series of neural networks, because human beings have hopes, fears, and morale. The characteristic of an organisation that I, as author of a book about evidence-based healthcare, would most like to see developed is the capacity to create, find, appraise, use, and store evidence in order to inform decision-making. The other prevailing management trends are all conducive to the realisation of this objective.

An evidence-based knowledge-rich learning organisation is one in which:

- the creation and use of knowledge is valued and the availability of knowledge is assured;
- there is a commitment to knowledge management to ensure that systems and skills for finding, appraising, and using evidence are developed and supported;
- both tacit and explicit knowledge are readily available when and where needed.

7.1.5.1 Kondratieff cycles on

Kondratieff was a Russian economist who developed a theory of long-cycle economics, in which he argued that the world's economy is dominated by certain commodities which tend to hold their value for up to 60 years. This cyclic pattern of dominant commodities can be clearly seen in Western civilisation over the last 200 years (see Table 7.2).

Table 7.2 Kondratieff cycles of dominant commodities

Era	Dominant commodity	Wealthiest individuals	Biggest companies
1800–1850	Land	Kings Archbishops Hereditary landowners	
1850–1910	Coal Steel	Carnegie Frick	Railroad, coal and steel
1910–1990	Oil	Getty Rockefeller Ford Nuffield	Oil refiners, car manufacturers, electricity generators
1990– ?	Knowledge	Gates Dell Clark	Computers, software, Internet, telephone

Knowledge is currently the dominant commodity, thus, it is not surprising that various theories of knowledge management have been formulated, some of which are described in this section. An evidence-based approach is only one aspect of the knowledge revolution, but all the different aspects act to sustain and support one another.

References

1. EXPERT GROUP ON LEARNING FROM ADVERSE EVENTS IN THE
    NHS (2000) *An Organisation with a Memory*. The Stationery Office,
    London. Available at: http://www.doh.gov.uk/orgmemrep/index.htm
2. SENGE, P.M. (1990) *The Fifth Discipline. The Art and Practice of the
    Learning Organisation*. Century Business.
3. MORGAN, G. (1998) *Images of Organisation*. Sage Publications.
4. STOCKER, K., WAITZKIN, H. and IPIART, C. (1999) *The exportation of
    managed care to Latin America*. N. Engl. J. Med. 340: 1131–6.

7.2   AN EVIDENCE-BASED HEALTH SERVICE

The key components in an evidence-based health service
are:

1. healthcare organisations designed with the capability to
    generate, and the flexibility to incorporate, evidence;
2. healthcare professionals who, as individuals and teams,
    are able to find, appraise, and use knowledge from
    research as evidence (see Chapter 9).

These two components are inter-related (see Fig. 7.1).

   For any healthcare organisation to increase the degree to
which decisions taken within it are evidence based, it is
important to develop the appropriate *systems* and *culture*; it
may also be necessary to change the *structure* of the
organisation (see Margin Fig. 7.1). Individuals and

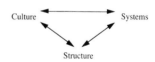

Margin Fig. 7.1

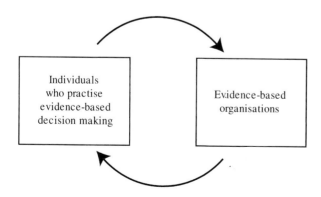

Fig. 7.1
The relationship between individuals and organisations within
an evidence-based paradigm

organisations need to be supported by systems that provide the best knowledge currently available when and where it is required, and to exist in an evaluative culture.

- The culture of an evidence-based healthcare organisation is evaluative – there is an obsession with finding, appraising, and using research-based knowledge as evidence in decision-making.
- In every system of an evidence-based healthcare organisation, research-based knowledge must be sought, appraised, and used as evidence when making decisions. Within that organisation, there must also be systems for managing knowledge, and for developing the skills of individuals who work in the organisation.
- The structure of an evidence-based healthcare organisation should promote and facilitate evidence-based decision-making.

The culture, systems and structure for evidence-based healthcare organisations are discussed in Sections 7.3, 7.4 and 7.5, respectively.

7.3   CULTURE

Gentle Reader,

Marvel at Ernest Schneider, responsible for one of the major sporting breakthroughs of the 20th century: the change in downhill skiing from reliance on the Nordic telemark technique to the fixed heel approach of the European Alps. In the Foreword to his book published in 1936, he said 'more than 29 years of experience as a teacher are behind the assertions I make here.'

Commentary

In general, there are two types of statement in decision-making

* propositions supported by evidence;
* unsubstantiated assertions, which tend to be subjective.

Ernest Schneider made the basis for his statement absolutely clear. How many healthcare decision-makers do the same?

7.3.1   The evidence-based chief executive

It is vital that the promotion of evidence-based decision-making is not a task assigned solely to the medical director or the director responsible for R&D or clinical development, although such personnel do have a central role in this activity; the chief executive must also be committed to evidence-based decision-making. S/he must be able, and be seen:

* to search for evidence, alone if necessary;
* to appraise evidence, having participated in a critical appraisal skills workshop;
* to store important evidence in a way that allows it to be retrieved using a computer;
* to use evidence to make decisions;
* to help those individuals accountable to the chief executive to develop evidence management skills and to change the systems for which they are responsible such that evidence can be incorporated into decision-making.

7.3.2 Evidence-based management

Gentle Reader,

Empathise with the medical director. He ground his teeth and bit his tongue: 'That's the third financial ledger system being introduced in less than 5 years, and there's no evidence to suggest that this system will be any better than the last two. They've spent hundreds of thousands of pounds, and no-one asked for evidence of effectiveness when the decisions were taken about which information systems to buy, particularly the financial information systems. All they kept banging on about was clinical effectiveness. What about some evidence-based management in this organisation!'

Commentary

There has been much emphasis on the need to improve clinical effectiveness and to promote evidence-based clinical practice. In this book, the need to be more scientific and to use evidence when making purchasing and managerial decisions about clinical services has been promoted, but what of the need to use evidence in managerial decisions about management?

- *What was the strength of the evidence on which the decision to introduce resource management was based?*
- *How good is the evidence used to justify investment in new IT?*

In this book I have focused primarily on decisions about clinical services, mainly because there is a paucity of evidence on the effectiveness, or cost-effectiveness, of different management arrangements. It is important, however, to ensure that a scientific approach is taken to all aspects of the work of a health service provider because cost pressures may be generated by the cumulation of many small changes, as the example below illustrates.

Barchester District General Hospital employs 140 consultants and has a turnover of £80 million – £570 000 per consultant per year. Over a year, about 3 000 000 clinical decisions are taken that will affect resource use. If each consultant were to change their clinical practice by increasing the volume or intensity of care at the cost of about £3000 (an increase of 0.52%), due to an increase in clinical and support costs, which may not fall within their clinical directorate, the Trust and its purchasers would face an increased cost of £420 000 a year. This would cause a major problem, yet which clinician would recognise a change of 0.52% in their practice?

7.4 SYSTEMS

The evidence-based organisation should comprise systems that are capable of:

- providing evidence;
- promoting the use of evidence;
- consuming and using evidence.

7.4.1 Systems that provide evidence

7.4.1.1 The 'evidence centre'

An evidence-based organisation needs an 'evidence centre', which has:

- access to the World Wide Web;
- subscriptions to the most relevant sources of data, such as MEDLINE and The Cochrane Library;
- a limited number of appropriate books and journals;
- arrangements in place for obtaining documents, or copies thereof, e.g. reprints of articles;
- personnel who can manage these resources and promote their use.

The evidence centre should not simply be a location that decision-makers can visit, but viewed as a resource that can be accessed to provide evidence when it is needed. To fulfil the latter function, it is important to consider not only what evidence is needed but also when it is needed, in what situations and in what form.

The commonest situations in which evidence is needed are:

- in a meeting;
- on a ward round/in a clinic.

At present, most decision-makers would have to walk to the library or, in the case of general practitioners, drive to the hospital, park the car (often a nightmare), then walk to the library, find the evidence and drive back to the health centre. The barriers to accessing evidence are often too great.

A series of systems for accessing evidence is shown in Table 7.3.

Table 7.3 Systems for gaining access to evidence and their associated drawbacks and advantages

System	Drawbacks	Advantages
Walk or drive to the library	Time	Break from work
Exit from patient record computer system and access the 'evidence centre'	Time	Possible within hospitals at present; no technology required
Consult 'evidence centre' through a parallel system while patient record is still running	Expensive; two systems needed	Possible at present; needs separate telephone line for primary care
Consult evidence base on lap top	Expensive (but getting cheaper)	Portable system
Cue cards appear on screen with evidence and guidelines when diagnosis, patient's name or test result is entered	None	Minimises time and facilitates incorporation of evidence

7.4.1.2 The National electronic Library for Health

In 1998, the UK Government published an Information Strategy[1] in which the National electronic Library for Health (NeLH) was introduced. The overall aim for the establishment of NeLH was to link all existing libraries or evidence centres. The governing objectives of NeLH are:

- to provide easy access to best current knowledge;
- to improve health and healthcare, clinical practice, and patient choice.

7.4.2 Systems that promote the use of evidence

7.4.2.1 Evidence-based clinical audit

The use of evidence should be incorporated into the audit cycle (see Fig. 7.2).

There are two ways in which this can be done:

1. by ensuring that the evidence of effectiveness or safety for the intervention subject to audit is of good quality;
2. by ensuring that the standards applied within the audit process are scientific and based on the best evidence available.

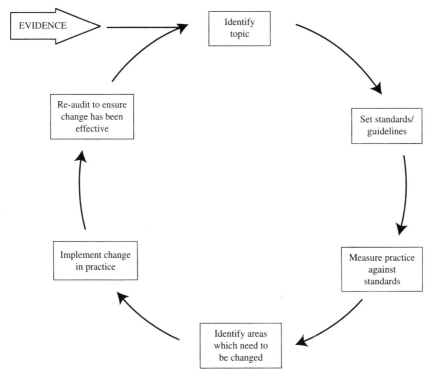

Fig. 7.2
The evidence-driven audit cycle

It is possible to select subjects for audit and suitable services for purchasing by analysing the research evidence. In the UK, the North Thames Regional Health Authority commissioned the London School of Hygiene and Tropical Medicine to undertake such an exercise; 10 topics were identified in a review of opportunities for evidence-based audit and purchasing (see Box 7.1).[2]

For each service or type of treatment, it is also possible to identify those interventions that are necessary in order to achieve a good outcome. This approach allows the identification of criteria that can be used to measure quality. A list of evidence-based criteria for the management of elderly patients with fractured neck of femur is shown in Box 7.2.[3-6]

Box 7.1 Evidence-based opportunities for audit (Source: Sanderson [2])

1. Prenatal steroids to prevent respiratory distress syndrome
2. Vacuum extraction vs forceps for obstetric delivery
3. Diagnostic D&C in young women
4. Systemic adjuvant therapy for breast cancer
5. Treatment of *Helicobacter pylori* to prevent recurrence of ulcer
6. Thromboprophylaxis for orthopaedic and general surgery
7. Management of mild hypertension
8. Cholesterol screening and use of cholesterol-lowering drugs
9. Aspirin, thrombolysis and anticoagulation after myocardial infarction
10. ACE inhibitors for chronic heart failure

Box 7.2 Evidence-based criteria for the management of elderly patients with fractured neck of femur (Source: refs 3–6)

1. Spending less than one hour in casualty
2. Receiving prophylactic antibiotics
3. Receiving pharmaceutical thromboembolic prophylaxis
4. Having surgery within 24 hours
5. Recording the grade of surgeon and anaesthetist performing the operation
6. Number of days after surgery by which 50% of patients were mobilised
7. Occurrence of pressure sores, urinary tract infection and pneumonia
8. Provision of a thorough medical and social assessment
9. Degree and effectiveness of joint working between orthopaedic surgeons and consultants in medicine for the elderly
10. Adequacy of discharge planning and implementation

7.4.2.2 Training for evidence-based decision-making

Within the training and development programme of any organisation, there must be strategies to develop the skills of all personnel such that they can practise evidence-based decision-making and thereby:

- search for evidence (Section 9.2);
- appraise evidence (Section 9.3);
- store and retrieve evidence (Section 9.4);
- use evidence.

Previously, health service managers were responsible for the organisation and the systems within it; it was the responsibility of the professions and the educational establishments related to the health service to influence individual clinicians. This division of responsibilities has now changed for two reasons:

1. the professions and the educational establishments are considered to have been too slow in promoting evidence-based clinical practice;
2. it has been recognised that the development of systems and of individuals are inter-related (see Fig. 7.1).

Moreover, as those who pay for and manage health services must identify the resources to invest in audit and continuing professional development, they are interested in which types of intervention are effective in bringing about change in professional practice. Although certain interventions have already been shown to be effective, more detailed work is being done, as part of The Cochrane Collaboration,[7] to review the effectiveness of the interventions shown in Box 7.3.

Box 7.3 Interventions under review for effectiveness (Source: Freemantle et al.[6])

- Audit and feedback
- Printed educational materials
- Opinion leaders
- Educational outreach
- The extended role of the pharmacist
- Nursing care planning
- Computerised drug information and dosage
- Reminders and prompts
- Guidelines and protocols
- Patient penalties
- Mass media strategies
- Conferences, seminars and training attachments (preceptorships)

7.4.3 Systems that consume and use evidence

7.4.3.1 Systems that should be more evidence based

Although evidence should be used to inform every decision, there are some aspects of healthcare for which the evidence is scanty. However, there are other aspects of healthcare to which evidence could and should be applied to a much greater extent than at present to ensure that the best value is obtained from the resources available, for example:

- drugs and therapeutics decision-making;
- equipment purchasing.

As decision-making about drugs is usually centralised within a hospital or primary care team, it is possible to exercise control over it. There are also good sources of information about the costs, safety and effectiveness of new drugs, which will provide a sound evidence base.

Decision-making about the purchase of equipment, however, is more problematic: there is less evidence available, and the available evidence is of poor quality, partly because RCTs of equipment are more difficult to organise and partly because there is no requirement to demonstrate efficacy before introducing new equipment, as is the case for the introduction of new drugs.

The introduction of new equipment usually follows one of two routes. The first is via the hospital 'equipment bank' or similar budget, the disbursement of which has to be undertaken with some degree of equity among different departments. A possible consequence of this arrangement is that a particular department may request a new piece of equipment because it is 'their turn', even if good evidence cannot be presented to support the application. The second is via public subscription and charitable appeals due to the constraints imposed on equipment budgets. In this situation, equipment is bought using money obtained directly from the public, for example, through a 'scanner appeal', the consequence of which is that the purchase often bypasses any form of evaluation (see Fig. 7.3).

A checklist of questions useful when appraising the evidence base for any proposals to change clinical practice

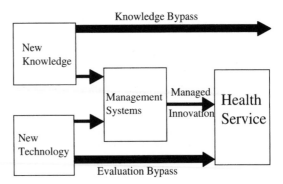

Fig. 7.3
The two main bypass routes for innovations in healthcare

is shown in Box 7.4; these questions can be applied to the introduction of new drugs or of new equipment, and should be incorporated into the system in which information is assimilated for decision-making.

Box 7.4 Checklist for the appraisal of proposals to change clinical practice

1. How did you search for evidence to support this proposal? (Please append the search strategy to this application.)
2. What is the best quality evidence supporting the proposal?
3. What will be the magnitude of the benefit compared with present practice? (Please give estimates based on the most optimistic and the most pessimistic estimate of the effect – the upper and lower confidence intervals.)
4. Compared with present practice, will there be any changes in:
   - patient safety?
   - acceptability and patient satisfaction?
   - cost:
     a) to your directorate?
     b) to any other directorate?
     c) to any other part of the health service?

For this type of appraisal to be effective when conducted on a local service, it must be complemented by a framework for, and system of, appraisal at a national level. At present, before a drug can be licensed and made available for prescription, it must have been demonstrated to be efficacious and safe. In some countries, notably Australia, there is greater control over the introduction of new drugs.[8] The approach developed in Australia is set out in the Guidelines for the Pharmaceutical Industry on Preparation of Submissions to the Pharmaceutical Benefits Advisory Committee (PBAC) (see Fig. 7.4).

In 1999, the National Institute for Clinical Excellence (NICE) was set up as a special health authority in the NHS for England and Wales. Its role is to provide patients, healthcare professionals and the public with authoritative, robust and reliable guidance on current best practice for:

- health technologies, including therapy, medical devices, diagnostic techniques, and procedures;
- clinical management of specific conditions.

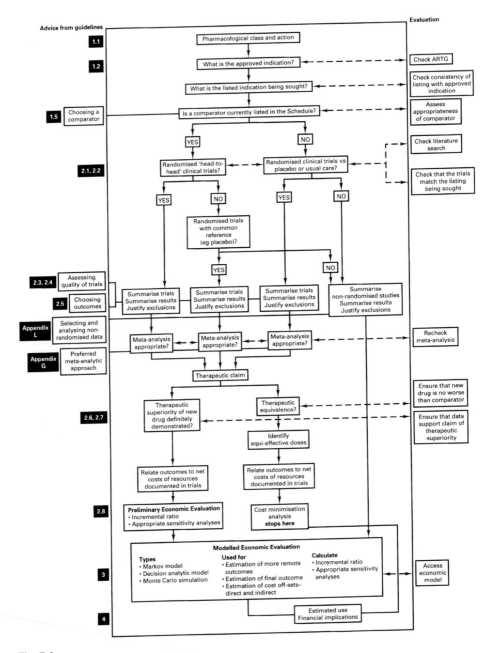

Fig. 7.4
Schema of key decisions in preparing and evaluating major submissions to the PBAC (Source: PBAC Guidelines)

7.4.3.2 Systems for managing innovation

A single issue of any journal might contain material that could prompt a clinician to make changes to his/her clinical practice; for example, take the issue of the *Annals of Internal Medicine* published on 15 August 1995 (see Box 7.5) in which there are as many as five innovations in knowledge and technology. Extrapolating from this figure, there may be more than 100 innovations a year in one journal alone. Given the large number of innovations being developed and published, it is essential to institute a system whereby the introduction of any innovation is managed.

Box 7.5 Innovations in knowledge and technology that appeared in the *Annals of Internal Medicine* of 15 August 1995

- An RCT of a drug in which it was found to reduce gastrointestinal complications in the treatment of rheumatoid arthritis
- A cost-effectiveness analysis of high-tech and low-tech strategies for managing suspected peptic ulcer disease
- The use of hepatic vein insulin measurement to diagnose an insulinoma
- A comparison of two different techniques for managing bleeding veins in the oesophagus
- Different strategies for managing chest pain in accident and emergency, including radioisotope single photon emission computed tomographic imaging and the proposal that a cardiologist be available to see all patients suffering from chest pain

---

There are two types of innovation: new knowledge and new technology. At present, new technology may enter directly into the service without evaluation, whereas new knowledge is not assimilated into clinical practice rapidly or systematically (see Fig. 7.3).

Those who purchase or provide healthcare must have systems to manage the introduction of innovation. For example, an implementation committee could be set up to decide:

- what action, if any, is needed in the light of new knowledge;
- what new technology should be introduced;
- what new technology should be prevented from entering the service, or removed from the service if it is currently being offered and yet known to be ineffective.

References

1. DEPARTMENT OF HEALTH, NHS EXECUTIVE (1998) *Information for Health: an Information Strategy for the Modem NHS 1998–2005 – a National Strategy for Local Implementation. Department of Health, London.* Available from: DH Distribution Centre, PO Box 410, Wetherby LS23 7LN.
2. SANDERSON, C. (1996) *Evidence-based candidates for the audit and purchasing agenda [Report].* North Thames Regional Health Authority, London. Cited in *Bandolier* 3(3) (Number 25): 5.
3. ROYAL COLLEGE OF PHYSICIANS (1989) *Fractured neck of femur, prevention and management: summary and recommendations of a report of the Royal College of Physicians.* J. Roy. Coll. Phys. 23: 8–12.
4. AUDIT CONMSSION (1995) *United They Stand: Co-ordinating Care for Elderly Patients with Hip Fracture.* HMSO, london.
5. TODD, C.J., FREEMAN, C.J., CAMILLERI-FERRANTE, C. et al. (1995) *Differences in mortality after fracture of the hip: the East Anglian audit.* Br. Med. J. 310: 904–8.
6. BEDFORD, M. (1996) *Broken hips – measuring performance.* Bandolier 25, Vol 3 (issue 3): 4
7. FREEMANTLE, N., GRILLI, R., GRIMSHAW, J.M. and OXMAN, A.D. (1995) *Implementing the findings of medical research: the Cochrane Collaboration and effective professional practice.* Quality in Health Care 4: 45—7.
8. FREEMANTLE, N., HENRY, D., MAYNARD, A. and TORRANCE, G. (1995) *Promoting cost-effective prescribing.* Br. Med. J. 310: 995–6

7.5 STRUCTURE

7.5.1 Creating a team for managing knowledge

Although more resources could be spent on the promotion of evidence-based management, it is possible to make better use of the resources currently allocated to one function but assigned among different directorates within a hospital, such as the library, audit resources, and educational resources. At some hospitals, these disparate elements are now being combined into directorates of clinical effectiveness; the checklist used in one NHS Trust is shown in Table 7.4.

7.5.2 Getting research into purchasing and practice

The Getting Research into Practice and Purchasing (GRiPP) Project was launched in Oxford in 1993. The aim of the

Table 7.4 The clinical development directorate: activities and roles (Source: Summerton [1])

How do we find information?	Literature searching	L, CE, A
Is the information of good quality?	Validation	CE, S (A, L, M)
Is it right for the population we treat?	Applicability	CE, S (A, L, M)
How do we tell people about it?	Dissemination/education	CE, M, PGME, A (?L)
How do we make it happen?	Implementation/change management	CE, A, M, PGME (?L)
Have we got the new treatment working?	Audit of process	A, CE
Is it doing what we wanted it to?	Audit of outcome	A, CE
Is appropriate evidence lacking?	Research questions	R, CE
Is it value for effort? Is it value for resources? Is it the best use of resources?	Economics and statistics	S, E

CE = clinical epidemiology and public health; M = management; A = audit; PGME = medical education; R = research; L = library; S = statistician; E = economist.

project was to take evidence about interventions and drive them into practice. In autumn 1995, it became the starting point for the PACE Programme – Promoting Action in Clinical Effectiveness – which was developed by the King's Fund and funded by the Department of Health. The PACE programme emphasis was on action learning, and the aim was to determine how health authorities could use research evidence to improve health when commissioning services for the local population. Sixteen local projects were supported to demonstrate the process of 'turning evidence into everyday practice'.[2] A wide range of different topics were selected – from the management of pressure sores to the eradication of *Helicobacter pylori*. The learning points from the various PACE projects are summarised in Box 7.6.

References

1. SUMMERTON, N. (1995) *The burden of proof.* Health Service J. 5481 (30.11.95), Vol 105: 33.
2. DUNNING, M., ABI-AAD, G., GILBERT, D., GILLAM, S. and LIVETT, H. (1998) *Turning Evidence into Everyday Practice. An interim report from the PACE programme, November 1997.* King's Fund Publishing.

Box 7.6   The lessons from PACE (Source: Dunning et al.[2])

A. Preparing the ground
Lesson A1: Base local guidelines on national reviews of evidence and guidelines.
Lesson A2: Acknowledge that evidence may be ambiguous and incomplete.
Lesson A3: Be clear about what needs to change.
Lesson A4: Link the work into local priorities.
Lesson A5: Consider the options available for securing change.
Lesson A6: Understand local issues and potential barriers to change.
Lesson A7: Take into account the needs and interests of GPs and primary health care teams.
Lesson A8: Establish data required to monitor progress.

B. Securing action
Lesson B1: Present the change in terms of benefits for staff and patients.
Lesson B2: Help people work together.
Lesson B3: Provide a local education and training programme.
Lesson B4: Give more than information to primary health care teams.
Lesson B5: A balanced approach across primary and secondary care is important.
Lesson B6: Decide how to engage pharmaceutical companies.

C. Managing the work
Lesson C1: Create a realistic timetable.
Lesson C2: Decide how to co-ordinate the work.
Lesson C3: Recognise that new skills may be required.
Lesson C4: Keep in touch with those affected by the work.
Lesson C5: Retain a balanced approach.
Lesson C6: Do not be too ambitious.
Lesson C7: Expect the unexpected and be able to respond.

7.6   EVIDENCE-BASED PRIMARY CARE

Primary care is care to which a patient can gain access directly. It comprises primary medical care, community nursing and those aspects of mental health and learning disability services that are delivered to people at home.

There are several important differences between the provision of primary care and that of hospital-based care (see Table 7.5).

Table 7.5   Differences in the provision of primary care and hospital-based care

Feature	Primary care	Hospital-based care
No. sites for healthcare provision per million population (UK)	250	3–4
No. work sites for individual professionals	100–200	1–2
No clinical decisions per million population (UK)	30 million	10 million
Health problems seen by individual professionals	Wide spectrum across numerous specialties	Narrow spectrum within one specialty
Site(s) of decision-making about patients	Primary care premises; patients' homes	Hospital
Access to a library/support of a librarian	Difficult	Available

In primary care, the provision of healthcare is undertaken over a large area at many scattered sites, and decision-making covers a wide range of health problems, sometimes in situations where it is not possible to access support. For these reasons, evidence-based decision-making is more difficult to organise in primary care. However, it is possible to distil the introduction of evidence-based decision-making in primary care to manageable proportions. Although the range of health problems encountered is wide, only a small number commonly occurs and the organisation of evidence for these common problems is feasible.

In a retrospective review of case notes at a suburban training general practice in the UK,[1] it was found that effective treatment for the health problems suffered by a large proportion of patients was based on evidence. Consecutive doctor–patient consultations ($n = 122$) conducted over two days were assessed to determine the proportion of interventions based on evidence from clinical trials; 21 were excluded because of insufficient data while the remaining 101 were assigned to one of three categories. The results are shown in Table 7.6. It can be seen that for a third of consultations, the intervention was based on evidence from RCTs, and for half of the consultations it was based on convincing non-experimental evidence.

Similarly, when making decisions about the provision of mental health and learning disability services, or about individuals who require such services, a small number of common problems recur, and therefore the relevant evidence base is of a manageable size.

Table 7.6 The nature of the supporting evidence for interventions undertaken in general practice (Source: Gill et al.[1])

Nature of substantiating evidence for intervention	No. consultations (*total = 101*)
Interventions substantiated by evidence from RCTs	31
Interventions substantiated by convincing non-experimental evidence, e.g. incision and drainage of an abscess	51
Interventions without substantial evidence	19

7.6.1 Improving access: promoting finding

Those whose job it is to provide evidence to decision-makers must:

- ensure easy access to information;
- provide relevant information, i.e. minimise the amount disseminated to the busy primary care professional.

7.6.1.1 *Ease of access to information* (Margin Fig. 7.2)

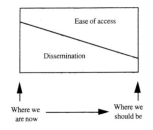

Margin Fig. 7.2

It can take hours for a primary care professional to reach and use a library and then return to base but, provided the service of a good librarian is available, access to that same information can be achieved by:

- phone;
- fax;
- Wide Area Network;
- the Internet.

Access to information can be facilitated by:

- using computer resources designated for management and administration to provide evidence to decision-makers;
- using a Web page, with access by a separate telephone line to protect the confidentiality of primary care information systems;
- regularly downloading information for storage on the primary care hard disks to minimise the dependence on slow Internet connections.

To be of use, information must be stored in convenient systems. Access to information can be promoted by:

- offering primary care professionals reference management software;
- providing information in various media, e.g.:
  - in Filofax size on paper;
  - in a form that can be downloaded to a personal organiser or other palm-top;
  - in hypertext files for a PC or Macintosh;
  - as cue card software will appear on screen when the primary care system is running patient record software.

7.6.1.2 Provision of relevant information

Although MEDLINE and EMBASE are excellent resources, they can generate a large volume of detailed information inappropriate to decision-making in primary and community care, principally because most of the articles indexed have been written by researchers for researchers. Primary care and community professionals need distillates of primary research that relate to the clinical problems they encounter, that is, evidence-based guidelines, supported by the facility to access the evidence directly if necessary (see Table 7.7).

Table 7.7 Need for, and accessibility of, different types of clinical information in primary care

Type of clinical information	Frequency of need	Accessibility
Evidence-based guidelines	++++	+
Written abstract of the systematic review on which the guideline is based	+++	++
Data from the systematic review	++	+++
Primary research on which the systematic review is based	+	++++

Other ways in which relevant information can be made available to primary care professionals include:

- providing every primary and community care site with a copy of The Cochrane Library (see Appendix I, I.2.1) or *Clinical Evidence*;
- ensuring on-line access to MEDLINE, for example, via the BMA library;

- disseminating in a systematic way, for instance, in a newsletter, new information of high quality needed by primary care decision-makers;
- ensuring that each professional has the support of a librarian for the development of searching and storing skills.

7.6.2   Improving appraisal skills

As primary care professionals have to deal with a wide range of health problems, they need to search a broad evidence base and must be taught the skills of appraisal. Although the approach that needs to be taken is no different from that for decision-makers in a hospital, primary care professionals may benefit from different examples.

Bandolier is a newsletter written principally to help clinicians, managers and purchasers develop their appraisal skills; one of the target audiences is general practitioners. The objectives of *Bandolier* are shown in Box 7.7.

Reference

1. GILL, P., DOWELL, A.C., NEAL, R.D., SMITH, N., HEYWOOD, P. and WILSON, A.E. (1996) *Evidence based general practice: a retrospective study of interventions in one training practice.* Br. Med. J. 312: 819–21.

Box 7.7   The objectives of the editors of *Bandolier*

To support any decision-maker in their ability to:

- find the best available evidence on tests and treatments;
- be conversant with the criteria used to appraise trials and systematic reviews on tests and clinical and cost effectiveness;
- define absolute and relative risk and be aware of the strengths and weaknesses of different methods of expressing research results;
- define, calculate and use NNT;
- list screening tests that do more good than harm;
- define odds ratios and know their value;
- define and interpret confidence intervals and power;
- distinguish sensitivity, specificity and predictive value of tests.

7.7 EVIDENCE-BASED PURCHASING AND COMMISSIONING

In health services world-wide, there is a trend to separate the function of purchasing healthcare from that of providing healthcare. Purchasers make decisions about which health services to buy; providers deliver healthcare to individual patients within the resources available. This separation of functions enables purchasers to focus on how best to use finite resources with respect to:

- particular groups of patients;
- particular diseases, such as heart disease;
- particular interventions, such as hip replacement.

The aim of those who pay for health services for different groups of people with, or at risk of, different diseases is to maximise the value obtained from the resources available by ensuring that:

- the resources are allocated to the groups in proportions that maximise value, i.e. it is not possible to achieve better health gain for the population by redistribution of resources;
- the healthcare professional responsible for managing each of these groups achieves maximum value from the resources allocated to the group by: offering only those interventions that do more good than harm at reasonable cost; ensuring that these interventions are offered to those who are most likely to be helped rather than harmed and, at the time, most likely to benefit; and ensuring that the interventions are given as well and as cheaply as possible.

Those who pay for healthcare can use their purchasing power to accomplish four evidence-based tasks:

- resource reallocation among disease management systems (Section 7.7.1);
- resource reallocation within a single disease management system (Section 7.7.2);
- managing innovation (Section 7.7.3);
- controlling increases in healthcare costs without affecting the health of the population.

However, in the current context of increasing involvement of patients and the general public in healthcare decision-making, those who pay for services should bear in mind that the aims of the public for resource allocation may be different to those of healthcare professionals.

- The aim of an individual patient is to ensure the maximum allocation of resources to treat his/her case.
- The aim of a group of patients or carers who have the same problem is to obtain more resources for the particular patient group, and openness and equity in the distribution of healthcare resources for that group.
- The aim of representatives of the general public is to ensure openness and equity in the distribution of resources across the entire range of patient groups.

Those who purchase healthcare in the UK experience certain advantages and disadvantages in comparison with purchasers elsewhere in the world. A major disadvantage is that in many parts of the UK there is no, or only limited, choice of providers when compared with the USA, for example. However, a major advantage is coverage of discrete populations; in the USA and in some European countries, the population of a single city may be covered by three or more nationwide purchasers.

The advantage of being able to focus on a discrete population has two important consequences:

1. it facilitates the process of population needs assessment;
2. it enables a purchaser to undertake the broader role of health 'commissioner', that is, being able to integrate the health services that are purchased with a broad range of public health measures to prevent disease, promote health, and reduce inequalities in a defined population.

1. Population needs assessment
A definition of health need that can be used in evidence-based purchasing is:

> a health problem for which there is an intervention about which there is strong evidence, based on good-quality research, that it does more good than harm.

Population needs assessment comprises:

- the estimation of the frequency of various health problems in a population;

- the appraisal of the evidence for the beneficial and harmful effects of the interventions used to treat each health problem, which is the focus of this book.

2. Commissioning

Commissioners have the ability to supplement what has been achieved by negotiation with providers during the contracting process with the following functions:

- the promotion of health in general;
- public and patient education;
- professional education, thereby exerting an influence through the resources invested in education;
- commissioning research where evidence is lacking, thereby exerting an influence through the Research and Development levy.

7.7.1 Resource reallocation among disease management systems

A disease management system consists of all those services and interventions designed to improve the health of individuals who have a particular disease (e.g. diabetes) or a group of diseases (e.g. cardiac disease). Such systems can be managed by the use of guidelines, for both the referral and discharge of patients (see 1–3 in Fig. 7.5), and for the treatment of patients (see A–D in Fig. 7.5). If all the elements of a system are governed by the use of guidelines, the care provided is often referred to as 'managed care' (see Section 1.7.1).

In the NHS, disease management systems are rudimentary because the service is still dominated by broad distinctions between primary and secondary care, or between hospital and community care. It is not possible to make an evidence-based decision about the balance of expenditure between primary and secondary care as a whole; it is possible only to make evidence-based decisions

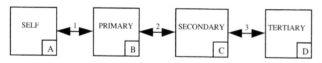

Fig. 7.5
Schematic representation of a disease management system showing routes for the care of patients

about the balance of expenditure on primary and secondary care for a particular disease. A comparison of the health outcomes arising from investment in different disease management systems requires information from studies of safety, effectiveness, and cost, for example, by comparing the cost per QALY.

However, purchasers are not usually asked to reallocate resources on the basis of specific diseases; the purchase of healthcare is usually founded on contracts for particular patient groups, and purchasers face demands to increase the amount of investment in the ENT, the oral surgery or the gynaecology contract (sometimes all three). If purchasers are able to address only the secondary care sector of these systems, it is worth asking the following questions.

- What would be the beneficial health effects of adding £200 000 to each of these three contracts?
- What would be the health effects of subtracting £200 000 from each of these three contracts?

In both cases, it is wise to elicit the evidence upon which any answers have been based.

7.7.2 Resource reallocation within a single disease management system

Any decision-maker trying to reallocate resources within a disease management system on the basis of evidence that resources could be better spent faces several problems.

- Increased expenditure in budget A, such as the drug budget, is required before there can be savings in budget B, the inpatient budget.
- The budgets may be in different compartments.
- The potential savings may appear to be large when calculated nationally; for instance, increasing the prescription of ACE inhibitors in general practice will reduce hospital costs for the treatment of heart failure, but for an individual hospital the actual reduction in the amount of resources used may not be sufficient to allow a facility, such as a ward, to be closed and 'real' cash to be released for reallocation into another part of the system.

These problems are particularly difficult for purchasers to address because:

- they are not able to reduce expenditure on hospital care and redirect it into primary care drug budgets;
- they may not have access to diagnostic service costs, which are not subject to external contract but allocated internally within a provider unit;
- professionals in any service in which savings from better management of one disease could be made can usually identify needs among a different group of patients under their care which they believe should be met with these savings; for example, professionals in a respiratory unit would argue that any savings on hospital care of asthma should be spent on sleep apnoea or cystic fibrosis.

Although the main opportunities for better disease management within a hospital are open to the managers at that hospital, it is possible for health 'commissioners' to promote investment in disease management systems by focusing on specific points on the primary/secondary care interface, rather than making broad generalisations about need for closer co-operation between the two sectors. Within a single disease management system, a purchaser will attempt to promote cost containment on the basis of research evidence and to minimise any adverse effects on the health of the population (Fig. 7.6).

7.7.3 Managing innovation

Innovation occurs continually. A purchaser must try to manage the introduction of innovation in the following ways:

- *starting starting right* – those innovations that do more good than harm, and which are *affordable*, are introduced at a defined standard of quality;
- *starting stopping* – those innovations that do more harm than good but have already entered the service are no longer offered;
- *stopping starting* – those innovations that do more harm than good are not introduced;
- *promoting trials* – innovations of unknown effect are investigated during trials;
- *slowing starting* – those innovations that require training and infrastructure are introduced in a planned way.

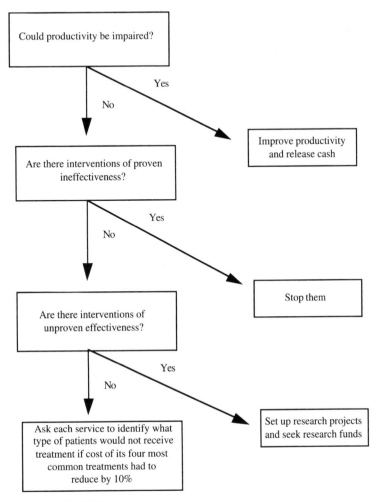

Fig. 7.6
Evidence-based cost containment or cutting

7.7.3.1 Promoting innovation – starting starting right

Promoting innovation has two facets:

1. promoting completely novel interventions;
2. changing the provision of an established service.

When promoting a novel intervention, for example, thrombolysis after acute myocardial infarction (AMI), it is possible for purchasers to be explicit about their requirements. It is more problematic when trying to change established professional practice, for instance, persuading gynaecologists to stop performing dilatation and curettage

(D&C) operations in women under the age of 40 years, or to perform fewer Caesarean sections.

Further means of promoting change can also be used to supplement a purchaser's specifications, namely:

- changing individual behaviour through professional education and audit, and public and patient education;
- the development of better systems of care.

The development of better systems of care is particularly important in situations in which a change in professional practice is not sufficient to ensure a better outcome for patients. As an example, for thrombolysis after AMI to be delivered effectively, a reconfiguration of the system of care is necessary to change the way in which patients with chest pain are managed:

- when they contact their GP;
- when they are in transit in the ambulance;
- and when they arrive at the A&E department.

Part of the management of innovation is to identify interventions that do more good than harm at affordable cost and drive them into the service quickly and effectively – starting starting right. It is no longer acceptable to allow important innovations to drift into practice in a piecemeal fashion.

An example of the problems that can be encountered in the introduction of a low-cost, highly effective and cost-effective intervention is the administration of antenatal corticosteroid therapy to women who go into labour prematurely. Good-quality RCTs conducted between 1972 and the 1990s demonstrated the benefit of this intervention in preventing the hazards of fetal immaturity, namely, death and cerebral palsy.[1] Incidentally, this series of RCTs forms the basis of the design for the Cochrane Collaboration logo (see Margin Figure 5.2).

However, despite this evidence of effectiveness, the use of corticosteroid therapy was relatively low during the 1990s.[2] Leviton et al.[3] evaluated two dissemination strategies to increase the appropriate use of this therapy. Twenty-seven tertiary care hospitals were randomly assigned to be subject to either 'usual dissemination of practice recommendations' ($n = 14$) or usual dissemination plus an active, focused dissemination effort ($n = 13$). Active dissemination comprised a one-year education programme led by an influential physician and a nurse co-ordinator in which the following mechanisms were used:

- grand rounds;
- chart reminder system;
- group discussion of case scenarios;
- monitoring;
- feedback.

These techniques had been identified as being effective by the Cochrane Effective Practice and Organisation of Care (EPOC) Group (see Appendix V, V.3.2).

It was found that active dissemination significantly increased the odds of corticosteroid use. It is clear from the results of this study that the promotion of innovation must be actively managed.

7.7.3.2 *Stopping starting, starting stopping and slowing starting*

When there is no evidence from good-quality research that an intervention does more good than harm, it should not be introduced – stopping starting (see Section 2.4.1.2). In such situations, it is vital for purchasers to be clear about innovations they do not want to purchase for a particular population due to the lack of evidence of effectiveness. The logic is easy for press and public to understand: all interventions are associated with risk; some people will suffer if any intervention is introduced; if there is no evidence of a beneficial effect, the harm done by the intervention will be greater than the good.

Interventions of proven ineffectiveness and unproven effectiveness should be clearly identified. If any intervention in the latter group is introduced, it must be only as part of a properly designed and ethically approved trial.

However, there are interventions already in routine use for which there is either no evidence of effectiveness or evidence of ineffectiveness. The strategy in such cases is to discontinue their use by starting stopping (see Section 2.4.1.2). However, as this can be a difficult objective to achieve, it may be easier in some cases to pursue a strategy of slowing starting (see Section 2.4.1.3).

7.7.3.3 Promoting trials

Interventions of unproven effectiveness should be tested within an RCT; purchasers should promote and support the performance of RCTs. One benefit of promoting trials is that it enables those who pay for healthcare to be categorical about which services/interventions will be supported.

For example, in the UK, the NHS Executive (NHSE) issued an Executive Letter (EL) about improving the effectiveness of clinical services [EL(95)105], as part of their strategy for improving clinical effectiveness. In Annex 1 of the EL, the NHSE was explicit about which interventions were included in the Health Technology Assessment Programme and gave clear advice as follows.

> The following interventions are currently under assessment (or studies will start in the next 12 months). Purchasers are advised to invest in these interventions in the context of the assessment but not as part of routine care. It is important that sufficient numbers of patients are recruited to these clinical studies to reduce areas of uncertainty. Purchasers should therefore play an active role and encourage providers to participate fully in recognised assessments.

> The following assessments include major clinical trials and systematic reviews. These studies are supported by the Medical Research Council, the Department of Health, charities and the NHS (including the NHS Health Technology Assessment Programme). These have been grouped together in broad service categories, for convenience.

> Briefing sheets for each of the interventions listed are available from the contact given at the end of this annex. This should place the assessment in context and better inform purchasing practice.

Included in Annex 1 were those screening tests that should not be offered as part of 'routine care' but should be supported 'in the context of the assessment', i.e. offered only as part of a high-quality research programme (see Box 7.8).

Box 7.8   Screening tests which should be offered only within the context of research (UK) (Initial source: EL(95)105; updated mid-2000)

- Screening for colorectal cancer by once only flexible sigmoidoscopy
- Screening for Down's syndrome, using ultrasound measurement of nuchal translucency
- Screening for fragile X
- Neonatal screening for inborn errors of metabolism, including use of tandem mass-spectrometry and DNA analysis
- Screening for abdominal aortic aneurysm
- Screening for ovarian cancer
- Breast cancer screening from the age of 40
- Yearly breast screening
- Identifying and monitoring osteoporosis, featuring use of:
  - dual-energy X-ray absorptiometry;
  - low frequency ultrasound;
  - biochemical markers

7.7.4 Evidence-based insurance

In the past, the source of finance has dictated the system of healthcare introduced. In countries in which systems of paying for healthcare develop, there are two main sources of finance:

1. insurance;
2. taxation.

In some countries, there may be complicated permutations of these two systems, for instance, government underwriting of insurance schemes. Insurance-based systems derive revenue from customers; in tax-based systems, health services are paid for directly from funds raised through taxation. The distinction between the two systems has changed dramatically in recent years. Some insurance companies provide their own healthcare, for example, in health maintenance organisations such as Kaiser Permanente. In tax-based systems, such as the NHS, the opposite trend is taking place, as demonstrated by the division between the purchase and provision of healthcare.

Insurance schemes operate in a different way from health authorities in the NHS. Instead of negotiating contracts for services for geographical populations, insurance companies develop health plans that cover those people (sometimes called the 'members') who pay premiums to the company. The contents of the health plan describe the interventions or benefits for which the company will pay. In the past, insurance companies paid for all the costs of treatment, but as costs have increased the services provided have been rationed. The plans insurance companies now offer are carefully couched in what Eddy calls 'benefit language'.[4] 'Benefit language' has three main components:

1. coverage categories describing the services that will be covered – for example, orthopaedic surgery is covered but not osteopathy;
2. patient responsibilities – the contribution the member may have to make to the cost of care;
3. coverage criteria.

Coverage criteria are the means by which the insurance companies fine-tune the categories of service covered, and seek to balance cost control with the range of services provided that they hope members will find attractive. It is upon these coverage criteria that guidelines, protocols and clinical policies are developed by insurance companies, and thus it is through coverage criteria that a system of managed care is created (see Section 1.7.1).

The coverage criteria will vary from one health plan to another. They relate not to services but to specific interventions, i.e. activities undertaken to prevent, diagnose, treat or improve a medical condition. The criteria that need to be met for an intervention to be included in a health plan are shown in Box 7.9.

Box 7.9 Coverage criteria (Source: Eddy[4])

- The intervention is used for a medical condition.
- There is sufficient evidence to draw conclusions about the intervention's effects on health outcomes.
- The evidence demonstrates that the intervention can be expected to produce its intended effects on health outcomes.
- The intervention's expected beneficial effects on health outcomes outweigh its expected harmful effects.
- The intervention is the most cost-effective method available to address the medical condition.

Coverage criteria are the means insurers use to promote evidence-based healthcare, in particular, through the requirement that 'sufficient evidence' is available. Sufficient evidence is the concept investigated in studies of the proportion of patients whose care it is possible to substantiate with evidence (see Tables 7.6 and 10.1). Sufficient evidence is defined as that evidence derived from RCTs and systematic reviews of trials, and convincing non-experimental evidence (e.g. there is convincing empirical evidence to support the decision to drain an abscess).

Clinicians in the UK have worked within a form of managed care since 1948. The development of a system of managed care has occurred rapidly in the USA. In less than two decades, American doctors have been taken from a tradition in which they worked as they chose to a system of care that is governed by stricter controls than are set out in UK commissioning contracts. In an editorial published in the *Annals of Internal Medicine*, the situation was described as follows:

> the physician has moved from Pegasus, soaring aloft on the heady excitement of biomedical science, to Sisyphus, condemned forever to push a boulder up a hill.[5]

7.7.5 'Black belt' decision-making

The approach described hitherto is relatively simple, but detailed flow charts can be used to describe a framework for more complex decision-making; an example of one prepared by Irwig et al.[6] is shown in Fig. 7.7.

7.7.6 The limits of structural reform

Faced by soaring healthcare costs, most governments took steps in the last decade of the 20th century to control the rate of increase of expenditure. The principal means of doing this, supported by the World Bank, has been the introduction of structural reform. The key components of structural reform are shown in Box 7.10.

Structural reform is essential for the control of costs. Some aspects of quality can be improved by structural reform. It is possible to use this type of structure to control the introduction of expensive innovations, for example, breast cancer screening for women under the age of 50 years, by instructing providers that there will be no

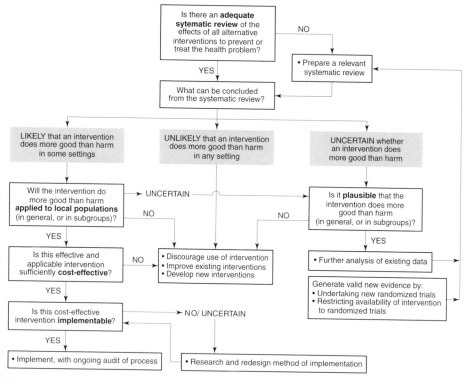

Fig. 7.7
Flow diagram of decision-making based on research synthesis (Source: Irwig et al.[6])

Box 7.10   Key components of structural reform

- Imposition of a limit to the amount of GNP or public expenditure allocated to health services.
- Separation of functions of purchasing (or commissioning) and providing care.
- Introduction of managed care.
- Shift to insurance-based funding of care.

---

reimbursement for such a service. It is also possible to tackle specific issues within a context of structural reform by using the appropriate levers in the system, e.g.:

- centralisation of services;
- improving patient satisfaction, for example, by reducing waiting lists;
- increasing productivity;
- enabling decisions to be made in a more open and explicit way.

However, it is difficult to ensure that maximum value is obtained from the resources invested in healthcare through structural reform because an increase in value is determined not only by a small number of big changes but also by a large number of small changes, as Eddy has identified (see Sections 1.2 and 2.5). For every million population, there may be a thousand healthcare professionals, each of them changing their practice in many small ways, most of which will be too small for managers to identify and control.

Thus, structural reform cannot be used in isolation to improve the value obtained from resources invested; cultural reform is also necessary such that every professional is asking the following questions:

- 'Does this intervention do more good than harm?'
- 'What is the evidence on which I should base this change in my practice?'

References

1. CROWLEY, P., CHALMERS, I. and KEIRSE MARC, J.N.C. (1990) *The effects of corticosteroid administration before preterm delivery: an overview of the evidence from controlled trials.* Br. J. Obstet. Gynaecol. 97: 11–25.
2. BRONSTEIN, J.M. and GOLDENBERG, R.L. (1995) *Practice variation in the use of corticosteroids: a comparison of eight datasets.* Am. J. Obstet. Gynecol. 173: 296–8.
3. LEVITON, L.C., GOLDENBERG, R.L., BAKER, C.S. et al. (1999) *Methods to encourage the use of antenatal corticosteroid therapy for fetal maturation. A randomised controlled trial.* JAMA 281: 46–52.
4. EDDY, D. (1996) *Benefit language. Criteria that will improve quality while reducing cost.* JAMA 275: 650–7.
5. LIPKIN, M. Jr. (1996) *Sisyphus or Pegasus? The physician interviewer in the era of corporatization of care.* Ann. Intern. Med. 124: 511–12.
6. IRWIG, L., ZWARENSTEIN, M., ZWI, A. and CHALMERS, I. (1998) *A flow diagram to facilitate selection of interventions and research for health care.* Bull. World Health Organ. 76: 17–24.

7.8   PROMOTING EVIDENCE-BASED MANAGEMENT

In the UK, the Department of Health set up an R&D programme in 1991 which had five main functions:

1. to ascertain the knowledge that NHS decision-makers need;
2. to ensure that knowledge was produced;
3. to make the knowledge available to decision-makers;
4. to promote the implementation of R&D findings;
5. to promote an evaluative culture.

   The key verb is 'to promote' in functions 4 and 5. Within the R&D Programme, the aim is primarily that of producing knowledge which is needed and making that knowledge available. To complement this activity, the Secretary of State for Health launched a Clinical Effectiveness Initiative, a simple and easily understood framework encompassing three main themes:

1. inform;
2. change;
3. monitor.

As the primary purpose of the NHS is 'to secure through the resources available, the greatest possible improvement to the health of the people', it was emphasised that the provision of effective services in terms of outcome and cost was central to achieving this purpose.

   For the Clinical Effectiveness Initiative, several separate projects and programmes were brought together. In the booklet produced for chief executives, the ways in which a wide range of Departmental initiatives within the service could be co-ordinated to increase the cost-effectiveness of the NHS are described. This bold programme of work was founded on the R&D initiative to ensure that research-based knowledge is not only produced and made available to decision-makers but also used as evidence in decision-making to improve the provision of health services and the health of the population.

7.8.1   Analysis of obstacles

A report of the progress that had been made in introducing evidence-based healthcare in England and Wales was prepared by staff at the Health Services Management

Centre (HSMC) at Birmingham University.[1] The key points that emerged from this report are listed in Box 7.11.

The authors also proposed a checklist of questions that could be used by managers in any organisation to ensure that all areas of possible action were being covered (see Box 7.12).

Box 7.11 Key findings about the introduction of evidence-based healthcare in England and Wales (Source: Appleby et al.[1])

- Many health authorities and most Trusts do not have a written strategy for improving clinical effectiveness, and therefore cannot claim to take the issue seriously.
- At more than half the health authorities and more than a third of Trusts which responded to the survey, clinical effectiveness initiatives were underway. Most of these initiatives concerned a single topic.
- Access to clinical information needs to be improved. Many hospital libraries restrict access and are not open outside office hours.
- Performance indicators should take effectiveness into account.

Box 7.12 A checklist of actions to ensure the incorporation of evidence-based healthcare into an organisation (Source: Appleby et al.[1])

- Is the board really involved in, and genuinely committed to, improving clinical effectiveness?
- Is there an executive director on the board who takes full responsibility for improving clinical effectiveness?
- Does the organisation have a formal strategy for clinical effectiveness?
- Is there a co-ordinating group responsible for leading on clinical effectiveness?
- Is there a senior individual working with the lead executive director to implement the strategy on clinical effectiveness?
- Has the organisation reviewed its structures in the light of its strategy for improving clinical effectiveness?
- Does the organisation have adequate access to information resources?
- How does the organisation disseminate and follow up information on effectiveness?
- Is appropriate training relating to clinical effectiveness being provided?
- Are health authorities incorporating evidence on effectiveness into their key roles in assessing healthcare needs and commissioning services to meet those needs?
- Are trusts incorporating evidence on effectiveness into their key roles in healthcare provision?
- Is the progress of efforts to improve clinical effectiveness and to foster evidence-based healthcare regularly monitored and reviewed?
- Are efforts to improve clinical effectiveness having a measurable impact?

7.8.2 Promoting implementation

Several different approaches are being adopted to promote the introduction of evidence-based healthcare and to ensure that research findings are adopted at a faster rate and in a more systematic manner.

In the UK, at a national level, one of the remits of the National Institute of Clinical Excellence (NICE) is to promote both clinical effectiveness and cost-effectiveness by issuing guidance to the NHS (see Section 2.4.1.2 for NICE's initial guidance about the prescription of Relenza).

In addition, the NHS Executive in England has introduced a performance development framework for assessing the work that is being done to promote clinical effectiveness. An example of the type of question being considered for inclusion in this framework is given below.

How does the Board of the Health Authority view its role in promoting clinical effectiveness?

One way in which it is possible for the board of a health authority to promote clinical effectiveness is to request evidence of effectiveness in support of bids for health authority funding. Dixon et al.[2] describe an attempt to introduce evidence of the effectiveness of interventions into the annual priority-setting process of a district health authority in England. Dixon et al. undertook literature searches on 144 applications for funding, appraised the literature, and then members of the department of public health scored the bids in terms of health gain. These scores were then fed into the priority-setting process. The main results of assessing the strength of evidence underpinning the bids are shown in Table 7.8; strong evidence to support the proposed service developments was found for only seven of the applications (6.2%). Dixon et al. observed that although this process did appear to influence the initial assessment of proposals, the strength of the research evidence was not reflected in the priority choices made by the health authority in its purchasing plan. They conclude that 'it is feasible, but difficult, to use information resources and critical assessment of research evidence as part of the priority-setting process of a DHA'.[2]

Table 7.8 Strength of evidence to support bids for funding to a health authority (Source: Dixon et al.[2])

		No. of bids	%
A	There is good evidence to support the use of the procedure	7	6.2
B	There is fair evidence to support the use of the procedure	24	21.2
C	There is poor evidence to support the use of the procedure	43	38.1
D	There is fair evidence to reject the use of the procedure	0	0.0
E	There is good evidence to support the rejection of the use of the procedure	0	0.0
	Insufficient details with which to conduct literature search	19	16.8
	No direct impact on patient care	17	15.0
	No evidence found	3	2.7
Total		113	100.0

References

1. APPLEBY, J., WALSHE, K. and HAM, C. (1995) *Acting on the Evidence: a Review of Clinical Effectiveness, Sources of Information, Dissemination and Implementation.* National Association of Health Authorities and Trusts, Birmingham.
2. DIXON, S., BOOTH, A. and PERRETT, K. (1997) *The application of evidence-based priority setting in a District Health Authority.* Public Health Med. 19: 307–12.

7.9 EVIDENCE-BASED POLICY-MAKING

Policy: 5. a course of action adopted and pursued by a government, party, ruler, statesman, etc.; any course of action adopted as advantageous or expedient. (The chief living sense.)

Shorter Oxford English Dictionary

To govern is to make choices.

Duc de Lévis, Politique

You can't do it all by sums, Adrian. We're not academics, we're civil servants. We have to deal with things as they are. We have to deal with people, with events.

John le Carré, The Looking Glass War, *1965*

7.9.1 The dominance of values in policy-making

There is nothing a politician likes so little as to be
well informed; it makes decision making so complex
and difficult.

J. M. Keynes

Politics tends to be driven by beliefs, and it is the values
politicians believe to be important that dominate decision-
making about policy. Although such decisions will be
tempered by the availability of resources, resource
allocation can also be based on beliefs and values. Evidence
can be used during policy-making, but some policies have
been formulated without consideration of the available
evidence.

7.9.2 The influence of budgetary pressures

However, a shortage of resources can force policy-makers
to consider the evidence and alter policy as a result. This is
illustrated by an eloquent letter written by Danial Patrick
Moynihan, Chairman of the US Senate Finance Committee.[1]

Dear Dr Tyson,

You will recall that last Thursday when you so
kindly joined us at a meeting of the Democratic
Policy Committee you and I discussed the
President's family preservation proposal. You
indicated how much he supports the measure. I
assured you I, too, support it, but went on to ask
what evidence was there that it would have any
effect. You assured me there was such data. Just
for fun. I asked for two citations.

The next day we received a fax from Sharon Glied
of your staff with a number of citations and a
paper, 'Evaluating the Results', that appears to
have been written by Frank Farrow of the Center
for the Study of Social Policy here in Washington
and Harold Richman at the Chapin Hall Center at
the University of Chicago. The paper is quite
direct: '. . . solid proof that family preservation
services can affect a state's overall placement rates
is still lacking.

Just yesterday, the same Chapin Hall Center released an 'Evaluation of the Illinois Family First Placement Prevention Program: Final Report'. This was a large-scale study of the Illinois Family First initiative authorized by the Illinois Family Preservation Act of 1987. It was 'designed to test effects of this program on out-of-home placements of children and other outcomes, such as subsequent child maltreatment.' Data on case and service characteristics were provided by Family First caseworkers on approximately 4,500 cases; approximately 1,600 families participated in the randomized experiment. The findings are clear enough. 'Overall, the Family First placement prevention program results in a slight increase in placement rates (when data from all experimental sites are combined). This effect disappears once case and site variations are taken into account.' In other words, there are either negative effects or no effects.

7.9.3 The growing influence of evidence in policy-making

What makes for a good health system? What makes a health system fair? And how do we know whether a health system is performing as well as it could?

Dr Gro Harlem Brundtland, Director General, WHO[2]

In any country, one of the factors affecting the health and well-being of individuals and populations is the quality of care provided within the health service (see Fig. 8.1). In turn, the performance of any health system is determined by the way in which it is designed, managed, and financed. In *The World Health Report 2000*,[2] the World Health Organization (WHO) has addressed health system performance for the first time as a determinant of health, and signals the Director General's intention to pursue this issue in all subsequent reports. Dr Brundtland sees health systems development to improve performance as increasingly central to WHO's work, arguing that the outcomes of health system failure can be measured in terms of death, disability, impoverishment, and despair. The need to assess health systems performance is made more pressing by the level of variation around the world, even among those countries that have similar levels of health spending.

To this end, the principal writers of the report have analysed the factors that affect health system performance using the best available evidence to date, while accepting that knowledge of health systems is hampered by the weakness of routine information systems and insufficient attention paid to research in this area. In addition to these limitations, the issue of health systems performance is complex.

In this report, a health system is defined as including: '… all the activities whose primary purpose is to promote, restore or maintain health'.[2]

All health systems are recognised as having three fundamental goals irrespective of the level of resources available for healthcare and the way in which each health system is organised:

1. to improve the health of the population they serve;
2. to respond to people's expectations;
3. to provide financial protection against the costs of ill-health.

The ways in which these goals can be attained are explored in the report, and measures are developed to assess how well a health system performs in relation to each of them. However, in order to act on measures of performance, it is necessary to understand the key functions of a health system. The principal writers identify four key functions, as follows:

- service provision;
- resource (human, material, and conceptual) generation and development;
- mobilisation and channelling of financing;
- stewardship, that is, ensuring that the individuals and organisations within the system act as good stewards of the resources and trust given into their care – described as being the 'most critical' function.

The report represents evidence-based policy-making at its best, and sets an agenda for future work that encompasses the following issues.

- The ultimate responsibility for the performance of a country's health system lies with government: careful and responsible management of the well-being of the population – stewardship – is the essence of good government; the health of the people is always a national priority, and government responsibility for health is continuous and permanent.

- In dollar for dollar spent on health, many countries are falling short of their performance potential, with the result that a large number of preventable deaths occur and lives are stunted by disability. The impact of this failure of performance is borne disproportionately by the poor.
- Health systems are not just concerned with improving people's health but with protecting them against the financial cost of illness. The challenge facing governments in low-income countries is to reduce the burden of out-of-pocket payment for health by expanding pre-payment schemes, which allow financial risk to be spread, and thereby reduce large healthcare expenditures.
- Within governments, many health ministries focus on the public sector, often disregarding the private finance and provision of care, which is frequently much larger. A growing challenge is for governments to harness the skills and resources in the private and voluntary sectors to improve health systems performance while at the same time offsetting the failures of the private sector.
- Stewardship is ultimately concerned with oversight of the entire system, avoiding short-sightedness, tunnel vision, and turning a blind eye to a system's failings.

7.9.4   Healthcare policy-making

Healthcare policies relate to the financing and organisation of health services. At the highest level, government takes decisions about the level of investment that will be made in a country's health services. Policy-makers also make decisions about the organisation of those health services, which are usually related to service financing. Organisational change may be instigated to fulfil one or more central government objectives, such as:

- to decentralise power;
- to involve more people in decision-making;
- to encourage cost control;
- to reduce the number of managerial staff;
- to encourage competition as a stimulus to reduce costs and increase quality.

In the NHS, examples of organisational policy-making include:

- the creation of health authorities in 1974, in which were combined the financing of the local authority health committee and the regional hospital boards;
- the introduction of the purchaser/provider split and the creation of GP-fundholding in 1991;
- the abolition of regional health authorities in 1996;
- the creation of primary care trusts (PCTs) in 2000.

In many of the organisational changes that have taken place since the inception of the NHS in 1948, power has changed hands, an outcome achieved principally by changing the responsibility for resources.

Although the idea underpinning the introduction of any organisational change may reflect the ideology of the political party in power, or that of an individual, pressure group or think tank, the decision taken can be based on evidence (Fig. 7.8). The nature of the evidence may be:

- the experience of what happened since the last change in service financing and organisation;
- derived from research findings.

However, the amount of research evidence available on which to base healthcare policy is often limited, and politicians may argue that the introduction of a particular policy is supported by common sense (Fig. 7.8).

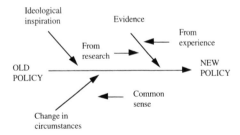

Fig. 7.8
Factors underlying healthcare-policy changes

GP-fundholding, for example, was introduced in 1991 as part of a series of changes designed:

- to increase competitive pressure on the providers of healthcare as a stimulus to improve productivity and quality;

- to increase the motivation of general practitioners to control expenditure on prescribing by allowing them to retain any 'savings' for other types of patient care.

Although there was no evidence on which to base such a policy, it would have been possible to design and manage an RCT of GP-fundholding, randomly allocating volunteer practices to be either fundholding or control practices. It was not practicable to perform such a trial because it would have taken three or more years to complete, and policy-makers operate on a timescale that does not generally admit of such delays. Although it would have been feasible to identify pilot practices as a 'simpler' trial design than an RCT, this strategy would have been unacceptable to policy-makers: it could have been interpreted as uncertainty about the policy of GP-fundholding, and uncertainty is not a characteristic that policy-makers like to display.

The policy of GP-fundholding has now been evaluated in several observational cohort studies, conclusions from two of which are given below.

> No evidence existed that budgetary pressures caused first wave fundholders to reduce referral rates, although the method of budget allocation may have encouraged general practitioners to inflate their referral rates in the preparatory year. Despite investment in new practice facilities, no evidence yet exists that fundholding encourages a shift away from specialist care.[3]

> Fundholding has altered practice prescribing patterns compared with those of non-fundholders, increasing generic prescribing and reducing the rate of increase of prescribing costs.[4]

Despite the usefulness of these studies, they are evaluations of a policy already in place; as such they are examples of policy-based research, not research-based policy. Similarly, a search for research evidence on purchasing healthcare in the UK[5,6] or on self-governing Trusts[7,8] will identify only articles on work done *after* the introduction of such policies.

7.9.4.1 The NHS Plan

The NHS Plan,[9] published in the year 2000, is a 10–year plan for:

- investment in the NHS;
- reform of the NHS.

The purpose of the plan is to develop a health service for the 21st century that is designed around the patient.

Within the plan, there is an acceptance, on the basis of the available evidence, that it is possible to improve the performance of the NHS. Mechanisms are outlined through which knowledge can be put into action, for example, the introduction of care pathways and systems of care for the treatment of various conditions based on the evidence of benefit that is currently available. In addition, it is recognised that traditional management techniques can be effective provided that a single message is used as the basis for change. However, some of the proposals, such as the establishment of a Modernisation Agency, are based on a belief, supported by some evidence, that the existing management structure has not been entirely effective and that a new approach is needed.

While accepting that the NHS is unique and that evidence arising from the assessment of other health systems cannot necessarily be applied without thorough critical appraisal, it is to be hoped that the changes proposed in *The NHS Plan* will be regarded as an 'N of 1' trial (see Section 5.4.1.3), and progress towards a set of objectives is to be measured and evaluated in an unbiased and systematic way.

7.9.5 Public health policy-making

For public health policy-making, there is a greater body of research evidence available on which to base decisions, and as such there is a greater tradition of using evidence in decision-making (see Section 3.5).

Public health has been defined as the improvement of health through the organised efforts of society – social interventions. Interventions that cannot be undertaken by individual members of the public or individual clinicians include:

- screening programmes;
- immunisation programmes;
- environmental protection.

Screening and immunisation programmes are simple public health interventions that can be considered as analogous to interventions in clinical practice. As such, the effectiveness of these interventions should be evaluated within systematic reviews of trials and RCTs (see Section 3.4). Environmental protection policies, however, are a different type of social intervention designed to remove or reduce risk. For these interventions, evaluation comprises a two-stage process:

1. establishing that a particular factor, or set of factors, increases the risk of a disease;
2. establishing that policies to reduce risk are feasible, effective, and affordable.

7.9.5.1   Does the evidence show an increased risk?

It is important to bear in mind throughout the following discussion that there is usually no qualitative difference between 'high' and 'low' risk.

In public health, risk factor analysis is commonly required to determine whether a cluster of cases of a particular condition has occurred by chance or constitutes an 'epidemic' that has an environmental cause. In epidemiological research, risk factors can be identified and quantified within cohort studies (Section 5.6) and case-control studies (Section 5.5); however, personnel in service public health departments are often asked about a health hazard which may have been publicised by the media – for example, the public perception that there has been a rapid increase in the incidence of childhood leukaemia related to, or reported in the media as 'caused by', electricity power lines.

It is relatively easy to answer such queries if evidence is available from cohort or case-control studies, or an expert is on hand who can give a scientific briefing based on the strength of evidence about the magnitude of the risk. It is more difficult when a director of public health is faced with the media eager to know if there is an epidemic of a particular cancer, what the cause is and what the health service is doing about it. The incidence of every non-communicable disease fluctuates with time; when the disease is uncommon and numbers of sufferers are small, fluctuations that would be unremarkable if large numbers of cases occurred regularly can appear to be dramatic. In this situation, a director of public health must decide whether the increase in incidence is greater than that which would be expected by chance.

Statistical techniques for the analysis of disease clusters can be exceptionally difficult to perform; indeed, the use of some techniques is limited to those who have degrees in mathematics and statistics. It is, however, essential for public health policy-makers to understand the application of various techniques in the analysis of clusters of disease – sometimes called 'extreme data'. The most accessible and comprehensible paper on the subject is by Palmer.[10] He describes a simple method that can be used to measure the 'degree of surprise' to patterns of data classified by time and place, which will help any decision-maker presented with such data to detect 'significant departures from random variation'.[8]

Palmer based this paper on a real health problem. In one health region of the UK (at a time when there was a configuration of 14 regional health authorities), one of the eight health districts in that region had the highest annual incidence of a particular disease on four occasions in six years. There was an obvious need to identify whether this was a cause for concern (a 'surprise') or simply due to chance. The approach Palmer took to determine this point will become increasingly important as league tables of performance are published: he reviewed conventional techniques used to analyse disease clusters, such as longitudinal data analysis and the Friedman two-way analysis of variance, and presented a simple, easily understandable alternative.

He warns against placing too much emphasis on the probability level of 0.05 – the 'surprise threshold' – because a probability below 0.05 is not impossible, it is simply less likely. Anyone responsible for the health of a population presented with either population-based data on mortality or data relating to the performance of different health services serving that population should either be able to carry out the type of analysis outlined in Palmer's paper or have access to personnel who can do so.

He also identified a trap into which most people fall: that of focusing solely on the performer at the 'wrong' end of any league table, depending upon whether appearance at the top or bottom indicates a problem. Palmer gives guidance on other statistical approaches that can be used, including the facility to take account of ranking over a period of time, such as the repeated appearance of a provider unit in the worst five of a league table.

7.9.5.2 Is it possible to reduce the risk?

Once a risk to the public health has been identified, a policy-maker must decide:

- if an intervention can reduce that risk;
- if it is possible to introduce the intervention(s) necessary to reduce that risk;
- whether the measures taken to reduce the risk that is the main cause of concern will increase other risks;
- what the cost would be to save a life or provide an added year of life (cost-effectiveness and cost-utility studies are of particular importance in public health policy-making because the costs of prevention can be surprisingly high – see Section 6.7).

7.9.5.3 The use of legislation to promote public health

The traditional role of law is to protect the individual from harm by third parties rather than to protect the public health.

There is an inverse relationship between the magnitude of a health problem and the strength of opposition to legislation framed to prevent it (see Fig. 7.9). When public concern about a problem exceeds public opposition to legislation, a threshold is crossed and it is possible to legislate for the implementation of a policy.

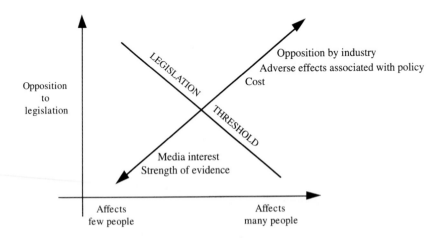

Fig. 7.9
Factors affecting the 'legislation threshold': those at the right-hand end of the double-headed arrow will raise the threshold whereas those on the left-hand end will lower it

However, the level of that threshold can be influenced by many factors other than the magnitude of the health problem; some of these factors raise the threshold while others lower it. Strong evidence is now a necessary prerequisite before any public health policy can be introduced, but the converse is not true: the existence of strong evidence indicating the need for a public health policy does not necessarily result in such a policy being introduced.

Greater obstacles are faced when using the law to implement a public health policy with the aim of protecting individuals from their own inclinations – the paternalistic role of law. Powerful evidence is needed to show that such legislation is not only effective but also safe. When legislation was being drafted to make the wearing of seat belts compulsory, a law that now seems uncontroversial, it was argued that the state should not introduce paternalistic legislation for the benefit of a large number of people if it resulted in the unnecessary harm of even one person. It was considered tantamount to sacrificing one person for the benefit of other people who did not wish to take protective action of their own volition.

There is evidence that controls on cigarette advertising can play a part in preventing teenage smoking, but that evidence is not regarded as strong enough to justify a policy of statutory, as opposed to voluntary, control of advertising. As so often occurs in policy-making, values can outweigh evidence.

7.9.6 Evidence-based policy-making in the developing world

Although most of the work referred to in Section 7.9 has been undertaken in developed countries, evidence-based policy-making is of paramount importance in developing countries. However, the availability of research evidence may be limited because the performance of RCTs in countries with limited resources can be problematic. Despite this, it is possible to carry out high-quality controlled trials in poor countries but it does require considerable commitment and skill. The Collaborative Eclampsia Trial,[11] in which the effects of different anticonvulsant regimens on recurrent convulsions and maternal mortality in women suffering from eclampsia were investigated, was designed such that:

- the results could be applicable to areas where maternal mortality is highest;
- it could be conducted within existing health services;
- treating women within the trial was easier and faster for clinicians than treating women outside it, to ensure that clinicians were not burdened and large numbers of women could be included.

The authors point to the low attrition, high compliance, and completeness of data collection in this study as indicators of the achievement of these aims.

In an excellent study to assess the impact of fly control on the incidence of childhood diarrhoea in Pakistan,[12] six villages were randomly allocated to one of two groups (A and B); two villages acted as controls. It was found that during the fly seasons (March–June) in both 1995 and 1996 the application of insecticide practically eliminated the fly population in the treated villages. Moreover, the incidence of diarrhoea was lower in the treated villages in both 1995 and 1996; the reduction in incidence was 23%. Baited fly traps were not effective in this setting (assessed according to fly density data). The authors conclude that fly control can have an impact on the incidence of diarrhoea similar to, or greater than, that of interventions currently recommended by WHO for inclusion in diarrhoeal disease control programmes.

In a study of the introduction of a community-based maternity-care delivery system in Matlab, Bangladesh,[13] it appeared that the new service had significantly reduced direct obstetric mortality when compared with the three years prior to the introduction of the programme. However, Ronsmans et al. investigated whether this effect was sustained over time. They found that although the introduction of the maternity-care programme coincided with a declining trend in direct obstetric mortality in the areas covered by the programme, a decline also occurred in one of the areas not covered by the programme. Therefore, it is necessary to exercise caution in the interpretation of a short-term trend in only one indicator in studies that have been designed without random allocation of the intervention to a treatment and a control group.

References

1. MOYNIHAN, D.P. (1995) The Congressional Record, 12 December 1995. Reproduced as *Congress builds a coffin*, New York Review of Books, January 11 1996, pp 33–6.
2. MUSGROVE, P., CRESE, A., PREKER, A., BAEZA, C., ANELL, A. and PRENTICE, T. (Principal writers) (2000) *The World Health Report 2000 – Health Systems: improving performance.* The World Health Organization, Geneva. Available at http//www.who.int/whr/2000/en/report.htm
3. SURENDER, R., BRADLOW, J., COULTER, A., DOLL, H. and STEWART-BROWN, S. (1995) *Prospective study of trends in referral patterns in fundholding and non-fundholding practices in the Oxford Region 1990–1994.* Br. Med. J. 311: 1205–8.
4. WILSON, R.P.H., BUCHAN, I. and WALLEY, T. (1995) *Alterations in prescribing by general practitioners: an observational study.* Br. Med. J. 311: 1347–50.
5. GHODSE, B. (1995) *Extracontractural referrals: safety valve or administrative paperchase?* Br. Med. J. 310: 1573–6.
6. KLEIN, R. and REDMAYNE, S. (1992) *Patterns of Priorities: A Study of the Purchasing and Rationing Policies of Health Authorities.* National Association of Health Authorities and Trusts, Birmingham.
7. SHIELL, A. (1991) *Competing hospitals: assessing the impact of self-governing status in the United Kingdom.* Health Policy 19(2–3): 141–58.
8. SPURGEON, P. (1994) *Purchaser/provider relationships: current practice and future prospects.* Health Service Manage. Res. 7: 195–200.
9. Department of Health (2000) *The NHS Plan. A plan for investment. A plan for reform.* The Stationery Office, London. Available at: http://www.nhs.uk/nationalplan/
10. PALMER, C.R. (1993) *Probability of recurrence of extreme data: an aid to decision making.* Lancet 342: 845–7.
11. THE ECLAMPSIA TRIAL COLLABORATIVE GROUP (1995) *Which anticonvulsant for women with eclampsia? Evidence from the Collaborative Eclampsia Trial.* Lancet 345: 1455–63.
12. CHAVASSE, D.C., SHIER, R.P., MURPHY, O.A., HUTTLY, S.R.A., COUSENS, S.N. and AKHTAR, T. (1999) *Impact of fly control on childhood diarrhoea in Pakistan: community-randomised trial.* Lancet 353: 22–5.
13. RONSMANS, C., VANNESTE, A.M., CHAKRABORTY, J. and van GINNEKEN, J. (1997) *Decline in maternal mortality in Matlab, Bangladesh: a cautionary tale.* Lancet 350: 1810–14.

7.10 EVIDENCE-BASED LITIGATION

7.10.1 'Evidence' in court

Although the word 'evidence' is much used in court, the nature of the evidence that is presented and appraised there, and upon which judgements are made, differs in quality to the nature of the evidence discussed in this book (see Table 7.9).

Table 7.9 The qualities of evidence in two different contexts

Evidence in court	Evidence used in an evidence-based approach
Opinion of experts	Evidence based on research
All or nothing	Probabilistic

In the judicial system of some countries, e.g. the UK and the USA, expert witnesses can be called to give 'evidence'. However, this evidence may merely reflect the expert's opinion rather than be based on evidence derived from research. Indeed, both the prosecution and the defence try to find an expert whose opinion will support their case. In the USA, an 'expert' industry has developed, in which big companies maintain and support experts in research institutions and ensure that their work is publicised (as opposed to published) in the media.

Furthermore, after an expert has given an opinion, its generalisability and relevance to the individual case under judgement appears to be treated with remarkable naivety.

Probabilistic thinking is inimical to a system in which the outcome is either 'guilty' or 'not guilty', and its potential contribution in this situation has been emphatically ruled out in the UK by the Bench of the Court of Appeal, as one President of the Royal Statistical Society described in his Presidential address.[1]

> Evidence of the Bayes Theorem or any similar statistical method of analysis in a criminal trial plunged the jury into inappropriate and unnecessary realms of theory and complexity, deflecting them from their proper task ... Their Lordships ... had very grave doubts as to whether that evidence was properly admissible because it trespassed on an area peculiarly and exclusively within the jury's province, namely the way in which they evaluated the relationship between one piece of evidence and

another. The Bayes Theorem might be an appropriate and useful tool for statisticians, but it was not appropriate for use in jury trials or as a means to assist the jury in its task.

The sometimes dramatic consequences of exploiting the potential of accepting 'expert' opinion as evidence in court in the USA are described by Marcia Angell in *Science on Trial*,[2] a brilliant book about the legal handling of the purported harmful effects of breast implants. Despite the lack of research-based evidence that breast implants increase the risk of autoimmune disease, an action totalling $4.25 billion evolved in which more than 400 000 women believed themselves to have been harmed by implants. This belief was fired by media and legal hyperbole, supported by the opinion of 'experts' who had published nothing of note on the subject. Apart from the fact that many lawyers have become fabulously rich working on such cases, the most dispiriting aspect of this saga is the lack of impact the type of evidence that readers of this book might accept actually had on the judges or the jurors. Prosecution lawyers even subpoenaed, and accused of conspiracy, the *New England Journal of Medicine*, of which Dr Angell is the Executive Editor, when it published the Food and Drug Administration's statement on breast implants[3] in conjunction with Dr Angell's editorial.[4]

In the UK, the matter of breast implants was dealt with somewhat differently. The departments of health commissioned an independent review group to conduct a systematic review of the evidence. The conclusion was that silicone gel breast implants 'are not associated with any greater health risk than other surgical implants' and there is 'no evidence of an association with an abnormal immune response or typical or atypical connective tissue disease or syndromes'.[5]

An interesting and important focus in the report is the need for evidence-based patient choice. In the chapter entitled 'Consent to medical treatment', the need to give patients full, clear and written information is emphasised. This is the first time the need for patients to be given 'full knowledge' has been made explicit in a document of this type, and, as knowledge becomes a dominant commodity in society (see Section 7.1.5.1), the provision of best current knowledge to patients must become standard practice.[6]

However, plaintiff lawyers are not always villains. In American society where the welfare safety net is gossamer thin, they can help the poor and disadvantaged obtain the resources they need to cope with the effects of disease. Such a situation is described by Peter Pringle in his book *Dirty Business*,[7] the story of the legal battle to hold American tobacco companies to account for the damage caused to the public health.

7.10.2 Death of an expert witness

The death of the expert witness may now be imminent. In a famous case brought to trial in America, *Daubert et al. v. Merrell Dow Pharmaceuticals*, concerning the role of Benedictin in causing birth defects, the judgement held that federal trial judges have the responsibility to ensure that an expert's testimony is reliable and relevant.[8] Judges are now required to undertake: 'a preliminary assessment of whether the testimony's underlying reasoning or methodology is scientifically valid and properly can be applied to the facts at issue.' (cited in ref. 8).

To fulfil this expanded responsibility for determining the validity of scientific evidence, the judiciary has made greater use of a long-held responsibility to appoint any expert witness agreed upon by the parties, and of its own selection. These panels are known as 'Daubert panels' and their functions are:

* to assess the qualifications of expert witnesses;
* to evaluate the evidence;
* to assess the nature of the issues.

Hulka et al.[8] report on their experiences as members of the National Science Panel appointed by Judge Pointer, who was responsible for overseeing all federal cases involving silicone gel-filled breast implants. The Panel was charged with providing the federal judiciary with unbiased scientific evidence on the relation between silicone breast implants and connective tissue diseases and autoimmune dysfunction. They believe that such panels should be used more frequently because they can bring unbiased information about complex scientific and medical matters into the courtroom.

This move has not been popular, particularly with those who make a good living as expert witnesses, but it marks the beginning of the end of opinion masquerading as evidence in court.

7.10.3 The influence of clinical guidelines in malpractice litigation

The application of medical practice guidelines in courts may also accelerate the decline of the use of expert witnesses.

In a survey of 960 randomly selected medical malpractice attorneys in the USA, Hyams et al.[9] investigated the lawyers' awareness of medical practice guidelines and the use of guidelines in malpractice litigation. The authors also conducted a computerised search to find cases in the US courts in which medical practice guidelines and standards had been used from January 1980 to 31 May 1994.

There was a 60% response rate to the survey. One half of the attorneys who responded were 'very' or 'somewhat' aware of the concept of medical practice guidelines. The search of the US courts' practice yielded 28 cases in which guidelines were used successfully: in 22 of these, the guidelines were used to support the plaintiff's case; in the remaining six they were used to support the defendant, i.e. the clinician. The search also disclosed seven cases in which plaintiffs were unsuccessful in using guidelines and two cases in which defendants were unsuccessful in using guidelines.

In reviewing the different perspectives on medical practice guidelines – professionals and the funders of healthcare see them as a 'one-way street' designed to favour clinicians, whereas the courts and attorneys for the plaintiff see them as a 'one-way street' in favour of the plaintiff – the authors conclude that guidelines have been applied as two-way streets, i.e. as evidence to support either side's case. However, it would appear that attorneys for the plaintiff are more active in finding and using guidelines than those for the defendant. Hyams et al. believe that 'on the whole practice guidelines are a rationalising force in malpractice litigation'.

7.10.4 Failure to act on the evidence

There is the possibility that failure of a health professional to act on evidence of effective forms of care might *ipso facto* be grounds for litigation brought by patients. In a debate about the importance of research and development conducted in *The Health Service Journal*, one correspondent urged patients and patients' organisations to consider using this strategy as an option for the future.

Five years ago I wrote to *The Lancet* speculating that parents might begin to sue the Royal College of Obstetricians and Gynaecologists because it had taken so long to promote use of prenatal steroids, which research had shown reduced the risk that premature babies would die or survive handicapped. I might have added that there would be a case for suing the health authorities and trusts which were acquiescing in under-use of prenatal steroids, particularly as they also reduce health service costs.

Both as a potential patient and a taxpayer, I was prompted by parts of Barbara Millar's article to ask when patients will begin to sue HAs and trusts for ignoring research. A mass of research evidence relevant to the wellbeing of NHS users is available, much of it through the NHS R&D Programme. Over two years ago, in the NHS Executive's paper *Promoting Clinical Effectiveness*, it was made clear that 'every NHS trust should have access to up-to-date sources of information such as the Cochrane and Centre for Reviews and Dissemination databases'. Yet last year an article in the *Journal* (Who's acting on the evidence?, 3 April 1997) made it clear that this advice was being widely ignored by trusts.

...

I urge patients and patients' organisations to consider suing HAs and trusts which are ignoring the important information available through the NHS R&D Programme. As a potential patient, I will certainly consider suing if I am not offered forms of care which have been shown to be effective for people experiencing heart attacks, strokes and trauma.[10]

References

1. SMITH, A. (1996) *Mad cows and ecstasy: chance and choice in an evidence-based society.* J.R. Stat. Assoc. A 159: 367–83.
2. ANGELL, M. (1996) *Science on Trial.* W.W. Norton, New York.
3. KESSLER, D. (1992) *The basis for the FDA's decision on breast implants.* N. Engl. J. Med. 326: 1713–15.
4. ANGELL, M. (1992) *Breast implants: protection or paternalism? [Editorial]* N. Engl. J. Med. 326: 1695–6.
5. INDEPENDENT REVIEW GROUP (1998) *Silicone Gel Breast Implants. The Report of the Independent Review Group.* Prepared for publication by Jill Rogers Associates, Cambridge. Available at: http://www.silicone-review.gov.uk/silicone_implants.pdf

6. GRAY, J.A.M. (1999) *Breast implants: evidence based patient choice and litigation. The only safety lies in providing patients with full information.* Br. Med. J. 318: 414.
7. PRINGLE, P. (1998) *Dirty Business. Big Tobacco at the Bar of Justice.* Aurum Press, London.
8. HULKA, B.S., KERKVLIET, N.L. and TUGWELL, P. (2000) *Experience of a scientific panel formed to advise the Federal Judiciary on silicone breast implants.* N. Engl. J. Med. 342: 812–15.
9. HYAMS, A.L., SHAPIRO, D.W. and BRENNAN, T.A. (1996) *Medical practice guidelines in malpractice litigation: an early retrospective.* J. Health Polit. Policy Law 21: 289–313.
10. CHALMERS, I. (1998) *Patients should sue when available research isn't put into practice [Letter].* Health Service J. 108(5599): 18.

7.11 THE ETHICS OF PRIORITISATION – THE INDIVIDUAL OR SOCIETY?

Any robust interrogation of the individual who wishes to do good for society highlights the problems of utilitarianism, the ethical system devised by John Stuart Mill in which the concept of 'the greatest good for the greatest number' was promoted.

Those who have to make decisions about groups or populations often adopt a utilitarian approach, but the utilitarian approach can lead to what Mill in his famous essay, *On Liberty,* called 'the tyranny of the majority'. In a health service, the application of the greatest good for the greatest number will always result in the provision of treatment for people who have common diseases, thus aggravating the problems of those who suffer from rare diseases. Moreover, although such patients certainly benefit from attracting the interest of their medical advisers, it is likely that therapies are few in number and expensive because the pharmaceutical industry is generally less likely to invest in R&D to find a therapy for a disease from which a thousand people suffer than for one from which a million people suffer.

During prioritisation, therefore, it is important to recognise that at the end of each decision there is an individual. This is an unpleasant and difficult fact to accept, but those who make decisions about groups and populations must remain continually aware of it.

Gentle Reader,

Empathise with the public health physician who had just put down Dickens' Bleak House with a strong sense of déjà vu. He had been reading Chapter 4 in which the young hero pays his first visit to the Jellybys to find Mrs Jellyby in great form, busily sorting out the problems of Africa.

'You find me, my dears,' said Mrs Jellyby, snuffing the two great office candles in tin candlesticks which made the room taste strongly of hot tallow (the fire had gone out, and there was nothing in the grate but ashes, a bundle of wood, and a poker), 'you find me, my dears, as usual, very busy; but that you will excuse. The African project at present employs my whole time. It involves me in correspondence with public bodies, and with private individuals anxious for the welfare of their species all over the country. I am happy to say it is advancing. We hope by this time next year to have from a hundred and fifty to two hundred healthy families cultivating coffee and educating the natives of Borrioboola-Gha, on the left bank of the Niger.'

Commentary

Mrs Jellyby was engaged in a great public health initiative; unfortunately she spent so much of her effort on Africa that her own house was in great disorder: the dinner was delayed 'in consequence of such accidents as the dish of potatoes being mislaid in the coal scuttle, and the handle of the corkscrew coming off, and striking the young woman in the chin'. Throughout dinner, Mrs Jellyby had continued to discuss her good works with a reforming zeal that was excellent. However, the dinner itself was not quite of the same standard, as Miss Summerson recorded: 'We had a fine codfish, a piece of roast beef, a dish of cutlets, and a pudding; an excellent dinner, if it had had any cooking to speak of, but it was almost raw'.

Public health professionals have been prominent in the promotion of evidence-based decision-making in healthcare but the evidence base of public health itself is not particularly well established. It would be appropriate if some of the energy of the public health establishment currently being directed at encouraging others to be more evidence based were used to strengthen the evidence base of public health itself.

CHAPTER 8

EVIDENCE-BASED PUBLIC HEALTH

More than any other branch of healthcare, decision-making in public health has been based on the application of guidelines and 'laws'. Indeed, the epistemology of public health has had a long evolution, starting with a basis in the scriptures and for many centuries in a combination of religion and magic. The Enlightenment led people to look for natural, rather than supernatural, explanations of disease causation and prevention. Once natural causes of disease gained acceptance, progress in public health was made during the 19th century, to which Victorian concerns for order and cleanliness contributed. However, in the second half of the 19th century, an empirical approach was adopted that led to the development and use of statistics, on which were founded the movements towards epidemiologically and evidence-based public health.

8.1.1 Scripturally based public health

Zoologists classify the rock badger as a member of the family *Melidae,* together with the skunk. Moses, however, classified it with the camel, the hare and the pig, and declared these animals to be 'unclean', prohibiting the consumption of their flesh. Animals that Moses did consider to be clean and whose flesh could be eaten were ruminants that have hooves. In her anthropological analysis of pollution, entitled *Purity and Danger,*[1] Mary Douglas points out that the type of animals approved by the Mosaic Law set out in Leviticus – oxen, sheep and goats – were thought of as almost human, even holy.

This law-giving earned Moses the accolade of the first public health legislator from some 19th century historians, but Moses had not proscribed the flesh of swine because he suspected it carried parasites but because pigs were not ruminants and as such were unclean. Those who argued that the proscription of pork provides an early example of public health legislation are guilty of 'medical materialism', a term coined by the American psychologist and philosopher William James, brother of the writer Henry. In his book *The Varieties of Religious Experience,*[2] James defined medical materialism as the retrospective attachment of medical meanings to acts undertaken for other purposes. Pork was proscribed by Moses not because of the prevalence of *Taenia solium* but because it was part of a social process that enabled the Jews to distinguish themselves from other peoples.

8.1.2 Supernaturally based public health

Before the Enlightenment, it was common for people to ascribe the causes of disease to supernatural rather than natural phenomena. Disease of either individuals or populations was perceived as the result of God's displeasure or as a manifestation of the malice of others. Religion and magic were used to explain both causation and outcome, as Keith Thomas so eloquently describes in his classic work, *Religion and the Decline of Magic.*[3] Although at this time certain interventions were implemented that might have limited the spread of disease, notably preventing the egress of people from towns and cities during episodes of the plague, and the shunning and isolation of lepers, these measures probably had little effect. They almost certainly originated from atavistic fears and an aversion to the sight of disability rather than a logical analysis of the natural causes of disease, and the identification of appropriate means of preventing and treating it.

8.1.3 Aesthetically based public health

After the Enlightenment, natural, rather than supernatural, explanations of the causation of disease began to be accepted, and a scientific approach to intervention became the prevailing paradigm.

The prevention of disease was a prominent social issue in the first half of the 19th century, partly because people were stimulated by the new scientific approach to disease but also because public attitudes were shaped by the diseases prevalent in society at that time.

8.1.3.1 Fear as an agent of social change

Tuberculosis was the commonest cause of death when Victoria came to the throne. In the first report of the Registrar General, 17.6% of all deaths were attributed to tuberculosis. Associated with poor diet and bad housing, tuberculosis, known as consumption or phthisis, was greatly feared, yet perhaps because it was ubiquitous it provoked much less public reaction than the epidemics of typhus and cholera.

Typhus had been endemic in the UK for hundreds of years, but during hard times the number of people affected by typhus increased very rapidly. Terrible though typhus was, it did not seem to create quite as much public concern as cholera. During the 19th century, cholera spread from its initial source in India along the trade routes through Afghanistan, Persia, and Europe. In 1831, William IV opened Parliament with a grave announcement of the 'continued progress of a formidable disease'. Four months later it had reached Hamburg, and the first officially recorded case in Britain was reported at the Port of Sunderland on 4 November 1831. Four great epidemics followed: in 1832, 1848–9, 1853–4, and 1866, throwing the whole country into turmoil. In his book *Cholera, 1832*, R. J. Morris suggests that the terror people felt during the first epidemic, and the lessons learnt, were soon forgotten; however, the repeated recurrence of cholera epidemics did contribute to a change in public opinion, and a realisation of the need to improve the environment, in part because cholera could be seen to affect rich and poor alike.[4]

The relative importance of typhus and cholera as agents of social change is difficult to assess. Although typhus was more frequently mentioned in the parliamentary debates leading to the enactment of the Public Health Act 1848, Norman Longmate's analysis[5] of the rioting that followed cholera epidemics indicated that cholera was at least as important a stimulus as typhus. This may be because cholera was perceived as alien, and evoked a range of emotional responses from the public which influenced their attitudes to health. Fear of disease, therefore, provided the stimulus for change, but on what basis did the Victorians decide which changes to make?

8.1.3.2 Knowledge as an agent of social change

The contribution of new knowledge to improving the public health during the 19th century is even more difficult to assess. Despite the fact that the 19th century saw the birth of bacteriology, pathology, and physiology, new knowledge appears to have been only a weak agent for change. For instance, Pasteur's theory of germs was not established until 1865, more than a decade after the first Public Health Act. Moreover, although John Snow had demonstrated the link between water and the spread of cholera by removing the handle from the water pump in Soho's Broad Street – no further cases of cholera occurred in the surrounding area which had hitherto been heavily affected – it took many years for Snow's hypothesis to be universally accepted over the popular view that cholera was carried by a miasma of foul air because of the dominance of the theory of 'nuisances'.

Legislators in the 19th century operated on the principle enunciated by Sir John Simon that: 'the interests of health and the interests of common physical comfort and convenience are in various cases identical'.

The title of the Nuisance Removal and Disease Prevention Act epitomises this principle which, however sound, was not based on scientific evidence.

As a consequence, public health measures were largely directed at increasing order and reducing the level of sensory insults, for example, removing or cleansing anything that was offensive, such as the accumulation of sewage, dwellings infested with vermin, or the keeping of pigs near human habitation. Two important themes began to emerge.

1. *Cleanliness is next to godliness.* One of the characteristics of middle class life in 19th century Britain was an increasing preoccupation with cleanliness and, as a corollary to this, the identification of the poor as a section of society who were unclean.

2. *Order is an enemy of disease.* The word 'nuisance' derives from the Old French word 'nuire', meaning to hurt or injure, and nuisances were considered to be offensive to the senses and, *ipso facto*, in 19th century thinking, dangerous to health. However, any threat to the health of individuals was also conceived of as a threat to the health of society. One of the aspects of 19th century life that alarmed the middle class, who by that time were important politically, was the disorder of the poor.

Action taken to tackle disorder, for example, improving housing or clearing slums, was seen as benefiting not only the health of the individuals directly concerned but also society as a whole by eliminating chaos and counteracting potential subversion or insurrection.

Although there was opposition to several of the public health measures proposed – for example, from some of the water companies – such conflict between certain sections of society and the authorities created a tension which probably furthered the prevention debate, and led to an acceptance of the need for public health legislation. Social change rarely takes place in an atmosphere of indifference.

However, by building on observation and occasional experiment, the Victorians were able to formulate a knowledge base to improve the public health that comprised three main tenets:

1. the supply of drinking water should be kept separate from the disposal of sewage;
2. good housing that has adequate ventilation is essential to health;
3. a good diet increases resistance to disease.

Using this simple knowledge base, significant gains in public health were made for about 100 years from 1850 to 1950.

8.1.3.3   The Siege of Krishnapur – miasmatists vs Snowites

In general, measures to create an orderly society and promote cleanliness were beneficial in improving health and preventing disease, but sometimes the application of the principle that cleanliness and order were the enemies of disease was completely erroneous. This is best exemplified by the debate about the cause of cholera. The infectious agent is the bacterium *Vibrio cholerae*, which is spread either directly between individuals or by drinking contaminated water. Indeed, one school of thought led by John Snow did believe contaminated water was the cause; however, adherents to another school of thought believed that the presence of an offensive smell was indicative of a miasma of foul air which was the principal cause of cholera.

In J. G. Farrell's novel, *The Siege of Krishnapur*,[6] this controversy was personified in the characters of Dr Dunstaple, a miasmatist, and Dr McNab, who believed that water, even if it looked, smelt and tasted pure, was the cause of the spread of cholera, a disease that was rife in the enclosed community besieged by mutineers.

Dr Dunstaple's miasmatist arguments are encapsulated in the quotation below.

> Let me now read to you the conclusion of Dr Baly in his *Report on Epidemic Cholera*, drawn up at the desire of the Royal College of Physicians and published in 1854. Dr Baly finds the only theory satisfactorily supported by evidence is that 'which regards the cause of cholera as a matter increasing by some process, whether chemical or organic, in impure or damp air' ... I repeat, 'in impure or damp air'. Dr Dunstaple paused triumphantly for a moment to allow the significance of this to seep in.

> Many supporters of Dr McNab exchanged glances of dismay at the words they had just heard. They had not realized that Dr Dunstaple had the support of the Royal College of Physicians ... and felt distinctly aggrieved that they had not been told that such an august body disagreed with their own man. Two or three of Dr McNab's supporters wasted no time in surreptitiously slipping their cards of emergency instructions from their pockets, crossing out the name McNab, and substituting that of his rival, before settling back to watch their new champion in the lists. The Magistrate noted this with satisfaction. How much more easily they were swayed by prestige than by arguments!

> Meanwhile Dr Dunstaple was continuing to disprove Dr McNab's drinking-water theories.

> 'Ladies and gentlemen, the fact that cholera is conveyed in the atmosphere is amply supported by the epidemic in Newcastle in 1853 when it became clear that during the months of September and October an invisible cholera cloud was suspended over the town. Few persons living in Newcastle during this period escaped without suffering some of the symptoms that are inescapably associated with cholera, if not the disease itself. They suffered from pains in the head or indescribable sensations of uneasiness in the bowels. Furthermore, the fact of strangers coming into Newcastle from a distance in perfect health ... and not having had any contact

with cholera case ... being then suddenly seized with premonitory symptoms, and speedily passing into collapse, proves that it was the result of atmospheric infection.

8.1.4 Statistically based public health

She found statistics 'more enlivening than a novel' and loved to 'bite on a hard fact'. Dr Farr wrote in January 1860: 'I have a New Year's Gift for you. It is in the shape of Tables.' 'I am exceedingly anxious to see your charming Gift,' she replied, 'especially those returns showing the Deaths, Admissions, Diseases.' Hilary Bonham Carter wrote that however exhausted Florence might be the sight of long columns of figures was 'perfectly reviving' to her.

Cecil Woodham-Smith,
Florence Nightingale 1820–1910[7]

Although in the early part of the 19th century public health measures had been based largely on the removal of any offence to the senses, in the latter part, the use of statistical information started to become influential in the response to disease. Indeed, the 19th century provided an empirical basis for public health.

One figure dominates this movement towards statistically based public health – Florence Nightingale. In January 1855, she documented in breathtaking detail not only the conditions of the wounded and dying at Scutari in Albania but also the process of care and the resources available (see, for example, Table 8.1). The mass of facts

Table 8.1 An example of one of Florence Nightingale's requisitions on the Purveyor for supplies required for Barrack Hospital (Source: Woodham-Smith[7])

Flannel shirts	Answer	None in store
Socks	"	None in store
Drawers	"	None in store

N.B. There are some tea-pots and coffee-pots.

Required for Barrack Hospital		
Plates	"	None in store
Tin drinking cups	"	None in store
Earthenware urine cups	"	Metal plenty
Bedpans	"	Some
Close stools	"	Plenty but frames missing
Pails for tea	"	None at present

and figures she collected led to the establishment of a Sanitary Commission which was sent from Great Britain to investigate the sanitary state of the buildings used as hospitals, and of the camps both at Scutari and in the Crimea.

Although some of Nightingale's general theories were wrong – she still believed in the harmful effects of 'poisonous gases' – her drive to create order out of disorder and improve sanitary conditions was beneficial. Following the orders of the Commissioners to clear the courtyard and precincts of the hospital, during the first fortnight of this work, 556 handcarts and large baskets full of rubbish were removed, as well as 26 dead animals, including two horses; indeed, the water supply for the greater part of the hospital was found to be passing through the decaying carcass of a horse.[7] Moreover, drinking water was stored in tanks next to the temporary privies that had been erected for the men suffering from diarrhoea.

In addition to her pioneering work at Scutari and in the Crimea, Nightingale published *Notes on Matters affecting the Health, Efficiency and Hospital Administration of the British Army*, which consists of almost 1000 closely printed pages packed with figures, tables, and statistical comparisons proving that the hospital was more fatal than the battlefield.[7] She also became involved in measures to improve civil hospitals, encouraged in this venture by Dr William Farr, a pioneer of the science of statistics. In 1859, she published *Notes on Hospitals*, and followed this up by drafting model hospital statistical forms which would:

> ... enable us to ascertain the relative mortality of different hospitals, as well as of different diseases and injuries at the same and at different ages, the relative frequency of different diseases and injuries among the classes which enter hospitals in different countries, and in different districts of the same countries.
>
> *Quoted in ref. 7*

St Mary's Hospital, Paddington, St Thomas's, St Bartholomew's, and University College Hospital agreed to use these forms immediately.[7] (For an interesting twist to this tale, see Section 6.8.1.2.)

However, much of the work to develop the science of statistics and its application in government was completed by statisticians of lesser profile. In Ian Hacking's book *The*

Taming of Chance,[8] he describes the development of the official use of statistics. Early originators of this approach included Leibniz, whose zeal in data collection and the presentation of statistics contributed to the pre-eminence of Prussia, and Sir James Sinclair, who published a *Statistical Account of Scotland*, in which he attempted to measure not only the quantum of sickness but also the quantum of happiness.

Despite this developmental work, in the 19th century the science of statistics was based on a few simple premises, and relied on only one method – inference. The collection of mortality and morbidity statistics did little to further knowledge of the causation of disease following the breakthroughs that led to the identification of clean drinking water, good housing and good food as foundations for disease prevention. More sophisticated methods were required to identify other causes of ill-health, and to assess the effectiveness of any measures designed to improve the public health.

8.1.5 Epidemiologically based public health

In the 19th century, the prevailing view was that the causes of diseases were known, and statistics were used to determine progress in limiting the spread of disease and altering the environmental conditions in which disease was thought to thrive. In the 20th century, novel methods of generating and testing hypotheses about disease causation were developed within the discipline of epidemiology.

However, in the first half of the 20th century, only a few outstanding epidemiological studies were conducted, notably Goldberger's analysis of pellagra. It was not until the 1940s, during the darkest days of the Second World War, that public health, or social medicine as it was often called then, began its academic development. In 1940, J. M. Macintosh resigned as Chief Medical Officer at the Scottish Department of Health to become Professor of Public Health and Social Medicine at Glasgow, and in 1943 Ryle was appointed to the first Chair of Social Medicine in England.

In the years immediately after the Second World War, a small group of academics – Bradford Hill, Jerry Morris, Archie Cochrane, Richard Doll, and Thomas McKeown – developed the practice of social medicine and the underlying science of epidemiology. They realised that observation could be biased, and that the findings of investigations might arise as a result of chance and not the aetiological factor or therapeutic intervention which is the subject of a study. During this time, various methods for identifying the causes of disease and for identifying effective and efficient treatments were developed, particularly the randomised controlled trial, a methodology popularised and promoted by Archie Cochrane in his Rock Carling Lectures .[9] The flavour of this early work can be appreciated by reading Jerry Morris's classic monograph on *The Uses of Epidemiology,*[10] first published in 1957, and Archie Cochrane's autobiography.[11]

Thus, a new rigour was brought to statistics, and epidemiology was used to find the causes of disease, particularly those that were social and behavioural. The same techniques were also used to determine whether interventions to treat disease were effective.

8.1.5.1 Epidemiology as the foundation for public health practice

In response to criticism of the Faculty of Community Medicine's syllabus, in which some highlighted an insufficient emphasis on environmental health and on management and too much emphasis on epidemiology, the President at the time, Sir John Brotherston, replied:

> Are community medicine and epidemiology interchangeable terms? Is epidemiology a monopoly of community medicine ... epidemiology is a prime diagnostic tool to identify problems and needs but community medicine has a therapeutic responsibility to go beyond diagnosis to achieve action for improvement.[12]

Brotherston's definition highlights the analytical function of epidemiology.

8.1.6 Evidence-based public health

Public health is different to epidemiology: the aim of public health medicine is to improve the health of populations through the organised efforts of society. Therefore, interventions need to be based on good evidence of effectiveness in promoting the health of populations. However, the skills of public health professionals – from classical epidemiology to health economics, managerial skills, politics and sociology – enable them to promote evidence-based decision-making in all sectors of health and

healthcare. Thus, public health practitioners have a
responsibility not only to be evidence based in the
promotion of health but also to promote evidence-based
healthcare.

8.1.6.1   The promotion of evidence-based healthcare

As it is not possible for any health service to provide
universal healthcare for the entire population on demand, it
is necessary for priorities to be set. Following the
publication of Cochrane's famous monograph, *Efficiency
and Effectiveness*,[8] the most obvious criterion for
prioritisation in the provision of healthcare was efficiency,
the most important prerequisite of which is effectiveness.
Since the inception of the NHS's Research and
Development Programme in 1993, the need to assess the
effectiveness of interventions on the basis of evidence has
been reinforced, and public health professionals have
contributed to the development of an evaluative culture
through their roles in strategic commissioning and
education.

The rigour and systematic approach applied within
evidence-based practice influence, and are influenced by,
two of the emerging trends in healthcare provision, namely:

- the information revolution, and the resulting need to
  cope with uncertainty;
- the involvement and participation of patients in
  decision-making.

In the process of introducing an evidence-based
approach, another important feature of decision-making
has emerged – that of explicitness. Until now, there have
been neither obvious incentives nor opportunities to make
extrinsic and explicit all the values, judgements and facts
that underpin the decisions made during the provision of
healthcare. However, the need for explicitness in the
allocation of resources has been reinforced by social trends,
particularly the rise in consumerism, which has led to
demands for openness in decision-making at all levels from
government through to clinical consultations. This pressure
for explicitness necessitates that medicine is de-mystified
and health de-medicalised, for professionals, patients, the
general public and politicians alike.

8.1.6.2 *Future challenges*

There remain many challenges for practitioners of an evidence-based approach to face, and public health professionals have the skills to facilitate and mediate appropriate responses to three of these challenges.

The first challenge is to broaden the concept of effectiveness using criteria and standards that have been developed by people other than doctors and researchers. What do we mean when we use the word 'effective' and whose definition are we using?

The second challenge is to extend the emerging culture of critical appraisal. Key criteria are likely to be equity, efficiency, and affordability, without all three of which the concept of effectiveness has little meaning.

The third challenge is to supplement and complement the use of evidence from quantitative research, especially that derived from RCTs, with that from good-quality qualitative research. As the primary determinant of the effective management of a healthcare system is the competence and behaviour of the professionals within it, there needs to be an increase in the amount of behavioural research conducted. A starting point for this strategy is to provide good-quality training in various research methodologies and their appropriate usage.

Thus, the application of epidemiology alone is too narrow a base for an evidence-based approach to public health. It will be necessary to draw evidence from a wide variety of disciplines if public health professionals are to continue to identify the causes of ill-health *and* to prevent disease and promote health through the organised efforts of society.

References

1. DOUGLAS, M. (1993) *Purity and Danger: an Analysis of Concepts of Pollution and Taboo.* Routledge.
2. JAMES, W. (1902) *The Varieties of Religious Experience.* Collier Books, New York. [Reproduced in 1961 by Collier Macmillan Publishers.]
3. THOMAS, K. *Religion and the Decline of Magic.* [In print in paperback, Oxford University Press, 1997.]
4. MORRIS, R. J. (1976) *Cholera, 1832: The Social Response to an Epidemic.* Croom Helm.
5. LONGMATE, N. (1966) *King Cholera: The Biography of a Disease.* Hamish Hamilton, London.
6. FARRELL, J. G. (1973) *The Siege of Krishnapur.* George Weidenfeld and Nicolson, London. [In print in paperback, Orion Books, 1993.]
7. WOODHAM-SMITH, C. (1955) *Florence Nightingale 1820–1910.* Penguin Books, London.
8. HACKING, I. (1990) *The Taming of Chance.* Cambridge University Press, Cambridge.
9. COCHRANE, A. (1972) *Effectiveness and Efficiency.* The Nuffield Provincial Hospitals Trust, London.
10. MORRIS, J. B. (1957) *Uses of Epidemiology.* Churchill Livingstone, Edinburgh.
11. COCHRANE, A. L. with BLYTHE, M. (1989) *One Man's Medicine.* The Memoir Club – BMJ.
12. WARREN, M. D. (1997) *The Genesis of the Faculty of Community Medicine.* Centre for Health Service Studies, University of Kent at Canterbury.

8.2   EVIDENCE-BASED PUBLIC HEALTH INTERVENTIONS

Any intervention to improve the public health must act on at least one of the main determinants of health, which are shown in Fig. 8.1.

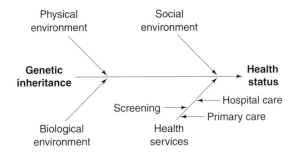

Fig. 8.1
The determinants of health

There are four types of intervention that can be used to improve public health:

- healthcare;
- educational;
- social;
- legislative.

However, before an intervention to improve the public health can be introduced, four factors – evidence, resources, and the needs and the values of the population – have to be taken into consideration, although the nature of the evidence required is different for each type of intervention.

8.2.1   Healthcare interventions

Most of the text of this book is about healthcare interventions in the way that they affect the health of populations rather than the health of individuals, for example, a screening programme or a new type of cancer care. Evidence of effectiveness of these interventions should meet the same requirements as that for the introduction of new treatments for individuals, with the systematic review of RCTs representing the gold standard.

8.2.2 Educational interventions

Educational interventions are currently subject to less
rigorous scrutiny than healthcare interventions. However,
the establishment of The Campbell Collaboration, a sibling
organisation to The Cochrane Collaboration, should ensure
that the degree of scrutiny will improve. The aim of The
Campbell Collaboration is to promote the development of
systematic reviews of evidence about educational and
social policy issues. Preliminary work to identify RCTs in
these fields has disclosed a large number. In future, it is
likely that there will be an increasing use of systematic
reviews of RCTs in decision-making about education,
including health education and the education of healthcare
professionals.

8.2.3 Social and community action

Interventions undertaken on particular communities are
difficult to evaluate through a randomised controlled trial
because the unit of intervention is the community as a
whole and *not* the individuals within it. Thus, if 16
communities are involved in an RCT (8 in the intervention
group and 8 in the control group), the trial is one of only 16
units and as such is very small despite the fact that many
thousands of people might be involved. Such a trial would
have very low power (see Box 5.8).

   If methods other than an RCT are used to evaluate
interventions on communities, it is necessary to be cautious
when interpreting the results lest any change observed is
attributed to a particular intervention when that change
might have occurred irrespective of whether the
intervention had been undertaken (see Section 7.9.6).

8.2.4 The use of legislative power to improve the public health

It is perhaps when pressing for legislation to improve the
public health that the public health professional has to be
most pragmatic about the influence of evidence during the
decision-making process (see also Section 7.9.5.3). The job
of the public health professional is to improve the health of
populations, in which task the use of evidence is
prerequisite. In contrast, the job of the politician is to
introduce legislative power for the public good, in which
task values may be more influential than evidence.

Although some healthcare professionals may feel indignant about the influence that politicians, and indeed the media, can have in public health decision-making, it is wholly appropriate for politicians and the public to take decisions in situations where values are dominant. In such cases, it is the role of the scientist to be clear about the evidence, and what it shows, including the balance of good to harm of an intervention for the population. However, this is the extent of the scientist's responsibility; it is the responsibility of those individuals who represent society to clarify the values of relevance in particular situations and make the appropriate decisions using those values.

8.2.4.1   Value-based policy-making

During 1999, there were frequent battles between the French Government on the one hand and both the European Union (EU) and the United Kingdom on the other over the issue of the contamination of British beef with BSE. Although a panel of experts convened by the EU reviewed the evidence about the infectivity of British beef and recommended that it was safe for consumption, the French politicians declared British beef to be unsafe. The principal reason for this, as they openly stated, was the French general public's lack of faith in the capacity of the political system to protect the public health following the scandal surrounding the use of blood contaminated with HIV for transfusion. As a consequence, the politicians deemed any risk, however slight, to be unacceptable. Thus, in this particular decision, values were dominant.

8.2.4.2   Evidence-based policy-making

For some decisions, in which resources are not a major determining factor and the values are relatively straightforward, policy-making can be based on evidence alone. In the UK, the Government based its decision not to introduce screening for prostate cancer on the results of two systematic reviews of the evidence (see Box 2.2), neither of which demonstrated any reduction in mortality from screening.[1,2] As screening always does some harm (see Section 3.4.1.1), policy-makers were able to conclude that screening would do more harm than good and therefore should not be introduced.

It could be argued that this decision represented the values inherent in British decision-making which many people, particularly in the USA, see as over-cautious and timid (see Prologue, 'The USA and the rest of the developed world'). However, it is interesting to note that the American Cancer Society, formerly renowned for its aggressive approach to cancer screening, is now more cautious and has suggested a 'third way' based on its review of the evidence. In response to an article, the American Cancer Society stated that:

> the casual reader of the article by Stern et al might erroneously construe that ACS supports 'mass' screening. Studies have shown that when men are provided with more formal information regarding early detection testing for prostatic cancer, many decline it. The ACS is concerned that men may be undergoing screening without proper pre-test guidance and education and agreed that routine serum prostate specific antigen (PSA) measurement is not appropriate without such education. As was the case with testing for the human immunodeficiency virus, serum PSA measurement should be bundled in among other routine blood studies that do not require any preamble discussion. The ACS is also concerned that clinicians who do not let men know that early detection testing for prostate cancer is available vitiate a man's right to choose to undergo a relatively simple test that could conceivably save his life.[3]

8.2.5 Evidence-based humanitarianism

> Accurate and unbiased information about health effects of policies, tactics, and weapons are rarely available, but act as an antidote to war propaganda and is essential to efforts to achieve a just peace.
>
> *MacQueen and Santa-Barbara, 2000*[4]

Few public health interventions are as complex as those designed to tackle the major emergencies faced by populations, whether they result from civil war or natural disaster. However, the commitment to evidence-based public health in this most difficult of arenas was highlighted in an article by Banatvala and Zwi in the *British Medical Journal* entitled 'Conflict and health: Public health and humanitarian interventions: developing the evidence base'.[5] The authors make the following points:

- It is necessary to base policies and practice on the best available evidence to maximise the value of available resources.
- The evidence base must comprise not only evidence of effectiveness and efficiency, but also evidence related to other dimensions of health interventions such as their humanity, equity, local ownership, and political and financial feasibility – Banatvala and Zwi feel that the way in which these relate to humanitarian principles of independence, impartiality, and neutrality warrants further analysis and debate.
- It is difficult to promote the uptake of good practice in the emergency aid sector due to rapid staff turnover, the perception that there is little time to learn lessons given that there is always another emergency, and the scarcity of resources available for encouraging evidence-based practice.
- Humanitarian organisations need to meet the challenges of institutionalising a sensitive and inclusive culture informed by evidence and of building sustainable mechanisms through which policy advice is crystallised from the vast and valuable foundation of field experience.

The authors of this bold and visionary paper demonstrate how evidence from experience can be incorporated with evidence from scientific studies to create evidence-based public health and humanitarian aid.

Evidence about outcome can also be complemented by evidence about the effectiveness of the process of humanitarian aid. In a study of war-related fatality rates among the Kosovar Albanian population in Kosovo during 1998–99, it was found that men aged 50 years and older had a relative risk of dying from war-related trauma 3.2 times greater than that experienced by men of military age (15–49 years).[6] This finding indicates that it was safer for a man to be in the army than to be a civilian in an era of ethnic cleansing. Of greater importance, however, is the indication this study provides of the violation of international standards of conduct during warfare. It has led to the hypothesis that evacuation programmes to assist older people find refuge 'may prevent loss of life'. Although this hypothesis needs to be tested, on the basis of the evidence available from routine data the case for action is strong.

References

1. SELLEY, S., DONOVAN, J., FAULKNER, A., COAST. J. and GILLATT, D. (1997) *Diagnosis, management and screening of early localised prostate cancer.* Health Technology Assessment 1(2).
2. CHAMBERLAIN, J., MELIA, J., MOSS, S. and BROWN, J. (1997) *The diagnosis, management, treatment and costs of prostate cancer in England and Wales.* Health Technology Assessment 1(3).
3. STERN, S., ALTKORN, D. and LEVINSON, W. (1998) *Detection of prostate and colon cancer.* JAMA 280: 117–18.
4. MACQUEEN, G. and SANTA-BARBARA, J. (2000) *Peace building through health initiatives.* Br. Med. J. 321: 1293–6.
5. BANATVALA, N. and ZWI, A.B. (2000) *Public health and humanitarian interventions: developing the evidence base.* Br. Med. J. 321: 101–5.
6. SPIEGEL, P.B. and SALAMA, P. (2000) *War and mortality in Kosovo, 1998–99: an epidemiological testimony.* Lancet 355: 2204–9.

Gentle Reader,

Empathise with Dr John Hall, son-in-law of William Shakespeare, a man of good intentions. He wrote a treatise entitled Select Observations on English Bodies of Eminent Persons in Desperate Diseases. *In the preface, he reflects, 'we must study all ways possible to find out and appoint medicines of cheap rate and effectual for money is scarce and country people poor ...'*

Despite the worthiness of his objectives, his observational epidemiology was weak – most of his observations are of single cases. By today's standards, his level of skill was inadequate to the task, but in the 17th century he would have been considered highly skilled for his time. Can this be said of all healthcare professionals practising today?

Commentary

Dr Hall's treatise provides an example of an early text on effectiveness.

CHAPTER 9

DEVELOPING THE EVIDENCE MANAGEMENT SKILLS OF INDIVIDUALS

No system can make a bad man good but a bad
system can frustrate the efforts of good men.

Gandhi

Although any health service will undergo numerous
system changes, it is wise to remember that management,
although supported by systems, is a human activity, and it
is the competence of individuals within any system that is a
major determinant of system performance. Nonetheless, a
high level of competence does not of itself guarantee good
performance; performance is also directly related to an
individual's motivation and inversely related to the barriers
that individual has to overcome.

$$P = \frac{M \times C}{B}$$

where: P = performance
C = competence
M = motivation
B = barriers

However, in order to practise an evidence-based
approach, individuals need to develop their competence in
the core skills of evidence management – searching,
appraisal and storage (SAS). The development of these
skills requires training, but with the advent of an evidence-
based approach there has evolved a new paradigm in
learning (Table 9.1) in which some of the methods of
conventional training, in which learners are passive, are
eschewed.

Table 9.1 Paradigms in learning

Old	New
Knowledge-based	Problem-based
Knowing what one should know	Knowing what one does not know
Intuition very powerful	Ability to generate and refine a question, and to search for, appraise and act on the evidence to solve it
Learning from received wisdom	Ability to question received wisdom
Learning almost 'complete' at end of formal training – only a finite amount of knowledge to be absorbed	Life-long learning – there is always new knowledge to be absorbed
Learning dominated by knowledge from experience	Learning involves complementing experience with knowledge from research

9.1 THE PRE-REQUISITE: BEING ABLE TO ASK THE RIGHT QUESTION

> Real education begins with a question in the life of the learner.
>
> *Leo Tolstoy*

The pre-requisite for evidence-based decision-making is the ability to ask the right question. Although this statement might appear to be self-evident, many people hasten to find the evidence and appraise it *before* defining precisely the question they wish to answer. Careful consideration of the question that needs answering is the foundation for evidence-based decision-making.

9.2 SEARCHING

The issues about which decisions must be made usually arise without warning or at inconvenient times. In an ideal world, a manager would request a search for evidence from a librarian; in reality, managers often have to find the evidence for themselves.

9.2.1 Competencies

Everyone who makes decisions about groups of patients or populations should be able:

1. to define and identify the sources of evidence appropriate to a particular decision that must be made;
2. to carry out a search of MEDLINE or EMBASE without the help of a librarian and find at least 60% of the reviews or research studies that would have been found by the librarian;
3. to construct simple search strategies on MEDLINE, using Boolean operators ('and' and 'or') for:
   (a) the following types of healthcare intervention:
      – therapy;
      – test;
      – screening programme;
      – health policy or policy-making.
   (b) the following service characteristics:
      – effectiveness;
      – safety;
      – acceptability;
      – cost-effectiveness;
      – quality;
      – appropriateness.
4. To download the end-products of a search onto reference management software (Section 9.4).

9.2.2 Training

All decision-makers should be given induction training on how to find research evidence. Initial training, however, is effective only if it is supplemented by refresher sessions. For instance, it is advisable for every decision-maker to complete a literature search and review it with a skilled searcher several times a year.

9.2.3 Scanning

Evidence can also be found by scanning, that is, regularly reading certain journals. As this process can be time-consuming, it is advisable to allocate a certain amount of time to reading each week and then develop an appropriate scanning strategy (see Box 4.2).

9.3 APPRAISING EVIDENCE

Increasingly, librarians are being trained to appraise evidence as well as to search for it, and to teach both skills. At present, the main source of appraisal skills when making decisions about groups of patients or populations is in departments of public health. As a consultant in public health may not always be available when an appraisal needs to be undertaken, all those who make decisions about populations or groups of patients must have the necessary skills to appraise research articles on healthcare, that is, take a scientific approach to healthcare management.

9.3.1 Competencies

Everyone who makes decisions about groups of patients or populations should be able:

- to appraise the evidence presented in a review article on the following types of intervention:
  - a therapy (see Section 3.2.3);
  - a test (see Section 3.3.3);
  - a screening programme (see Section 3.4.3);
  - a health policy (see Section 3.5.3).
- to appraise the quality of the following research methodologies:
  - systematic review (see Section 5.3.3);
  - RCT (see Section 5.4.3);
  - case-control study (see Section 5.5.3);
  - cohort study (see Section 5.6.3);
  - survey (see Section 5.7.3);
  - decision analysis (Section 5.8.3);
  - qualitative research (see Section 5.9.3).
- to assess the population outcomes of an intervention against the following criteria:
  - acceptability (see Section 6.6.1.1);

- equity (see Section 6.3);
- effectiveness (see Section 6.4);
- safety (see Section 6.5);
- patient satisfaction and patients' experience of care (see Section 6.6);
- cost-effectiveness (see Section 6.7);
- quality (see Section 6.8);
- appropriateness (see Section 6.9).

It is vital to appraise the evidence found in the context of local circumstances: a decision-maker must consider not only the applicability of the findings to a particular population, but also the local factors that may affect the outcomes of applying those findings.

For those who do not appraise research evidence regularly, the checklists provided at the book's website may be used as prompts whenever appraisal is undertaken. http://www.shef.ac.uk/~scharr/ebhc/Intro.html

9.3.2 Training

The skills of appraisal should be developed during the basic training of all healthcare professionals. At present, these skills are virtually ignored; very few decision-makers have been taught how to be systematic in their appraisal of a report or a research project.

A critical appraisal skills programme is necessary to the development of any healthcare organisation (see Appendix III, III.3.5).

9.4 STORING AND RETRIEVING

> My storage system? I've got a foot and a half of papers torn out of the *BMJ* in a pile on my dining-room table.
>
> *A physician, 2 years after graduation*

Storing paper is easy, at least for the short term. However, the young doctor quoted above could have storage problems in 20 years' time if his rate of acquisition continues at 9 inches (22.86 cm) per year. It is highly likely that he could maintain a storage system of three four-drawer filing cabinets, filing papers alphabetically by surname of the first author, for example. The drawback with such a system, however, is the difficulty of retrieval unless the user has a good memory or the author of the paper has a memorable name. Retrieval from an alphabetically or chronologically ordered paper storage system is compounded when the user wants to retrieve all the papers on a particular subject. Although it is possible to store papers or reference cards by disease grouping, concepts or patient groups, it is impossible to combine any of these, e.g. to retrieve all the papers describing trials of coronary heart disease prevention on one occasion and all the papers investigating coronary heart disease in women on another. Only computer-based storage systems have the potential to store useful information in a form that will allow retrieval from several different 'entry' points.

9.4.1 Competencies

Everyone who makes decisions about groups of patients or populations should be able:

- to enter references and abstracts, using self-selected keywords, into one of the electronic systems for reference management (see Appendix IV, IV.2);
- to search for references within a reference management system;
- to download sets of references from a reference management system.

   As there are several different types of reference management software available and healthcare professionals are highly 'mobile', it is important that librarians are able to support staff who use any of the common reference management software systems, irrespective of that used in the library.

9.4.2 Training

After a short period of induction training, anyone who is intelligent enough to be a decision-maker in a health service should be able to use reference management systems.

9.4.3 Aphorisms on storage and retrieval

➤ Less than one in a hundred healthcare decision-makers have reference management software.
➤ Filing cabinets will always be full to capacity.

> A photocopier is a machine for creating storage problems.
> Only highly obsessional healthcare professionals can store paper in a system that will enable them to find what they need when they need it by themselves.
> One of the few ways in which computers have made life easier for healthcare professionals is the development of reference management software.

9.5   LEARNING BY DOING

Formal training has certain connotations for people: seminar rooms, overhead projectors, one person being active, many people being passive. In fact, formal training in which only one person is active while the learners are passive is relatively ineffective. Although some formal training is necessary, for example, to introduce people to critical appraisal, the best way to learn is to learn by doing. Learning by doing involves using skills on the job to face practical decisions and then reflect upon the theory and/or training received. The learning by doing cycle is shown in Fig. 9.1.

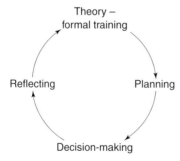

Fig. 9.1
The learning by doing cycle

9.5.1   Informatics support for staff who are learning by doing

Often, the need for evidence arises in meetings or on a ward round, during a debate, discussion or differences of opinion. However, in these situations, it is almost always impossible to resolve the matter by going to the library to carry out a search, appraise the articles found, and assemble the evidence on which a decision could be based. Although this strategy may sometimes be necessary, particularly when clinicians are making decisions in a life-or-death situation, a more realistic scenario is for staff to have ready access to a computer – at a clinical work station, or in a meeting – at which a search could be performed. At present, this is not a common occurrence. New developments in technology will facilitate the uptake of such a strategy.

For optimal decision-making when learning by doing, healthcare professionals should have access to The Cochrane Library at every clinical work station and in every Chief Executive's office. Another valuable source of support would be to provide all junior medical staff with a palmtop which would give them the facility to call a central point from anywhere in the hospital and obtain up-to-date guidelines and evidence to complement that which they carry in their filofax or in the junior doctor's *vade mecum*, the *Oxford Handbook of Clinical Medicine*.[1]

9.5.2 Support for staff learning by doing: the educational prescription

As certain developments in informatics are not widely available at present, it is necessary to find viable alternatives. Questions raised during debate, discussion or differences of opinion in meetings or on the ward round can be used as a starting point to drive the learning process. In the absence of a mechanism to capture such questions, and monitor progress toward finding the answers, it is more than likely that these opportunities to learn will be lost due to pressure of work.

One low-technology alternative that can be used to capture questions that arise during learning by doing is the educational prescription (see Fig. 9.2). Educational prescriptions were devised by Dave Sackett and co-workers at the Centre for Evidence-Based Medicine, Oxford, in order to keep track of a learner's progress from the formulation of an appropriate ('right') question about a patient's needs to a clinically useful answer.[2] The use of an educational prescription helps both learners and teachers in five ways:

1. it specifies the clinical problem that generated the questions;
2. it states the question in all of its key elements;

R✗ Educational Prescription

Patient's Name   Learner:

3-part Clinical Question
Target Disorder:

Intervention (+/- comparison):

Outcome:

Date and place to be filled:

Presentations will cover:
1. search strategy;
2. search results;
3. the validity of this evidence;
4. the importance of this valid evidence;
5. can this valid, important evidence be applied to your patient;
6. your evaluation of this process.

Fig. 9.2
The educational prescription: a suggested proforma (Source: Sackett et al.[2])

3. it specifies who is responsible for answering it;
4. it provides a reminder of the deadline pertinent to answering the question (taking into account the urgency of the clinical problem from which the question was generated);
5. it furnishes an *aide memoire* of the steps necessary for searching, critically appraising, and relating the answer back to the patient.

Educational prescriptions have been incorporated into various inpatient teaching settings from work rounds and attending consultant rounds to morning reports and noon conferences. They have also been used in outpatient teaching settings. A group of general practitioners has also been using the technique to determine their learning needs, and to review those needs periodically with colleagues in the partnership in order to identify recurrent themes.

References

1. HOPE, R.A., LONGMORE, J.M., HODGETTS, T.J. and RAMRAKHA, P.S. (1993) *Oxford Handbook of Clinical Medicine*. 3rd Edition. Oxford University Press, Oxford.
2. SACKETT, D.L., STRAUS, S.E., RICHARDSON, W.S., ROSENBERG, W. and HAYNES, R.B. (2000) *Evidence-based Medicine: How to Practice and Teach EBM*. 2nd Edition. Churchill Livingstone, Edinburgh.

The philosophers have only interpreted the world in
various ways; the point is to change it.

Karl Marx

Although searching, appraising and storing skills are
necessary, they are not sufficient; decision-makers also
need to practise and improve their skills of implementing
research findings if they are to change the organisation of a
health service and the patterns of delivery of clinical care.

Although the focus of this book is primarily on
developing searching, appraisal and storing skills, the skills
of implementing the changes that evidence dictates are of
equal importance. Many of these are general management
skills, such as those necessary for project management or
effective teamwork. Most managers already have these
skills because they are developed during management
training. As we embark upon the 21st century, it is the
combination of these two sets of skills that will fit any
healthcare manager for the challenges that lie ahead.

General management skills
+
Skills for evidence-based decision-making
=
The 'compleat' healthcare manager

Gentle Reader,

Empathise with Stephen Jay Gould.

'In July 1982, I learned that I was suffering from abdominal mesothelioma, a rare and serious cancer usually associated with exposure to asbestos. When I revived after surgery, I asked my first question of my doctor and chemotherapist: 'What is the best technical literature about mesothelioma?'. She replied, with a touch of diplomacy (the only departure she has ever made from direct frankness), that the medical literature contained nothing really worth reading.

Of course, trying to keep an intellectual away from literature works about as well as recommending chastity to Homo sapiens, *the sexiest primate of all. As soon as I could walk, I made a beeline for Harvard's Countway medical library and punched mesothelioma into the computer's bibliographic search program. An hour later, surrounded by the latest literature on abdominal mesothelioma, I realised with a gulp why my doctor had offered that humane advice. The literature couldn't have been more brutally clear: mesothelioma is incurable, with a median mortality of only 8 months after discovery. I sat stunned for about 15 minutes, then smiled and said to myself: so that's why they didn't give me anything to read.*

Then my mind started to work again, thank goodness.

The problem may be briefly stated: what does 'median mortality of 8 months' signify in our vernacular? I suspect that most people, without training in statistics, would read such a statement as 'I will probably be dead in 8 months' – the very conclusion that must be avoided, both because this formulation is false and because attitude matters so much.'

Stephen Jay Gould,
'The median isn't the message' in
Adam's Navel, 1995

Commentary

Stephen Jay Gould, world-class geologist, baseball guru and beautiful writer, is not perhaps the average patient, but neither should his experience, attitude and skills be disregarded. As the 21st century progresses, patients will become more literate, better organised and better educated, and many of them will be better at finding, but not necessarily appraising, knowledge using the World Wide Web. The relationship between clinician and patient will continue to evolve, and clinicians should be prepared to encounter more patients like Stephen Jay Gould in future.

CHAPTER 10

THE EVIDENCE-BASED CONSULTATION

Every year, for every million population receiving health services, many decisions are made, including:

- hundreds of purchasing decisions;
- thousands of managerial decisions;
- millions of clinical decisions.

Clinical decisions are of direct and immediate importance to patients. They are also of importance to those who manage or pay for health services because one of the outcomes of clinical decision-making is expenditure on health services. In a system in which resources are not finite, changes in the volume and intensity of clinical practice are the major factors driving the increase in healthcare costs that can be controlled,[1] and over which managers can exert considerable influence (see Section 2.4).

In order to exercise this influence, it is essential for those who make decisions about groups of patients or populations to understand how clinicians, in consultation with their patients, make and take decisions.

Reference

1. EDDY, D.M. (1993) *Three battles to watch in the 1990s.* JAMA 270: 520–6.

10.1 TYPES OF CLINICAL DECISION

10.1.1 'Faceless' decision-making

'Faceless' decisions are those in which the decision is based on either a specimen taken from or an image taken of a patient. Such decisions are the clinician's interpretation of a test result, sample or image; there is no discussion with the patient or their relatives. As the clinician is a human being and not a mechanical instrument, the decision will be influenced not only by what can be seen or measured but also by other variables (see Fig. 10.1, left-hand side).

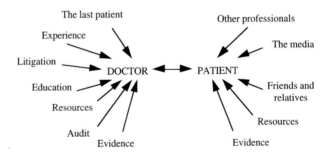

Fig. 10.1
The decision drivers

Owing to the influence of these other variables, 'faceless' decisions are always characterised by:

- interobserver variability, in which different clinicians interpret the same image or test results in different ways;
- intraobserver variability, in which the same clinician interprets the same image or test results differently on separate occasions.

These characteristics of 'faceless' decision-making can be observed among even the best clinicians; moreover, the level of variability increases as the image or test result approaches 'borderline'. Although certain levels of inter- and intraobserver variability are unacceptable and must be eradicated through clinical audit, inter- and intraobserver variability are inevitable consequences of using human beings as measuring and decision-taking instruments (p. 77).

10.1.2 Face-to-face decision-making

The principal characteristic of face-to-face decision-making is the dialogue between clinician and patient, to which the patient will bring his/her own set of beliefs, attitudes and values. Consequently, there are many more variables involved when face-to-face decisions are made (see Fig. 10.1, right-hand side).

The numerous interactions that take place during face-to-face decision-making may be classified as either non-verbal or verbal communication. Although non-verbal communication is important, the focus in this book is on verbal communication because it is upon words and numbers that evidence-based clinical decisions are made.

10.2 PATIENT COMMUNICATION

'You have an exorbitant auditory impediment,'
replied the doctor, ever conscious of the necessity for
maintaining a certain iatric mystique, and fully aware
that 'a pea in the ear' was unlikely to earn him any
kudos. 'I can remove it with a fishhook and a small
hammer; it's the ideal way of overcoming *un embarras
de petit pois.*' He spoke the French words in a
mincingly Parisian accent, even though his irony was
apparent only to himself.

Louis de Bernières,
Captain Corelli's Mandolin, *1994*

Communication with patients is a complicated topic that
has many aspects, some of which are contentious, such as
the issue of disclosure – how much should be revealed to
patients, especially to those who are terminally ill?[1] In this
chapter, the focus is on verbal communication in face-to-
face decision-making, which comprises three elements (see
Fig. 10.2):
1. the provision of evidence-based information to the
   patient by the clinician after a diagnosis has been made;
2. interpretation of that information by the patient;
3. discussion between clinician and patient.

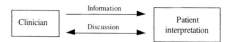

Fig. 10.2
The interaction between patient and clinician during face-to-
face decision-making

10.2.1 The provision of evidence-based information

For the clinician, steps in the provision of evidence-based
information to a patient include:

- finding all the available research evidence using the best
  possible searching techniques;
- appraising that research evidence systematically to
  identify the best evidence available;

- determining whether the best evidence available is relevant to the individual patient currently under care.

Determining the relevance of the best evidence available to an individual patient includes the following calculations:

- the probability that the patient will benefit;
- the magnitude of any benefit;
- the probability that the patient will suffer from any adverse effects of treatment;
- the magnitude of any adverse effects.

When giving evidence-based information to a patient, the clinician must present it in a form that patients will find useful. For example, in one study in which patients chose the therapy for lung cancer, it was found that patients would prefer the results to be expressed in terms of life-expectancy rather than in terms of the probability of surviving.[2]

It is also important to tailor the information to individual patient's needs. In a study of 1012 women who had a confirmed diagnosis of breast cancer,[3] one of the objectives was to identify the women's priorities for information. It was found that:

- for women over 70 years of age, their priority was to have information about the chance of cure, and the spread of the disease;
- for women less than 50 years of age, their priority was for information about the effect of treatment on their sexuality;
- for women who had positive family histories, their priority was for information about family risk.

10.2.1.1 Other sources of information for patients

Clinicians are not the only source of information for patients. Other sources of information include:

- relatives, friends, and acquaintances;
- the World Wide Web;
- the pharmaceutical industry.

Many patients are now able to access medical information from the World Wide Web. However, as there is no mechanism to control the content of material put up on the Web, the information that patients are able to find can vary widely in quality. It is important, therefore, that healthcare professionals contribute to providing good-quality information on the Web, i.e. information that is easy to find, easy to read, and free from bias.

The pharmaceutical industry sometimes uses the media to provide information directly to patients. In 1991, for example, the results of one study showed that a new drug for high blood pressure had less of an effect on a patient's metabolism than the traditional treatment. The company that manufactured the drug immediately called a press conference and received front-page coverage in the *New York Times* and many other newspapers. Although no evidence on outcomes was presented, only that on intermediate variables such as the level of insulin sensitivity, patients were targeted directly with success.[4]

10.2.2 Interpretation

Once a patient has been given the information, s/he has to interpret it, and may require time for reflection.

A patient will seek to interpret the information in two ways.

1. How the evidence provided applies to his/her particular case: this is difficult for a patient, who may need guidance. It is the responsibility of the clinician to assess the relevance of the evidence to the particular patient who is consulting.
2. How the outcomes, good and bad, sit within the context of his/her values. For example, a patient who has deep vein thrombosis and is offered treatment needs to weigh up two risks:
   - that of complications or death as a result of treatment;
   - that of experiencing complications or death if treatment is refused.

   It is possible to delineate these values using decision analysis techniques. In one study, all patients suspected of having venous thrombosis preferred to follow a course in which the risk of an early death from treatment was reduced rather than a course in which the risk of long-term complications from the disease was reduced.[5]

The provision of written information (patient leaflets) can be used to support the verbal communication, and aid the process of interpretation. Such leaflets can be used to give a clear indication of the strength of the evidence (see Fig. 10.3), for instance, by highlighting which statements are

❏ Aims

The guidelines# aim to improve the quality of stroke care by providing recommendations that are both scientifically valid and helpful in clinical practice for professionals caring for stroke patients in the community. They are consistent with the available scientific evidence [E] (at least one good randomised controlled trial) or, without such evidence, best clinical judgement [C]. A detailed systematic review of the literature can be obtained from Northamptonshire Health Authority.[1] Possible points for audit are indicated [AQ].

♦ Transient ischaemic attack (TIAs) will be discussed in relation to stroke prevention. The management of subarachnoid haemorrhage is not covered as it is clinically often regarded as a separate entity.

1. BLAIS, M.J. (1994) GRiP. *Using the evidence, Literature Review: Stroke.* Northampton: Northamptonshire Health Authority.

❏ How should patients / carers be supported?   [C]

(Please refer to guidelines on 'Stroke Rehabilitation and Aftercare following Hospitalisation' (no. 3)).

❏ Primary prevention   [E] [C] [AQ]

♦ Prevention must concentrate on the management of multiple risk factors:

➢ *Hypertension* (affected by diet, obesity, inadequate physical activity, excess alcohol, etc).

All patients should be given non-pharmalogical advice

- Reduce energy intake
- Reduce salt intake
- Avoid high saturated fat intake
- Avoid excessive alcohol
- Stop smoking
- Take regular exercise

#2. *Management of Stroke in Hospitals*
 3. *Stroke Rehabilitation and Aftercare Following Hospitalisation*

Fig. 10.3
Northamptonshire stroke leaflet

➢ *Hypertension.* Overall thresholds for intervention with drugs of ≥ 90 mm Hg, diastolic BP, and ≥ 160 mm Hg systolic BP are accepted, but with subgroups, e.g. younger age without coexisting risk factors, older age > 80 years, observation is indicated. *(Please refer to interim recommendations produced by the 'Second Working Party of the British Hypertension Society' for further details.)*

Thresholds of diastolic BP for intervention with drugs in younger patients

- ≥ 100 mm Hg – Treat
- 90–99 mm Hg – dependent on additional factors

Elderly patients

- Benefit from drug treatment
- Threshold ≥ 160 mm Hg systolic BP or ≥ 90 mm Hg diastolic BP, or both

○ Repeated measurement

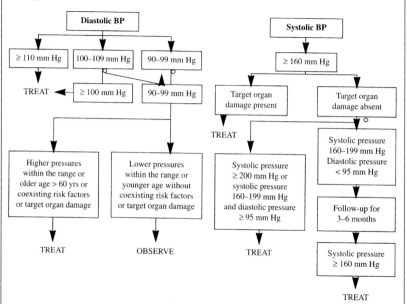

♦ Newer classes of drugs should be considered as 'alternative' first line agents when diuretics and β blockers are contraindicated or ineffective or when side effects occur.

Routine use of aspirin cannot be recommended in patients with important risk factors such as hypertension, hypercholesterolaemia or diabetes uncomplicated by vascular disease.

IF presence of atrial fibrillation, consider anticoagulation according to assessment of medical problems and risk of haemorrhage. *Please refer to long-term secondary prevention for further details.* [E] [AQ] supported by research and which by opinion or anecdote. Tools, such as DISCERN, have been developed to enable those who produce information for patients to ensure that the information provided is based on the best current knowledge, and takes into account the needs of patients and carers.[6]

10.2.3 Discussion

The quality of a discussion between clinician and patient is determined not by the quality of the evidence or the patient's knowledge of medical terms but primarily by the relationship between clinician and patient. If a patient feels powerless, the discussion will be stilted, inconclusive and unsatisfactory. If a patient feels empowered to participate with the clinician in decision-making, a satisfactory discussion will take place.

Skelton and Hobbs[7] have taken a novel approach to analysing the language used during the doctor–patient consultation. They applied the technique of computer concordancing, a methodology established in linguistic research but rarely applied to professional language, which enables both a quantitative and qualitative study of language. Skelton and Hobbs investigated the language of 40 doctors (native English speakers) and their patients during 373 primary care consultations to determine:

- the use of jargon by doctors;
- the use of the language of power, and that of the absence of power;
- the ways in which language was used to diminish the potential threat of the presenting disorder.

The authors found that doctors did not use jargon, which suggests that they are aware of the need to avoid it. However, some doctors did use language associated with social power, and some patients used language associated with absence of power, which could imply that consultations may be less democratic than is appropriate. Finally, there was substantial evidence that doctors used language to express emotions, to diminish threats, and to reassure patients, which Skelton and Hobbs feel denotes a therapeutic use of language.

References

1. ANNAS, G.J. (1994) *Informed consent, cancer and truth in prognosis*. N. Engl. J. Med. 330: 223–5.
2. McNEIL, B.J., PAUKER, S.G., SOX, H.C. and TVERSKY, A. (1982) *On the elicitation of preferences for alternative therapies*. N. Engl. J. Med. 306: 1259–62.
3. DEGNER, L.F., KRISTJANSON, L.J., BOWMAN, D. et al. (1997) *Information needs and decisional preferences in women with breast cancer*. JAMA 277: 1485–92.
4. MOSER, M., BLAUFOX, M.D., FRIES, E. et al. (1991) *Who really determines your patients' prescriptions?* JAMA 265: 498–500.
5. O'MEARA, J.J., MCNUTT, R.A., EVANS, A.T. et al. (1994) *A decision analysis of streptokinase plus heparin as compared with heparin alone for deep-vein thrombosis*. N. Engl. J. Med. 330: 1864–9.
6. COULTER, A. (1998) *Evidence based patient information*. Br. Med. J. 317: 225–6.
7. SKELTON, J.R. and HOBBS, F.D.R. (1999) *Concordancing: use of language-based research in medical communication*. Lancet 353: 108–11.

10.3 EVIDENCE-BASED PATIENT CHOICE

For a patient to exercise choice based on the available evidence, all three elements of patient communication must occur.

When patients are given information, their preferences for treatment may change. In one study of people aged between 60 and 99 years who were asked if they wished to receive cardiopulmonary resuscitation (CPR), 41% said yes initially; when they were apprised of the evidence and realised that survival after CPR was lower than their expectations, the proportion of those wishing to receive it dropped to 22%.[1] However, the nature of the information provided may also affect patient preference. Mazur and Hickam[2] compared the preference for intubation and ventilatory support (IVS) in two groups of patients randomly assigned to alternative explanations of the purpose of the intervention. One group considered IVS in an unspecified medical condition (general explanation); the other considered IVS in the context of severe pneumonia. They found that those patients who had been given a general explanation were willing to accept significantly fewer days of intubation (65 days vs 96 days; $P = 0.009$), and significantly fewer of them wanted to continue IVS when the probability of a successful outcome was less than 50% (30% vs 64%; $P < 0.0001$).

The provision of information to patients about new interventions can vary in difficulty depending on the treatment. The introduction of a new drug is usually easy; the means of administration will probably not be different to those of established drugs and therefore it is more likely to be acceptable to patients. In contrast, the introduction of a new operation is much more difficult; patients may want evidence about both the operation and the skill of the operator. There are two inter-related questions the patient may ask:

- 'Should I have this operation?';
- if the answer is in the affirmative, 'Whom should I ask to perform this operation?'.

A patient's decision about whether to have an operation is usually determined by the level of confidence the patient has in a particular operator. This is wise because the evidence on which any clinician's advice is based has been derived from trials in which high-quality professionals work within stringent criteria on a carefully defined and often relatively healthy subset of patients.

To resolve this situation, a patient can ask for evidence about those characteristics of the process of care that have been demonstrated as leading to good outcomes. For example, any American patient considering laparoscopic cholecystectomy is advised by Nenner et al.[3] to ask the questions shown in Box 10.1.

Box 10.1   Questions a patient contemplating laparoscopic cholecystectomy should ask about the operator (Source: Nenner et al.[3])

- Is the surgeon board-certified?
- Does the surgeon have hospital privileges to do open cholecystectomy?
- Was the surgeon formally trained in a recognised program in laparoscopic cholecystectomy?
- How many laparoscopic cholecystectomies did he or she do and what were the frequency and types of complications?

10.3.1   Factors inhibiting evidence-based patient choice

There are several factors that may prevent a patient exercising evidence-based choice about treatment options:

- clinical ignorance;

- the emphasis clinicians place on the beneficial effects of intervention;
- lack of full disclosure by clinicians.

10.3.1.1 Clinical ignorance

Clinical ignorance will limit patient choice and might impede the delivery of effective care. The causes of clinical ignorance are shown in Box 10.2. As can be seen, clinicians are not always aware of the best evidence available. For instance, in a study in which doctors' beliefs about the treatment of high blood pressure were compared with the treatment known to be effective based on the best evidence available,[4] it was found that doctors thought treatment should be commenced at a level of blood pressure that increased with the age of the patient whereas the evidence shows that treatment is indicated at lower levels of blood pressure as a patient grows older (Fig. 10.4).

Box 10.2   Causes of clinical ignorance

- There may be no knowledge to know.
- There may be knowledge not known to the clinician.
- There may be knowledge known to the clinician, but that knowledge does not allow the clinician to assess the probabilities of the outcomes of the different options available to the clinician and the patient.

10.3.1.2 Emphasising the benefits of intervention

Clinicians tend to emphasise the beneficial rather than the adverse effects of intervention, as this harrowing account of a person treated for myeloid leukaemia illustrates.

> We were told that the condition was serious, but in 50% of cases people were cured. When it was discovered there were sideroblasts the success rate was reduced to 25%. It was not until the second course of chemotherapy that the head of the department, B, saw Jeffrey and said that only 15% of patients can be treated successfully and for someone of Jeffrey's age a remission was impossible.[5]

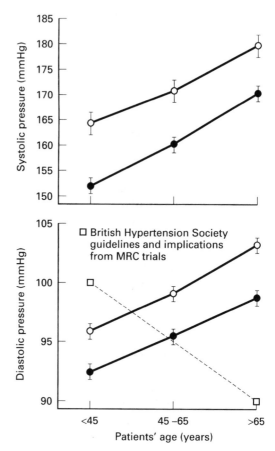

Fig. 10.4
Lowest systolic and diastolic blood pressure at which 125
general practitioners would define (●—●) and treat (○—○)
hypertension. Values are means (95% confidence intervals);
MRC = Medical Research Council (Source: Dickerson and
Brown,[4] with permission, BMJ Publishing Group)

10.3.1.3 Disclosure

It can be argued that any patient should have full
disclosure of the evidence from a clinician, much as they
would expect to be fully informed by a lawyer or television
engineer who was working for them. Indeed, one speaker
at a conference on bioethics in the USA said, 'I trust my
lawyer more than I trust my doctor', meaning that she
trusted the lawyer to tell her all the options available and
execute the one she chose, whereas she would not have this
confidence in her doctors if she were terminally ill.

In a survey in the USA in 1982,[6] it was found that:

- 85% of Americans wanted a realistic estimate of 'how long they had to live if their type of cancer' usually leads to death in less than one year;
- only 41% of physicians if asked by a patient with 'a fully confirmed diagnosis of lung cancer at an advanced stage' would give either a straight statistical prognosis (13%) or 'say that you can't tell how long the patient might live but stress that in most cases people lived no longer than a year' (28%).

Owing in part to the fear of litigation, clinicians are now more open and frank, particularly with patients who have a severe illness where a decision to proceed with treatment may expose the patient to interventions that have major side-effects but carry little prospect of cure. It is most common for this type of decision to be faced when there is a choice between further treatment for a malignancy or palliative care.

References

1. MURPHY, D.J., BURROWS, D., SANTILLI, S. et al. (1994) *The influence of the probability of survival on patients' preferences regarding cardiopulmonary resuscitation.* N. Engl. J. Med. 330: 565–9.
2. MAZUR, D.J. and HICKAM, D.H. (1997) *The influence of physician explanations on patient preferences about future health-care states.* Med. Decis. Making 17: 56–60.
3. NENNER, R.P., IMPERATO, P.J. and WILL, T.O. (1994) *Questions patients should ask about laparoscopic cholecystectomy [Letter].* Ann. Intern. Med. 120: 443.
4. DICKERSON, J.E.C. and BROWN, M.J. (1995) *Influence of age on general practitioners' definition and treatment of hypertension.* Br. Med. J. 310: 574.
5. ANONYMOUS (1994) *Dying for palliative care.* Br. Med. J. 309: 1696–9.
6. ANNAS, G.J. (1994) *Informed consent, cancer and truth in prognosis.* N. Engl. J. Med. 330: 223–5.

10.4 EVIDENCE-BASED CLINICAL PRACTICE

10.4.1 Definitions and dimensions

Evidence-based clinical practice or evidence-based medicine is:

> … the conscientious, explicit and judicious use of current best evidence in making decisions about the care of individual patients. The practice of evidence-based medicine means integrating individual clinical expertise with the best available external clinical

evidence from systematic research. By individual clinical expertise we mean the proficiency and judgement that individual clinicians acquire through clinical experience and clinical practice.[1]

This process of evidence-based decision-making described above can be represented diagrammatically, as shown in Fig. 10.5.

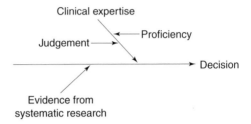

Fig. 10.5
Evidence-based decision-making

The use of the adjective 'judicious' signifies that the clinician must take into account a patient's condition, baseline risk, values, and circumstances when making a decision (Fig. 10.6); evidence-based clinical practice is not cookbook medicine.[1] In itself, the possession and provision of the current best evidence does not constitute a decision; the evidence must be interpreted in the context of the individual patient's needs, which requires clinical judgement and good communication skills.[2]

In evidence-based clinical practice, a clinician must also link the evidence to the other activities that promote the exercise of evidence-based patient choice (see Fig. 10.7).

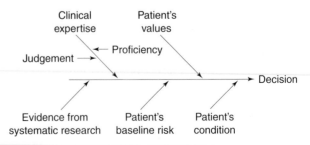

Fig. 10.6
The 'judicious' use of evidence in relation to a patient's baseline risk, condition, and values during decision-making

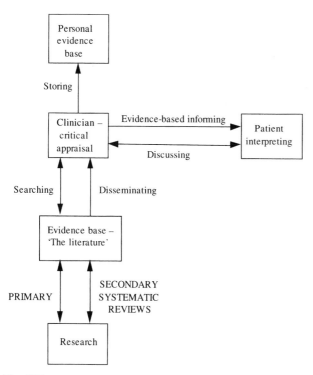

Fig. 10.7
Factors in the promotion of evidence-based patient choice

Contrary to the widely held belief that only 15–20% of clinical practice is based on good research evidence, it has been found that in the specialties of general medicine,[3] psychiatry,[4] and surgery[5] the majority of patients are treated on the basis of good evidence (Table 10.1; see Table 7.6 for the evidence base of consultations in general practice; visit http://www.shef.ac.uk/~scharr/ir/percent.html for that in haematology [clinical and malignant], paediatric surgery, and Medicare coverage).

Table 10.1   The nature of the evidence supporting the use of interventions in the specialties of general medicine, psychiatry, and surgery (Sources: refs. 3–5)

Nature of evidence supporting	% of total patients		
intervention	General medicine[3]	Psychiatry[4]	Surgery[5]
Evidence from good-quality RCTs	53	65*	24
Convincing non-experimental evidence	29	Not applicable	71
Interventions without convincing evidence	18	35	5

* Evidence from RCTs and systematic reviews

10.4.2 Failures in clinical decision-making

When evidence is not used during clinical practice, important failures in clinical decision-making occur:

- ineffective interventions are introduced;
- interventions that do more harm than good are introduced;
- interventions that do more good than harm are not introduced;
- interventions that are ineffective or do more harm than good are not discontinued.

When considering the reasons why these failures happen, it is helpful to remember the three factors that influence clinical performance:

$$P = \frac{M \times C}{B}$$

Performance (P) is directly related to a professional's competence (C) and motivation (M) and inversely related to the barriers (B) that the professional has to overcome. There is no evidence that clinicians lack motivation, but some skills (competence) do need to be improved (see Chapter 9) and many barriers need to be removed.

Of those factors that contribute to the existence of barriers, some are external (Table 10.2), over which clinicians have very little control, and others are internal (Table 10.3), over which clinicians can take action.

10.4.3 Clinical freedom

Isaiah Berlin's ebullient personality dominated Oxford, and much of the London intelligentsia, in the second half of the 20th century. From a brilliant career in Intelligence during the Second World War to his death in 1997, Berlin's irresistible flow of ideas enlivened many a dull academic and establishment meeting. In one of his most interesting essays, *Two Concepts of Liberty*, Berlin distinguished between what he called 'negative liberty', the freedom to do what we want (to wear a seat belt or not, to smoke cannabis or not), and 'positive liberty', the freedom to decide how much negative liberty we have.

Very often healthcare professionals, particularly doctors, will fight for negative liberty, namely the freedom for

Table 10.2 External factors contributing to the barriers that impair a healthcare professional's performance, and their solutions

External causes	Solutions outwith the power of clinicians
Poor quality of research producing biased evidence	Better training of research workers and more stringent ethics committees
Studies too small to produce unequivocal results	Promotion of systematic reviews
Unpublished research unavailable to clinicians	Publication of all research findings by pharmaceutical companies
Publication bias towards positive findings	Prevention of publication bias
Articles that cannot be found because of inadequate indexing	Better indexing
Failure of research workers to present evidence in forms useful to clinicians	Tougher action by journal editors
Inaccessible libraries	Extension of access to the World Wide Web to all clinicians

Table 10.3 Internal factors contributing to barriers that impair a healthcare professional's performance, and their solutions

Internal causes even a busy clinician can modify	Solutions for the busy clinician
Out-of-date textbooks	Don't read textbooks for guidance on therapy
Biased editorials and reviews	Don't read editorials and reviews for guidance on therapy except Cochrane Collaboration reviews and reviews in DARE (see Appendix I)
Too much primary research (the average clinician needs to read 19 articles a day to keep up)	Read good-quality reviews rather than primary research
Reviews difficult to find	Improve searching skills (Sections 4.3.2 and 9.2)
Inability to spot flaws in research	Improve appraisal skills (Sections 4.3.3 and 9.3)
Difficulty in retrieving evidence identified as useful	Develop skills to use reference management software (Section 9.4).
Translating the data about groups of patients in research papers into information relevant to an individual patient	Develop/improve understanding of baseline risk and NNT (Section 6.4.3.1) and ability to explain how research results apply to an individual patient (Section 10.2.1)[6–8]
Insufficient time	Be more discerning about what to read by developing a good scanning strategy (Box 4.2)

individual clinicians to do anything they see fit. However, in fighting to preserve negative liberty, clinicians have failed to recognise the change in public attitudes, which has influenced political attitudes, and the increasing concern felt about variations in the quality of professional practice (see Fig. 10.8). Thus, there is a desire among the public and politicians, usually supported by the media, to introduce controls on the behaviour of the profession as a whole but

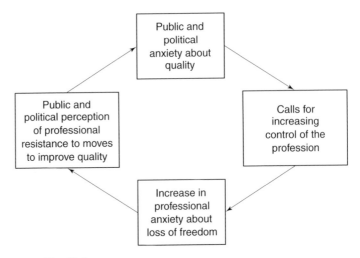

Fig. 10.8
The interaction of public anxiety about the quality of healthcare and professional anxiety about the loss of freedom

particularly on that of the worst members. It is ironic that the clinicians who call for the retention of negative liberty are often the most responsible members of the profession who base their clinical decisions on good evidence and best practice. However, by emphasising the need to maintain negative liberty, the profession is in danger of losing the trust of the public and the politicians, which may lead to greater controls on the profession. In this situation, healthcare professionals need to embrace the concept of evidence-based decision-making and, where systems of care can be developed, the introduction of guidelines and audit (see Fig. 1.4).

In the UK, the establishment of the National Institute for Clinical Excellence (NICE) and the Commission for Health Improvement (CHI) probably represents the best balance between positive and negative liberty that could be obtained. The overall aims for NICE are to manage the introduction of innovation in healthcare provision and to promote good-quality care, whereas CHI is empowered to identify failures in the quality of care and to take action to remedy them. The initial response of healthcare professionals to this development has been positive; it is viewed as an important opportunity for the professions to maintain positive liberty even though it will mean some diminution of negative liberty.

10.4.4 Clinical governance

The debate about the nature of liberty acceded to the professions is not new. In his book *Decline of the Guilds*, Elliott Krause[9] analyses the steady decline in prestige of the medical and several other professions in five countries – Italy, Germany, France, the UK and the USA. Krause discusses how the influence of the Guilds, precursors of the professions, waned, sometimes as a result of capitalism, sometimes as a result of State action, but usually as the result of joint action by the two forces. He also emphasises that there is now a third force affecting the status of the professions – consumerism. Throughout this process, the professions seem to have been relatively unaware of what was happening or unable to take a strategic view.

In the UK, the concept of clinical governance has been introduced. Clinical governance, which could have been termed 'clinical self-governance', gives clinicians the responsibility to monitor and manage their performance as part of the general management of healthcare organisations; this concept is central to preserving positive liberty. However, in clinical governance, chief executives have been given the responsibility for the quality of clinical care, which could be seen as a loss of negative liberty, except for the understanding that this responsibility can be fulfilled only with the full involvement of clinicians.

The range of views about clinical governance can be represented on a spectrum, as shown in Fig. 10.9. At one end are those who believe that clinical freedom has been abused and professionals need to be policed; at the other are those who believe that education is the key to improved performance. However, it is necessary to reconcile these two views because both approaches are complementary. For any professional activity, performance can be measured and categorised according to quality standards. The policing function is necessary to identify those individuals who fall below the minimal acceptable standard, but

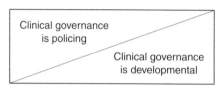

Fig. 10.9
The spectrum of views about the function of clinical governance

quality assurance is not simply a matter of identifying poor performance. The aim is to help all professionals improve their performance, which can be achieved through continuing professional development. As performance improves, it is important to re-set standards to ensure that healthcare professionals do not become complacent but are motivated to seek further improvement.

10.4.5 To whom should the clinician be loyal – patient or State?

The concepts of clinical freedom and clinical governance beg the question of how the individual clinician relates to the State on the one hand and to the patient on the other.

Patients want to trust that clinicians will give them the best possible care, but it is often not feasible for clinicians to do this because the majority work in health systems in which resources are finite and limited. Some people believe that clinicians should play no part in resource allocation or rationing; some, however, argue that the definition of evidence-based medicine is misguided to absolve clinicians of concerns about the resource consequences of each and every decision.

The approach that was taken in the development of the concepts of evidence-based medicine and evidence-based healthcare was that decision-making for groups of patients or populations was qualitatively different to that in clinical practice, even though the evidence used for both would be the same. This distinction enables the clinician and the patient to focus on incorporating the best current evidence with the patient's values and baseline condition without worrying about cost.

As an example, consider the ethical problems that might be raised when considering the use of either tissue plasminogen activator (tPA) or streptokinase for patients who have suffered an acute myocardial infarction (AMI). Both are clot-busting drugs: tPA may be marginally more effective than streptokinase (see Fig. 5.2), but it is very much more expensive. One possible approach in this situation is for the clinician to be responsible for deciding whether to administer tPA or streptokinase to each individual patient. However, if tPA is the drug of choice in the majority of cases because it may be slightly more effective, as the financial year progresses the budget will be under increasing pressure, and the clinician's decision-making becomes dominated by the availability of resources. A better approach is for those who pay for, purchase or commission health services, e.g. in the UK, a health authority, to decide whether tPA or streptokinase should be used. Although there are some minor additional benefits with the use of tPA, the population as a whole would be better served if the additional money necessary to fund the use of tPA were spent on improving the quality of care within the service, for example, the introduction of programmes to reduce the door-to-needle time for the administration of streptokinase, known to be a key factor influencing survival after AMI. If a clinician does not agree with the decision made by those who pay for the healthcare, in the UK, s/he can lobby his/her member of parliament for more money to be given to the health service to fund the use of tPA. However, it is better to make decisions about money, and marginal differences in effectiveness of interventions, at a population level.

This example highlights the nature of the ethical problems that clinicians practising evidence-based medicine, working in organisations practising evidence-based healthcare, may encounter. Thus, there can be conflict between the patient and the clinician, with the consultation as the focal point of that conflict, in which clinicians must balance the needs of the individual and the needs of society at large. If society has to limit the resources expended on healthcare and ensure those resources are used to best effect, rules and controls are essential, but so too are wise clinicians who can interpret those rules with wisdom and discretion.

Clinicians are able to see the need for wisdom and discretion most clearly when they become patients, as Chad Koller[10] describes in the *Annals of Internal Medicine* series 'On Being A Patient'. He had had major surgery and wanted analgesics for postoperative pain. The surgical intern and senior resident prescribed famotidine, 'according to the book', but the pain was worsening. Two and a half hours later, when Koller was told by the nurse his blood pressure was normal, he thought, 'Normal unless you consider my history of hypertension and my current pain. Mildly worrisome, actually'. He then asked what his last haemoglobin level was, to which the nurse replied, 'It was 7.1 mg/dL this morning, I think. I told the surgical intern, but he said that the book says you don't need a transfusion'. However, Koller knew his preoperative haemoglobin level had been 13.6 mg/dL, and was concerned that it had dropped from the postoperative level measured that morning.

The pain continued to worsen, and when the anaesthesia resident arrived, she discovered that owing to a kink in the line the epidural had not been administered by the pump, even though the readout indicated that it had. When Koller informed the anaesthesia resident of his last-measured haemoglobin level and she wondered why he had not been given any blood, the surgical intern said, 'Not unless the hemoglobin level is less than 7.0 mg/dL'. The patient then outlined his concerns, giving the entire clinical picture and strongly recommending that the intern consider giving a blood transfusion immediately. The intern paused and 'chanted', 'The book says your hemoglobin level has to be less than 7.0 mg/dL before we give you blood'. However, the intern did agree to consult the senior resident, who responded that 'the book says no transfusion'. Koller then pleaded to have his haemoglobin level re-checked. At this point, his blood pressure had dropped to 72/50 mmHg, and he felt very weak and everything 'looked dark and fuzzy'. The next thing he was aware of was the arrival of 2 units of blood. His last haemoglobin level had dropped to 6.6 mg/dL, and as the surgical intern said, 'The book said to give you blood'. In this case, the book was nearly the death of the man.

10.4.6 Remember the multiple goals of therapy

Gentle Reader,

Empathise with the clinician facing this dilemma: it is 11.30 pm and he is responsible for the care of a woman who is bleeding and near to death. However, she cannot accept she is dying and is desperate to see her son, who is five hours away but coming as quickly as he can to her bedside. Blood is scarce; the clinician knows that; he also knows that blood given to this woman will merely postpone the inevitable. There is no evidence that it will make her feel better or increase her life-expectancy, it will simply use blood that could be transfused into patients undergoing surgical interventions for which there is good evidence of effectiveness. However, the clinician chose to give the woman six units of blood over five hours. The woman was reconciled with her son and died peacefully when the transfusion was stopped.

Commentary

One of the problems faced by people suffering from cancer is that the clinicians caring for them can be confused about whether the principal goal of therapy is life extension or control of symptoms. When a decision has been made jointly with the patient that the principal goal of therapy is control of symptoms, a different pattern of care can be instituted which may be just as active and equally as, or even more, expensive than life-extension therapy.

The clinician involved in this case was accused of acting unethically by a health economist who thought he had wasted society's resources on a patient who was clearly close to death. A jury would probably have found for the clinician on grounds of humanity, but the ability of the clinician to act in this way was greatly strengthened by the fact that he happened to be one of the healthcare professionals most active not only in his hospital but also in the UK in the promotion of an evidence-based approach to decision-making. Indeed, he has championed the need for the profession to take a much more systematic, explicit and judicious approach to the use of evidence in the care of patients, whatever the objectives of therapy might be.

10.4.7 Shared decision-making

One of the aims of the provision of healthcare in the 21st century should be to promote shared decision-making. In shared decision-making, it is recognised that:

- the evidence-based clinician's contribution to the decision must take into account the patient's preferences and values;
- the consultation is no longer the only source of information – for example, patients can download information from the World Wide Web and relate that to their own preferences and values (see Margin Fig. 10.10).

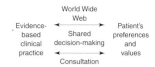

Margin Fig. 10.1

The results of a poll run in 1999 by the *British Medical Journal* to coincide with a theme issue on 'Embracing Patient Partnership' are shown in Matrix 10.1.[11] Visitors ($n = > 850$) to the website from 17 September to 4 October were asked who should make treatment decisions. As can be seen, the majority of patients preferred shared decision-making. When asked which consulting style will

	Doctor decides	Doctor and patient decide together	Patient decides
As a patient, which consulting style do you prefer?	56	737	54
Which consulting style predominates today?	503	298	43
Which consulting style do you think will predominate in 10 years' time?	75	546	223

Matrix 10.1

predominate in 10 years' time, 65% of visitors responded that it would be shared decision-making; however, it is interesting to note that 26% of visitors thought that the patient would be making the decision.

However, it is important to be aware that different patients may want different levels of control and participation in decision-making. In the study of 1012 women who had a confirmed diagnosis of breast cancer (see also p. 342), Degner et al.[12] investigated the level of control and participation the women desired in decision-making about their treatment, and the degree to which their desired level of control had been achieved. They found that:

- 22% wanted to select their own treatment;
- 44% preferred a collaborative approach;
- 34% wished to delegate the responsibility to the clinician.

The best single predictor of preference was a woman's educational status.

It can be seen that the majority of women did want to participate in the decision-making about their treatment, however, only 42% of the women felt that they had achieved their preferred level of control. From this study, it would appear that clinicians should not make assumptions but actively determine each individual patient's preferred level of control and participation in decision-making about treatment options, and tailor their approach accordingly. It is possible also that a patient's preference about participation may change during the course of an illness, and it is advisable to review this at suitable points during treatment.

A website devoted to the promotion of shared decision-making is available at:

http://www.shared-decision-making.org/

References

1. SACKETT, D.L., ROSENBERG, W.M.C., GRAY, J.A.M. et al. (1996) *Evidence-based medicine: what it is and what it isn't [Editorial]*. Br. Med. J. 312: 71–2.
2. McALISTER, F.A., STRAUS, S.E., GUYATT, G.D. and HAYNES, R.B. (2000) *Users' guides to the medical literature: XX. Integrating research evidence with the care of the individual patient*. JAMA 283: 2829–36.
3. ELLIS, J., MULLIGAN, I., ROWE, J. and SACKETT, D.L. (1995) *In-patient general medicine is evidence based*. Lancet 346: 407–10.
4. GEDDES, J.R., GAME, D., JENKINS, N.E., PETERSON, L.A., POTTINGER, G.R. and SACKETT, D.L. (1996) *What proportion of primary psychiatric interventions are based on randomised evidence?* Quality in Health Care 5: 215–17.
5. HOWES, N., CHAGLA, L., THORPE, M. and McCULLOCH, P. (1997) *Surgical practice is evidence based*. Br. J. Surg. 84: 1220–3.
6. GUYATT, G.H., COOK, D.J. and JAESCHKE, R. (1995) *How should clinicians use the results of randomized trials?* ACP Journal Club Jan–Feb: 122(1): A12–13
7. GUYATT, H.G., COOK, D.J. and JAESCHKE, R. (1995) *Applying the findings of clinical trials to individual patients [Editorial]*. ACP Journal Club Mar–Apr: 122(2): A12–13.
8. GLASZIOU, P.P. and IRWIG, L.M. (1995) *An evidence based approach to individualising treatment*. Br. Med. J. 311: 1356–9.
9. KRAUSE, E. (1996) *Decline of the Guilds: Professions, States and the Advance of Capitalism, 1930 to the Present*. Yale University Press, New Haven and London.
10. KOLLER, C. (1997) *What the book says*. Ann. Intern. Med. 127: 238–9.
11. e-BMJ (1999) *Poll results*. Br. Med. J. 319: 1026.
12. DEGNER, L.F., KRISTJANSON, L.J., BOWMAN, D. et al. (1997) *Information needs and decisional preferences in women with breast cancer*. JAMA 277: 1485–92.

10.5 CLINICIANS: WITCH DOCTORS OR SCIENTISTS? – DEALING WITH ANXIETY

Gentle Reader,

Empathise with the eminent American surgeon and his son, both of whom were prominent gastroenterologists. The surgeon was suffering from stomach cancer. Father and son searched and appraised the literature to determine what was the best course of action. They went to see expert after expert, each of whom gave different advice or behaved so cautiously that they merely re-stated the evidence, saying that it was inconclusive. Weary and dispirited, the son said to the last expert, 'What more do we need to get a good decision?'. To which the expert replied, 'You need a good doctor'.

Commentary

Throughout most of this book, it has been argued that there is a need for a scientific, evidence-based approach to decision-making. However, there are situations in which clinical decisions are not clear-cut, in fact only a small proportion ever are; as such, the relationship between clinician and patient is of central importance in decision-taking. Although evidence is influential in decision-making, in decision-taking the fears, anxieties and values of the patient may predominate.

Although patients do want to be treated as rational beings, that is, offered evidence, helped to assess the various options and left to take the decision, this approach does not take account of the effect of an important aspect of any consultation, that of anxiety. Anxiety may be felt by both clinician and patient. Patients can be anxious about many aspects of illness and disease, such as the diagnosis, when it is unknown, or the treatment options and outcomes when it is; clinicians may feel anxious about the possibility of misdiagnosis.

Anthropologists have defined magic as an intervention designed to reduce anxiety in times of uncertainty; a rain dance does not bring rain but it does relieve anxiety during the wait. Witch doctors use only magic, although they can proffer what they may call 'evidence': for example, rain did fall after the rain dance. A witch doctor's role, therefore, is not to cure disease but to minimise anxiety in times of uncertainty.

Clinicians do use certain techniques to control patient anxiety, either consciously or unconsciously. One technique is to appear to be more certain, or to state or imply that the evidence of effectiveness is certain when, as is usually the case, it indicates only a probability of success. This is done with the best of intentions. Indeed, some patients want the clinician to deal with their anxiety, and they look for reassurance and comfort; in fact, they require both a witch doctor and a clinician in the same consultation and in one and the same person.

There is usually a dilemma associated with every clinical decision, not simply those that are associated with a choice between palliative care and interventions that have a low probability of success and a high risk of side-effects. Patients have to make decisions about which treatment option to choose, e.g. mastectomy or breast-conserving treatment (lumpectomy), or about whether to opt for preventive intervention or risk acceptance, e.g. treatment for high blood pressure or no action.

In one study of decisions made between two types of treatment, Fallowfield et al.[1] investigated the association between being offered a choice of treatment and a patient being anxious or depressed after treatment. No difference was found in the prevalence of anxiety and depression between the patients who had been offered a choice of treatment and those to whom a firm recommendation had been made about a treatment option. What is striking about this result is that it is impossible to generalise about patients and their preferences. For example, of the 62 women offered choice, eight refused to choose, whereas a proportion of patients who were not offered choice expressed a wish for more autonomy.

Reference

1. FALLOWFIELD, L.J., HALL, A., MAGUIRE, P. et al. (1994) *Psychological effects of being offered choice of surgery for breast cancer.* Br. Med. J. 309: 448.

10.6 ACCELERATING CHANGE IN CLINICAL PRACTICE

Clinical practice is changing all the time. Over the last two decades, the medical profession as a whole has performed well in discarding ineffective therapies and adopting effective ones. However, in the current economic climate, the evolution of clinical practice must be telescoped. At present, the process of evolution is marked by the following characteristics:

- overenthusiastic adoption of interventions of unproven efficacy or even proven ineffectiveness;
- failure to adopt interventions that do more good than harm at a reasonable cost;
- continuing to offer interventions or services demonstrated to be ineffective;
- adoption of interventions without adequate preparation such that the benefits demonstrated in a research setting cannot be reproduced in the ordinary service setting;
- wide variation in the rates at which interventions are adopted or discarded.

10.6.1 Educate to influence

Within the numerous RCTs of different interventions designed to improve clinical practice, patient outcome has been taken as the end-point and not a professional's knowledge or level of skill. The results of such trials, which measure the outcomes that matter most to patients, should be of interest to educators and those who provide funds for education.

In continuing medical education, the following interventions have *not* been shown to be effective:

- standard lectures;
- the provision of knowledge alone;
- written information.

It has been shown that, for clinicians, educational needs assessment and framing of learning objectives are necessary precursors to the identification of topics about which an individual needs to learn.[1] Formal training can then improve performance with respect to these topics. However, for those topics individuals want to study, knowledge base and performance improves irrespective of training.

In a systematic review of 150 RCTs of different methods of continuing medical education,[2] the following interventions were found to be effective in changing behaviour.

- Mini-sabbaticals – allowing clinicians to go and work in units practising high-quality evidence-based healthcare.
- Sensitive personalised feedback on an individual's performance, either in comparison with that of others or against explicit standards, as part of a learning process.
- Patient education.
- Computer-assisted decision-making providing reminders and easy access to evidence-based guidelines and to knowledge itself.
- On-the-job training of practical skills.
- The use of opinion leaders or 'educational influentials', i.e. a colleague whose performance is respected.

It could be argued that these interventions will increase cost. However, it is also important to consider the cost of failing to offer effective education and of the current level of expenditure on continuing professional education using techniques of unproven effectiveness.

10.6.2 Carrots or sticks?

Two schools of thought have culminated in a polarisation of views: there are those who believe in incentives (the carrot) and those who believe in disincentives (the stick) as a means of achieving change. An interesting permutation that one commentator advocated was to hit people with the carrot!

The evidence of whether an incentive or a disincentive is more effective is difficult to interpret, in part because of the problem in defining what constitutes an incentive and what constitutes a disincentive. The introduction of incentive payments for cervical screening for general practitioners played a part in increasing the coverage of cervical screening. Was the money a carrot or was the threat of a drop in income a stick? Financial incentives are difficult to manage and it is easy for perverse incentives to be introduced into any system. The simplest system in which to operate evidence-based healthcare is one in which clinicians are salaried and receive no financial reward for increased volume or intensity of care, as George Bernard Shaw so elegantly articulated.

> It is not the fault of our doctors that the medical service of the community, as at present provided for, is a murderous absurdity. That any sane nation, having observed that you could provide for the supply of bread by giving bakers a pecuniary interest in baking for you, should go on to give a surgeon a pecuniary interest in cutting off your leg, is enough to make one despair of political humanity. But that is precisely what we have done. And the more appalling the mutilation, the more the mutilator is paid. He who corrects the ingrowing toe-nail receives a few shillings: he who cuts your inside out receives hundreds of guineas, except when he does it to a poor person for practice.
>
> *From 'Preface on Doctors',*
> *in* The Doctor's Dilemma, *1911*

If healthcare is delivered within a fee-based service, for example, in a private insurance scheme, it is easy to influence practice by stopping paying for a particular procedure. The response is usually marked and quick.

In systems in which finance is not a strong motivator, external pressures can be applied through the use of guidelines and other aspects of 'managed care' (Section 1.7). However, even in the preparation of guidelines, external pressures, whether as carrots or sticks, are relatively ineffective. In an evaluation of guidelines as a means of influencing clinical practice,[3] a wide variation was found ranging from nationally produced guidelines, which are evidence-based but relatively ineffective, to locally produced guidelines, in which local practitioners have been involved, which can be effective but may also be unscientific.

10.6.3 Growing carrots

The use of a simplistic carrot and stick metaphor implies that the only change that needs to take place is a change in clinical practice. However, to take such a narrow focus will have only a limited impact, even if all of the interventions shown to be effective in changing clinical practice are used.

Change is happening at an exponential rate, thereby increasing the pressure on professionals within a context of decreasing availability of resources. In this situation, it is essential to appreciate the wider context,[4] otherwise it will not be possible to overcome what has been called 'the subtle sabotage of withheld enthusiasm'.[5]

The most important step in facilitating change is to ensure that professionals want to change. The most effective way of encouraging professionals to change is to help them see evidence-based decision-making not as a management imperative but as an intellectual challenge. It is much more effective to stimulate professionals to grow their own carrots than to force them into behaving like donkeys, enticed by a carrot dangling in front and threatened by a stick held behind.

References

1. SIBLEY, J.C., SACKETT, D.L., NEUFELD, V.R. et al. (1982) *A randomized trial of continuing medical education.* N. Engl. J. Med. 302: 511.
2. DAVIS, D.A., THOMSON, M.A., OXMAN, A.D. and HAYNES, B.P. (1995) *Changing physicians' performance.* JAMA 274: 700–5.
3. GRIMSHAW, J.M. and RUSSELL, I.T. (1993) *Effect of clinical guidelines on medical practice: a systematic review of rigorous evaluations.* Lancet 342: 1317–22.
4. BACKER, T.E. (1995) *Integrating behavioral and systems strategies to change clinical practice.* J. Quality Improvement 21: 351–3.
5. KAEGI, L. (1993) *Using guidelines to change clinical behavior: dissemination through Area Health Centers and Geriatric Education Centers.* Quality Review Bulletin May: 165–9.

EVIDENCE-BASED HEALTHCARE IN THE POST-MODERN ERA

EVIDENCE, ECONOMICS AND ETHICS

If you want to learn people's values, present them a choice.

Roger Neighbour, The Inner Apprentice.

People making decisions about health and healthcare policy face three great challenges:

- population ageing;
- new technology and new knowledge;
- rising consumer expectations, which are being stimulated and driven by the explosion of information on the World Wide Web.

In some countries, particularly those in Africa, the prevalence of AIDS in the general population can be considered as a fourth challenge.

As a result of these challenges, the need and demand for healthcare are increasing at a rate that is greater than the rate at which resources are being made available. As a consequence, it is necessary for decision-making to be open, explicit, and evidence based.

The use of an evidence-based approach makes it possible to differentiate between a proposition that is supported by evidence and one made on unsubstantiated assertion or opinion (Fig. E.1). However, any evidence-based decision, whether being made in clinical practice or healthcare management or policy-making, is influenced by values. The clinician has to take into account the condition and values of the individual patient; the policy-maker has to take into account not only best current knowledge but also the needs of the population, the values of that population, the resources available, and the opportunity costs of any decision.

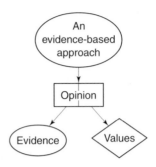

Fig. E.1
An evidence-based approach clarifies the basis of a
proposition

In evidence-based policy-making and management, it is
important also to distinguish between decision-making and
decision-taking. For effective decision-making in
healthcare, scientists have a responsibility to ensure that the
best current knowledge is available, but decisions need to
be taken by the public or their representatives, because all
healthcare decisions involve the allocation of finite
resources and have significant opportunity costs. In
general, the provision of information improves the quality
of decision-making, but it is important to bear in mind
Maynard Keynes' proverb that there is nothing that a
politician likes so little as to be well informed because it
makes decision-taking even more complicated and difficult.

Although it is sometimes possible to make a sharp
distinction between evidence and values, it is important for
the evidence-based decision-maker to bear in mind that
values are all pervasive. The assumption made throughout
this book that evidence and values can be distinguished
like oil and water is a necessary convenience. The reality is
that our values influence the way we ask questions, collect
information, interpret data, and express the results.

DOING BETTER, FEELING WORSE

Although *Doing Better and Feeling Worse* is the title of a
collection of essays about the American healthcare system,
it describes how many people felt about clinical practice
and healthcare during the 1990s. This feeling of unease is
experienced by those within the service, who feel criticised
as never before, and those who use the service, who feel
that health services are not as good as they were. Yet never
has the provision of healthcare been so effective or so
efficient, never have clinicians been trained to communicate
so well, nor has more attention been given to the needs and
aspirations of patients and carers. New complaint systems
have been introduced, and the clinical professions are open
to scrutiny as never before. Finally, and most recently,
clinicians are practising evidence-based decision-making,
and managers are making open and explicit decisions
about health services based on best current evidence.

As proponents of an evidence-based approach, we must
ask ourselves two profound questions.

- Why is it that as healthcare professionals, although we
  have become so effective, and concerned with
  communication and the patient's experience, we have
  never been so unpopular?
- Why is it that as healthcare professionals, although we
  have never been more self-critical, more scientific and
  more thoughtful, we have never been more insecure or
  less certain?

It may be that the phenomenon we are witnessing is simply
a widening gap between consumer expectations and the
delivery of a health service subject to increasing pressure
exerted by the population ageing and the advent of new
technology and new knowledge. However, there is the
possibility that in clinical practice and healthcare
management other more complex factors are at work,
which may stem from the marked ambivalence that society
has to the advances of science and technology.

THE MODERNISATION OF MEDICINE

It is possible to divide the practice of medicine into three main eras.

First era: *pre-modern medicine,* in which the enthusiasm and conviction of the individual clinician, and of the profession as a whole, was sufficient to bring about change.

Second era: *modern medicine,* which was based on science and characterised by scepticism and uncertainty. This era began not with the technological developments after the Second World War but in the 1960s when the new breed of epidemiologists, epitomised by Archie Cochrane with his conceptualisation of effectiveness and efficiency, sowed the seeds of doubt in the minds of once-confident clinicians.

Third era: *post-modern medicine,* the current era, which while retaining the characteristics of modern medicine needs to take account of and adapt to the following social concerns and trends:

- for many patients, the process of care is as important as the outcome;
- the process of care can influence the outcomes of care, not only with respect to patient satisfaction but also in terms of the patient's state of health and the effectiveness of treatment;
- modern medicine and complementary medicine can be used together in what Dr Andrew Weil, the leading protagonist of this movement, has called 'integrative medicine';
- the involvement of patients as *partners* in clinical decision-making, although it is important to be aware that different patients will require different degrees of involvement (see Section 10.4.7).
- the public are more concerned about the risks of modern medicine than the medical establishment which, until now, has emphasised the benefits.

Die Risikogesellschaft

Ulrich Beck, Professor of Sociology at Munich, is one of the leading figures in his discipline. In his book, *The Risk Society*, he proposed that:

> the scientists are entirely incapable of reacting adequately to civilisational risks since they are prominently involved in the origin and growth of those very risks. Instead – sometimes with a clear conscience of 'pure scientific method', sometimes with increasing pangs of guilt – the science has become the legitimising patrons of a global industrial pollution and contamination of air, water, foodstuff, etc.[1]

Beck castigates the sciences as 'a branch office of politics, ethics, business and judicial practice in the garb of numbers' and the scientists have, in his opinion, 'squandered until further notice their historic reputation for rationality'. Beck's main concerns, and his arguments, derive from his study of risk and pollution. He points out that it would be more honest to replace the phrase 'permitted maximum levels' of a harmful substance with another – 'collective standardised poisoning'.

His arguments are powerful, both as an analysis of the public views of science and as a trenchant stimulus to those involved in the sciences to re-think their claim to objectivity and rationality. Medicine, in strengthening its scientific base, and through its claim to be a branch of science, exposes itself to the general public's distrust of science. It is also worth considering what medicine may have lost in moving away from a style of practice based on the personal opinion of the physician to one based on 'impersonal' scientific evidence.

Beck has one further important message for evidence-based decision-makers, whether clinicians or managers: the 21st century will be one dominated by concerns about risk and the adverse effects of intervention, whereas scientists, including clinical scientists and epidemiologists, have hitherto emphasised the positive aspects of science and the benefits to be gained from intervention.

Evidence-based risk management

As evidence accumulates about the prevalence of medical errors, public concern about the quality of healthcare provision will increase. This could lead to an exponential rise in the number of complaints and in the level of litigation. However, it is possible to adopt a pro-active approach to risk management.

In a review of the implementation of a 'humanistic risk management policy' at the Veterans Affairs Medical Center in Lexington, Kentucky, from 1990 to 1996,[2] Kraman and Hamm assessed the impact of introducing 'a policy that seems to be designed to maximize malpractice claims'. The policy included:

- early injury review;
- steadfast maintenance of the relationship between the hospital and the patient;
- proactive full disclosure to patients who have been injured because of accidents or medical negligence;
- fair compensation for injuries.

From their analysis, Kraman and Hamm judged the financial consequences of full disclosure to be 'moderate', and the liability payments were found to be comparable with those of similar facilities. They concluded that an honest and forthright policy in which the patient's interests come first may be relatively inexpensive because it enables healthcare institutions to avoid lawsuit preparation, litigation, court judgement, and settlements at trial. Important additional advantages of such a policy are goodwill and the maintenance of the caregiver role. In an accompanying Editorial in the *Annals of Internal Medicine*, Wu states:

> only by changing the expectations of both patients and physicians can we achieve the solutions that will decrease medical errors and their devastating consequences.[3]

POST-MODERN CLINICAL PRACTICE

'…a primordial image', as Jacob Burckhardt once called it – the figure of a physician or teacher of mankind. The archetypal image of the wise man, the saviour or redeemer, lies buried and dormant in man's unconscious since the dawn of culture; it is awakened whenever the times are out of joint and a human society is committed to a serious error. When people go astray they feel the need of a guide or teacher or even of the physician.

Carl Gustav Jung,
Modern Man in Search of a Soul

It is likely that the 21st century will be one in which there will be greater uncertainty – economic, social and environmental. Against this background, it will be necessary for the clinician to practise evidence-based medicine (although the term may fall into disuse as evidence-based medicine becomes part of the accepted paradigm).

Anxiety and disease

There are several interesting trends that should give the proponents of evidence-based medicine cause to stop and think.

- The sector in healthcare undergoing the fastest growth is complementary medicine.
- Bookshops contain more books about alternative medicine than those about what might be termed scientific, evidence-based, or conventional medicine.
- Vitamin and nutritional supplements, for which there is no evidence of effectiveness, are two of the fastest growing retail lines – new 'health' shops are opening more rapidly than new healthcare facilities.

As proponents of an evidence-based approach, we must ask ourselves what it is that people want that they are not getting from conventional health services.

Perhaps it is certainty they need, and uncertainty is undoubtedly the hallmark of evidence-based healthcare and a critical approach to decision-making. In the past, a doctor was always certain, always had a diagnosis, and always had a treatment in which s/he believed, or at least appeared to believe. The modern doctor is sceptical, uncertain, and participate. Some patients welcome this development, but many do not. More confusing for the clinician, some patients apparently welcome the change but also want a doctor who is certain.

Thus, it is important to recognise that many patients want more than uncertainty from a consultation. People who are ill are anxious, and they want their anxiety assuaged as well as their disease treated. Many patients, however, do not have a disease that doctors can recognise; they simply bring to the doctor their feelings of unwellness and anxiety. Sometimes, reassurance that they do not have a disease is sufficient, but this is not always the case.

Dealing with anxiety: medicine or magic?

Evidence-based medicine, although a very good way of dealing with disease, is not necessarily a good way of dealing with anxiety. In fact, for some people, it may increase the level of anxiety which is why they might seek complementary care. Complementary therapists are rarely as uncertain as practitioners of evidence-based clinical practice, and are sometimes absolutely certain both about the theory on which they base their practice and about the advice they give an individual patient. Although some practitioners of evidence-based medicine are good at alleviating anxiety and some patients are not anxious, currently there is no mechanism through which the anxieties of individual patients can easily be identified and met by a busy clinician; moreover, a clinician's style of practice stems from his/her personality as well from a learned skill.

Anthropologists define magic as a technique used to allay anxiety when no effective interventions are available, and we are probably moving into an era in which people want magic as well as science.

The 21st century clinician

Three things which judgement demands:

- wisdom
- penetration
- knowledge

Ninth Century Irish Triad

David Pencheon has suggested that the three most important words for the clinician of the 21st century should be 'I don't know'. Openly admitting to patients that no-one can keep abreast of all the information being generated and taking on the role of and working as a knowledge manager is the most appropriate strategy for a clinician, rather than trying to retain a status as the fount of all knowledge, which was how physicians were viewed (and sometimes portrayed themselves) in the past.

In his book *Business @ the Speed of Thought*,[4] Bill Gates identified one of the important debates for the digital age as the need to identify the function of the human being; nowhere will this be more important than in clinical practice.

Conclusion

The challenge for the future will be to develop the scientific approaches described in this book while at the same time appreciating that individual patients are anxious and will need help and support to cope with that anxiety. Evidence-based decision-making emphasises probability and uncertainty. In a world that is increasingly uncertain, clinicians and managers of health services who evince an evidence-based approach may be faced not by patients and populations who welcome this uncertainty, and bravely tackle the epidemiological and economic issues involved, but by patients and populations who resort to magic. It is vital to think carefully about how we use evidence-based decision-making in future to ensure that it does not increase the unknowing use of magic in clinical practice and patient choice.

References

1. BECK, U. (1986) *The Risk Society* Sage.
2. KRAMAN, S.S. and HAMM, G.H. (1999) *Risk management: extreme honesty may be the best policy* Ann. Intern. Med. 131: 963–7.
3. WU, A.W. (1999) *Handling hospital errors: is disclosure the best defense? [Editorial]*. Ann. Intern. Med. 131: 970–2.
4. GATES, B. (2000) *Business @ the Speed of Thought*. Penguin, London.

INTRODUCTION TO APPENDICES

Evidence-based healthcare is a rapidly changing field. Although every effort has been made to provide information that is current at the time of going to press, it must be emphasised that the reader should also check the contents of resource guides to establish the availability of new resources and any recent changes to the coverage of existing resources. The two foremost resource guides for evidence-based healthcare may be found at:

- *Netting the Evidence: A ScHARR Guide to Evidence Based Practice on the Internet*
  http://www.shef.ac.uk/~scharr/ir/netting.html

- *CASPFew Sources of Evidence*
  http://www.ihs.ox.ac.uk/caspfew/sources.html

FINDING THE EVIDENCE

I.1   RESOURCE OVERVIEW

The search for evidence follows two main routes:

1. a reliable and well-conducted *systematic review* can provide a clinical bottom-line from the pooled result of several studies;
2. a comparative *primary study*, preferably of randomised controlled design, of sufficient power and robustness can provide an indication of clinical effectiveness.

In the absence of such published research, the search will be extended to registers of *ongoing research*. Research in progress indicates outstanding issues to be answered and may be used to set a review date for previously taken decisions in the light of new evidence.

Systematic reviews may be commissioned as separately funded research projects and issued as a report, published in the journal literature or, increasingly, made available in an electronic form. Randomised controlled trials are traditionally disseminated through the journal literature and can be identified through bibliographic databases. Recent interest in clinical trials has led to the development of an increasing number of trials registers whereby trials are tracked from their initiation rather than from publication. Finally, the notoriously elusive nature of research in progress is being countered by collection of data on research projects direct from the funding source.

I.2   RESOURCES

I.2.1   The Cochrane Library

The Cochrane Library is an electronic publication designed
to supply high-quality evidence to:

- those providing and receiving care;
- those responsible for research, teaching, funding and
  administration at all levels.

It is published quarterly on CD-ROM and the Internet, and
is distributed on a subscription basis. The abstracts of
Cochrane Collaboration Reviews are available without
charge and can be searched.
   The Cochrane Library includes:

- The Cochrane Database of Systematic Reviews –
  regularly updated reviews of the effects of healthcare;
- Database of Abstracts of Reviews of Effectiveness –
  critical assessments and structured abstracts of good
  systematic reviews published elsewhere;
- The Cochrane Controlled Trials Register – bibliographic
  information on controlled trials;
- other sources of information on the science of reviewing
  research and evidence-based healthcare.

Also included in The Cochrane Library are:

- The Cochrane Review Methodology Database – a
  bibliography of articles and books on the science of
  research synthesis;
- The NHS Economic Evaluation Database, produced by
  the NHS Centre for Reviews and Dissemination in York
  (see I.4.2);
- a handbook on critical appraisal and the science of
  reviewing research;
- a glossary of methodological terms;
- contact details for Cochrane Collaborative Review
  Groups and other entities in The Cochrane
  Collaboration;
- *Netting the Evidence* – where to find information on the
  Internet on using evidence in practice.

   The CD-ROM version requires a PC with 386SX processor
or higher, with minimum 4MB RAM. This represents an
absolute minimum and The Cochrane Library will run
much faster on machines with at least a 486DX processor

and 8MB RAM. The Cochrane Library CD-ROM is currently produced only as a Microsoft Windows program.

The Cochrane Library Online is an installation of the complete Cochrane Library that may be accessed using a standard Internet browser, such as Internet Explorer, or Netscape. The Cochrane Library Online is available directly from Update Software, who produce and publish it on behalf of The Cochrane Collaboration and manage subscriptions both directly and through licensed distribution partners. To subscribe directly through Update Software contact:

Update Software Ltd.
Summertown Pavilion
Middle Way
Summertown
Oxford, OX2 7LG
United Kingdom

Tel: +44 (0) 1865 513902

Fax: +44 (0) 1865 516918

e-mail: info@update.co.uk

http://www.update-software.com/ccweb/cochrane/cdsr.htm

I.2.1.1 The Cochrane Database of Systematic Reviews

The Cochrane Database of Systematic Reviews (CDSR) is a rapidly growing collection of regularly updated systematic reviews of the effects of healthcare. Entries are divided into completed reviews, available in full-text, and protocols which are expressions of intent and include a brief outline of the topic and a deadline for submission. These reviews and protocols are prepared by contributors to The Cochrane Collaboration (see I.3.1). New reviews are added with each issue of The Cochrane Library, so that eventually all areas of healthcare will be covered. In Issue 1 2000, there are 52 new reviews and 98 new protocols in the Cochrane Database of Systematic Reviews, bringing the total entries for this database up to 1338. These cover areas such as pregnancy and childbirth, diabetes, subfertility, stroke, schizophrenia, acute respiratory infections, airways, diabetes, musculoskeletal injuries, neonatal care, peripheral vascular disease and parasitic diseases among others.

The systematic reviews are prepared, and maintained, according to standards set out in *The Cochrane Collaboration: The Reviewers' Handbook.* (*The Reviewers' Handbook* is the official document which describes in detail the process of creating Cochrane systematic reviews. It is revised frequently to ensure that it remains up-to-date. The current version is 4.0, updated July 1999.) They are based on hand-searching of journals and prepared by personnel who will also be responsible for identifying and incorporating new evidence as it becomes available.

I.2.1.2 Database of Abstracts of Reviews of Effectiveness

Complementing the information on CDSR, the Database of Abstracts of Reviews of Effectiveness (DARE) provides pointers to over 2700 good-quality systematic reviews from around the world, all of which have been quality-filtered by reviewers at the NHS Centre for Reviews and Dissemination (NHS CRD) at the University of York, England (see I.3.2). Some of these are structured abstracts providing a brief appraisal of the review, others are briefer records for background information or abstracts of reviews produced by the *American College of Physicians (ACP) Journal Club.*

I.2.1.3 The Cochrane Controlled Trials Register

The Cochrane Controlled Trials Register (CCTR) is a bibliography of nearly 300 000 controlled trials (Issue 1 2000) identified by contributors to The Cochrane Collaboration and others as part of an international effort to create an unbiased source of data for systematic reviews. CCTR includes reports published in conference proceedings and in many other sources not currently listed in MEDLINE or other bibliographic databases. As its name suggests, this database is a register of trials found through systematic hand-searching and database-searching of the world's journals (a consequence of which is that a high proportion of references are duplicated having come from more than one source).

I.2.1.4 The Cochrane Review Methodology Database

The Cochrane Review Methodology Database (CRMD) is a bibliography of articles on the science of research synthesis and on practical aspects of preparing systematic reviews. This is an invaluable source of information on RCTs, and the strengths and weaknesses of systematic reviews.

I.2.2 Best Evidence

Best Evidence is a CD-ROM, launched in 1997, which contains the full text of two major journals of secondary publication:

- *ACP Journal Club*;
- *Evidence-Based Medicine*.

These two journals cover reviews from more than 90 journals world-wide, and articles are included only if they meet strict selection criteria for study design. Each article is summarised in a structured abstract, with expert commentary putting the information in clinical perspective. The database also includes:

- editorials about critical appraisal and clinical application of evidence;
- a reference glossary of statistical terms with examples.

Best Evidence is available from BMJ Publishing. Full details are available at:
http://www.bmjpg.com/data/ebm.htm

I.2.3 EBM Reviews, Best Evidence

EBM Reviews, Best Evidence is a database from Ovid that contains the full-text reviews of clinically relevant articles from *Evidence-Based Medicine* and *ACP Journal Club*, and full-text topic overviews from the Cochrane Database of Systematic Reviews (see I.2.1.1) to provide Internet access to both systematic reviews and critically appraised reviews of individual articles. A unique feature is the database's links both to a fully searchable version of Ovid's MEDLINE product and to the full-text of journals in Ovid's Biomedical Collections:

http://www.ovid.com/products/databases/

I.2.4   NHS Centre for Reviews and Dissemination (CRD) publications

I.2.4.1   CRD Reports

CRD Reports are produced by the NHS Centre for Reviews and Dissemination at the University of York. The following reports have been published to date:

1. Which way forward for the care of critically ill children?
2. Relationship between volume and quality of health care: a review of the literature .
3. Review of the research on the effectiveness of health service interventions to reduce variations in health.
4. Undertaking systematic reviews of research on effectiveness: CRD guidelines for those carrying out or commissioning reviews.
5. Ethnicity and health: reviews of literature and guidance for purchasers in the areas of cardiovascular disease, mental health and haemoglobinopathies.
6. Making cost-effectiveness information accessible: the NHS economic evaluation database project: CRD guidance for reporting critical summaries of economic evaluations.
7. A pilot study of informed choice leaflets on positions in labour and routine ultrasound.
8. Concentration and choice in the provision of hospital services (summary report, and three parts).
9. Preschool vision screening: results of a systematic review.
10. Systematic review of interventions in the treatment and prevention of obesity.
11. A systematic review of the effectiveness of interventions for managing childhood nocturnal enuresis.
12. *Screening for Speech and Language Delay: a Systematic Review of the Literature.* (Available only from HTA.)
13. *Screening for Ovarian Cancer: a Systematic Review.*
14. *Women and Secure Psychiatric Services: a Literature Review.*
15. *Systematic Review of the International Literature on the Epidemiology of Mentally Disordered Offenders.*
16. Scoping review of literature on the health and care of mentally disordered offenders.
17. Therapeutic community effectiveness: a systematic international review of therapeutic community

treatment for people with personality disorders and mentally disordered offenders.

18. Systematic review of the efficacy and safety of the fluoridation of drinking water.

http://www.york.ac.uk/inst/crd/crdrep.htm

The NHS CRD website also lists in-house and commissioned reviews, including reviews that are completed but not yet published, and reviews in progress or due to start:
http://www.york.ac.uk/inst/crd/

I.2.4.2   Effective Health Care bulletins

Effective Health Care (EHC) is a bi-monthly bulletin for decision-makers in which the effectiveness of a variety of healthcare interventions is examined, based on a systematic review and synthesis of research on clinical effectiveness, cost-effectiveness and acceptability. Reviews are carried out by a research team using established methodological guidelines, found in CRD Report No.4[1] with advice from expert consultants for each topic. The bulletins are subject to extensive and rigorous peer review.

In the UK, over 55 000 copies of *Effective Health Care* are distributed free within the NHS. Health Authorities also receive copies to distribute to GPs in their area. The contents of each volume are shown in Table I.1.

EHC bulletins are published by The Royal Society of Medicine Press Ltd. All orders and enquiries regarding subscriptions for EHC bulletins should be addressed to:

Publications Subscription Department
The Royal Society of Medicine Press Ltd.
PO Box 9002
London
W1A 0ZA

Tel: +44 (0)171 290 2927/8

Fax: +44 (0)171 290 2929

Bulletins from Volume 2 onwards are downloadable from the World Wide Web:
http://www.york.ac.uk/inst/crd/ehcb.htm

I.2.4.3   Effectiveness Matters

Effectiveness Matters is produced to complement *Effective Health Care*, and provides updates on the effectiveness of

Table I.1　Contents of *Effective Health Care* bulletins by volume

Volume 1	Volume 2	Volume 3	Volume 5
• Screening for Osteoporosis to Prevent Fractures	• The Prevention and Treatment of Pressure Sores	• Preventing and Reducing the Adverse Effects of Unintended Teenage Pregnancies	• Getting evidence into practice
• Stroke Rehabilitation	• Benign Prostatic Hyperplasia: Treatment for Lower Urinary Tract Symptoms in Older Men	• The Prevention and Treatment of Obesity	• Dental restoration: what type of filling?
• The Management of Subfertility		• Mental Health Promotion in High Risk Groups	• Management of gynaecological cancers
• The Treatment of Persistent Glue Ear in Children			• Complications of diabetes: screening for retinopathy; management of foot ulcers
• The Treatment of Depression in Primary Care	• Management of Cataract	• Compression Therapy for Venous Leg Ulcers	• Preventing the uptake of smoking in young people
• Cholesterol: Screening and Treatment	• Preventing Falls and Subsequent Injury in Older People	• Management of Stable Angina	
• Brief Interventions and Alcohol Abuse	• Preventing Unintentional Injuries in Children and Young Adolescents	• The Management of Colorectal Cancer	• Drug treatment for schizophrenia
• Implementing Clinical Practice Guidelines		**Volume 4**	
• Management of Menorrhagia	• Management of Primary Breast Cancer	• Cholesterol and coronary heart disease: screening and treatment	**Volume 6**
	• Total Hip Replacement		• Complications of diabetes: renal disease and promotion of self-management
	• Hospital Volume and Health Care Outcomes, Costs and Patient Access	• Pre-school hearing, speech, language and vision screening	• Promoting the initiation of breastfeeding
		• Management of lung cancer	• Psychosocial interventions for schizophrenia
		• Cardiac rehabilitation	
		• Antimicrobial prophylaxis in colorectal surgery	
		• Deliberate self-harm	

important health interventions for practitioners and decision-makers in the NHS. It covers topics in a shorter, more journalistic style, summarising the results of high-quality systematic reviews. In the UK, 60 000 copies of each issue are distributed throughout the NHS.

Volume 1 (1995)

1. Aspirin and myocardial infarction.
2. *Helicobacter pylori* and peptic ulcer.

Volume 2 (1996–97)

1. Influenza vaccination and older people.
2. Screening for prostate cancer (accompanied by a patient information leaflet: 'Screening for prostate cancer: the evidence. Information for men considering or asking for PSA tests').

Volume 3 (1998)
1. Smoking cessation: what the health service can do.
2. Prophylactic removal of impacted third molars: is it justified?

Volume 4 (1999)
1. Treating head lice and scabies.
2. Drug treatment of essential hypertension in older people.

Effectiveness Matters is a free publication available on subscription. To subscribe, contact CRD Publications: Tel: +44 (0)1904 433648. The full text of most of the *Effectiveness Matters* series can be viewed at: http://www.york.ac.uk/inst/crd/em.htm

I.2.5   Other good-quality reviews

There are other sources of reviewed evidence which, although they do not meet the standards of The Cochrane Collaboration or NHS CRD, can be recommended as a source of information.

I.2.5.1   Health Technology Assessment reports

The Health Technology Assessment reports are produced at the Wessex Institute for Research and Development. They contain abstracts, and in many cases full text, for the completed reviews from the NHS Health Technology Assessment (HTA) Programme. Health Technology Assessment is the largest single programme of work within the NHS Research and Development Programme. A broad interpretation of 'Health Technology' covers all interventions, including the use of devices, equipment, drugs, procedures and care across the whole spectrum of medical, nursing and health practices. The aim for the programme is to address the questions of purchasers, providers and users of health services on the effectiveness and cost-effectiveness of interventions. Reports are available in a variety of formats from the website at: http://www.hta.nhsweb.nhs.uk/htapubs.htm

I.2.5.2   Clinical Standards Advisory Group reports

The Clinical Standards Advisory Group (CSAG) was established in April 1991 and dissolved in 1999. The CSAG reports are usually based on the findings from a combination of commissioned research on the provision of specific services and visits made by senior clinicians to a sample of NHS units throughout the UK, and include the Government's response to the findings. They are published by The Stationery Office and distributed widely in the NHS. The following reports are available.

- Access to and availability of specialist services (summarising the following four reports).
- Coronary artery bypass grafting and coronary angioplasty: access to and availability of specialist services.
- Childhood leukaemia: access to and availability of specialist services .
- Neonatal intensive care: access to and availability of specialist services.
- Cystic fibrosis: access to and availability of specialist services.
- Back pain.
- Epidemiology review: the epidemiology and cost of back pain.
- Dental general anaesthesia.
- District elective surgery.
- Specialised services.
- Standards of clinical care for people with diabetes.
- Urgent and emergency admissions to hospital.
- Women in normal labour.
- Schizophrenia (2 volumes).
- Community health care for elderly people.
- Cleft lip and / or palate.
- Clinical effectiveness, using stroke care as an example.
- Services for patients with pain.
- Services for patients with epilepsy.
- Services for outpatients.
- Services for patients with depression.

I.2.5.3   The epidemiologically based needs assessment reviews

This series of healthcare needs assessment reviews was developed out of the NHS Management Executive's (now NHS Executive) District Health Authority project. Twenty topics were selected against the following criteria:

- the 'burden of disease' (i.e. mortality and morbidity) and the financial implication for the health service;

- the scope for changing purchasing patterns in the future;
- the need to test the method used for needs assessment using a wide range of topics.

These reviews provide guidance for purchasers about the incidence and the prevalence of certain health problems, and effective means of tackling those problems on the basis of a review of the evidence.

The first series of reviews was published in a compilation volume:

> STEVENS, A. and RAFTERY, J. (Eds) (1994) *Health Care Needs Assessment: The Epidemiologically Based Needs Assessment Reviews.* Radcliffe Medical Press, Oxford.

A second series extended coverage to a further eight topics. In a departure from the first series, these were published individually as well as in a second compilation volume:

> STEVENS, A. and RAFTERY, J. (eds.) (1997) *Health Care Needs Assessment: The Epidemiologically Based Needs Assessment Reviews: second series.* Radcliffe Medical Press, Oxford.

The contents of both series of epidemiologically based needs assessment reviews are shown in Table I.2.

I.2.5.4   Health Evidence Bulletins, Wales

The *Health Evidence Bulletins, Wales* are a new initiative in the field of health information because they act as signposts to the best current evidence across a broad range of evidence types and subject areas. Where information from RCTs is available, it is included. However, many health issues do not lend themselves easily to investigation, or

Table I.2   Contents of both series of epidemiologically based needs assessment reviews

First series Volume 1	First series Volume 2	Second Series
• Introduction	• Hernia repair	• Accident and emergency departments
• Diabetes mellitus	• Varicose vein treatments	
• Renal disease	• Prostatectomy for benign prostatic hyperplasia	• Child and adolescent mental health
• Stroke (acute cerebrovascular disease)		• Low back pain
• Lower respiratory disease	• Mental illness	• Palliative and terminal care
• Dementia	• Dementia	• Dermatology
• Coronary heart disease	• Alcohol misuse	• Breast cancer
• Colorectal cancer	• Drug abuse	• Genitourinary medicine services
• Cancer of the lung	• People with learning disabilities	• Gynaecology
• Total hip replacement	• Community child health services	
• Total knee replacement	• Family planning, abortion and fertility services	
• Cataract surgery	• Reflections and conclusions	

have not yet been studied, by this method. In these cases, high-quality evidence has been sought from observational and other studies. Bulletins that are available include: cancers, cardiovascular diseases, healthy environments, healthy living, injury prevention, learning disability, Maternal and early child health, Mental health, oral health, pain, discomfort and palliative care, physical disability and discomfort, and respiratory diseases.

http://www.uwcm. ac.uk/uwcm/lb/pep/index.html

I.2.6   MEDLINE

MEDLINE is the bibliographic database of the National Library of Medicine (NLM) in the USA. It includes such topics as microbiology, delivery of healthcare, nutrition, pharmacology, and environmental health. The categories covered in the database include anatomy, organisms, diseases, chemicals and drugs, techniques and equipment, psychiatry and psychology, biological sciences, physical sciences, social sciences and education, technology, agriculture, food, industry, humanities, information science and communications, and healthcare. Abstracts are available for 70% of entries.

Coverage: 1966 to date.

MEDLINE, together with other NLM databases, is available free of charge via the World Wide Web either through the PubMed or Internet Grateful Med interfaces:

http://www4.ncbi.nlm.nih.gov/PubMed/
http://igm.nlm.nih.gov/

Both of these Internet-based versions include PreMEDLINE, the weekly updated version of MEDLINE, which makes them more up-to-date than commercial alternatives.

I.2.7   EMBASE

EMBASE is the European equivalent of MEDLINE. The *Excerpta Medica* database focuses on drugs and pharmacology, over 40% of entries being drug-related. Other aspects of human medicine covered include health policy, drug and alcohol dependence, psychiatry, forensic science and pollution control. It provides world-wide coverage with a European focus.

Coverage: 1974 to date.

I.2.8 Subject specialist databases

There are a large number of specialist bibliographic databases that cover specific areas, for example, cancer, or nursing and allied health disciplines. Your local librarian will be able to help you to identify and find these. The main databases of relevance to health service managers are listed below.

I.2.8.1 Health Management Information Consortium

The Health Management Information Consortium (HMIC) database consists of the combined catalogues of the Department of Health and the King's Fund and the back catalogue of the Nuffield Institute for Health. The HMIC CD-ROM brings together the bibliographic databases of these three libraries whose main subject focus is healthcare management in the UK. The data are updated quarterly. A future aim is to incorporate a common thesaurus of health management subject headings to facilitate cross-database searching. The database is available via SilverPlatter.

I.2.8.2 HealthSTAR

HealthSTAR contains citations to the published literature on health services, technology, administration and research. It is focused on both the clinical and non-clinical aspects of healthcare delivery. The following topics are included:

- evaluation of patient outcomes;
- effectiveness of procedures, programmes, products service and processes;
- administration and planning of health facilities, services and manpower;
- health insurance;
- health policy;
- health services research;
- health economics and financial management;
- laws and regulation;
- personnel administration;
- quality assurance;
- licence;
- accreditation.

HealthSTAR is produced co-operatively by the National Library of Medicine and the American Hospital Association. The database contains citations and abstracts

when available to journal articles, monographs, technical reports, meeting abstracts and papers, book chapters, government documents and newspaper articles from 1975 to the present. HealthSTAR is updated monthly. It is available on CD-ROM from SilverPlatter and via Internet Grateful Med:
http://igm.nlm.nih.gov/

I.2.8.3 HEALTH-CD

HEALTH-CD is a database from the Stationery Office which contains the full-text of many publications and documents from the Department of Health. The database is split into three sections:

1. main collection;
2. acts of parliament;
3. statutory instruments.

The database is marketed by SilverPlatter.

I.2.8.4 Other databases

Other databases, together with their subject coverage and focus, are listed below.

- AMED – alternative medicine including complementary medicine, physiotherapy, occupational therapy, rehabilitation, podiatry and palliative care (UK);
- ASSIA – applied aspects of the social sciences including sociology, psychology, cultural anthropology, politics and economics (UK);
- British Nursing Index – nursing, midwifery and health visiting (UK);
- CANCERLIT- cancer including treatment together with information on epidemiology, pathogenesis and immunology (US);
- CINAHL – nursing and allied health database including health education, occupational therapy, emergency services, social services in healthcare (US);
- PsycLIT – psychology and related disciplines together with behavioural information from fields such as sociology, linguistics, medicine, law, physiology, business, psychiatry, and anthropology (US);
- SIGLE – 'grey' literature, i.e. literature that cannot be acquired readily through normal bookselling channels and therefore is difficult to identify or obtain (European).

I.2.9 Registers of published research

It is also important to be alert to the publication of registers of published research. *The Register of Cost-effectiveness Studies*, produced by the Economics and Operational Research Division of the Department of Health in 1994, is an excellent example of this type of resource.

I.2.10 Unpublished Evidence: Registers of Research in Progress

It is very important to identify research in progress. There are two major registers of research in progress, each of which point to other specialist research registers.

I.2.10.1 National Research Register

The National Research Register (NRR) is a register of ongoing and recently completed research projects funded by the UK's National Health Service. The first release contains information on over 28000 research projects, as well as entries from the Medical Research Council's (MRC) Clinical Trials Register, and details on reviews in progress collected by the NHS Centre for Reviews and Dissemination. Now available on the Internet at: http://www.doh.gov.uk/nrr.htm

I.2.10.2 Health Services Research Projects in Progress (HSRProj)

This register contains descriptions of research projects on health services including health technology assessment, and the development and use of clinical practice guidelines. Although it primarily covers the USA, coverage is currently being extended to include international research. About 350 projects are added for each quarterly update; the file now contains about 5000 records.

HSRProj provides project records for research in progress funded by federal and private grants and contracts. Records include:

- project summaries;
- names of performing and sponsoring agencies;
- names and addresses of the principal investigator;
- beginning and ending years of the project;
- when available, information about study design and methodology.

Records are indexed with NLM's Medical Subject Headings (MeSH), and the database is searchable using the NLM's Internet Grateful Med service: http://igm.nlm.nih.gov/

I.3   ORGANISATIONS

I.3.1 The Cochrane Collaboration

The Cochrane Collaboration was established in response to Archie Cochrane's call for systematic, up-to-date reviews of all relevant RCTs of healthcare. The NHS Research and Development Programme provided funds to establish a UK 'Cochrane Centre' in Oxford in October 1992. In October 1993 – at what was to become the first in a series of annual Cochrane Colloquia – 77 people from eleven countries co-founded 'The Cochrane Collaboration'.

The Cochrane Collaboration has evolved rapidly since its inauguration but its basic objectives and principles have remained the same. It is an international organisation set up with the aim to help people make well-informed decisions about healthcare by preparing, maintaining and ensuring the accessibility of systematic reviews of the effects of healthcare interventions. Preparation and maintenance of Cochrane reviews is the responsibility of international collaborative review groups. By mid year 2000, the existing and planned review groups numbered over 50 and covered most of the important areas of healthcare.

Other important Cochrane Collaboration entities include:

- Methods Groups – 16 in existence;
- Fields, i.e. Cochrane groupings that focus on dimensions such as the setting of care, the type of consumer, the type of provider, or the type of intervention – 10 in existence;
- 15 national or regional Cochrane Centres.

It has been said that: 'The Cochrane Collaboration is an enterprise that rivals the Human Genome Project in its potential implications for modern medicine'.[2]

UK Cochrane Centre
Summertown Pavilion,
Middle Way
Oxford OX2 7LG
UK

Phone: +44 (0)1865 516300

Fax: +44 (0)1865 516311

email: general@cochrane.co.uk

http://www.update-software.com/ccweb/default.html

I.3.2 NHS Centre for Reviews and Dissemination

The NHS Centre for Reviews and Dissemination (NHS CRD) is a facility commissioned by the NHS Research and Development Directorate. The aim of the NHS CRD is to identify and review the results of good-quality health research and to disseminate the findings to decision-makers within the NHS and to consumers of health services.

The reviews cover:

- the effectiveness of care for particular conditions;
- the effectiveness of health technologies;
- the evidence on efficient methods of organising and delivering particular types of healthcare.

University of York,
York YO1 5DD

email: revdis@york.ac.uk

http://www.york.ac.uk/inst/crd/dissem.htm

I.3.3 InterTASC

InterTASC is a collaboration of organisations that has been established to provide commissioners in health authorities and primary care groups/trusts (PCGs/PCTs), and NHS Trusts with research knowledge about the effectiveness and cost-effectiveness of acute service interventions. Members include:

- Development and Evaluation Service at the Wessex Institute for Health Research and Development, which supports the South and West Development and Evaluation Committee (DEC);
- the Working Group for Acute Purchasing of the Trent Institute for Health Services Research/School of Health and Related Research (ScHARR);
- the Development and Evaluation Service team at the Department of Public Health and Epidemiology, University of Birmingham
http://www.bham.ac.uk/WMidsDES/
InterTASC% 20home.htm

By far the largest collection of reports from InterTASC are those from the South and West DEC. These technology assessment reports can be found on the website of the South and West Regional R&D Programme of the NHS: http://cochrane.epi.bris.ac.uk/rd/publicat/dec/index.htm

I.3.4 Aggressive Research Intelligence Facility

The Aggressive Research Intelligence Facility (ARIF) is a specialist unit based at the University of Birmingham, set up to help healthcare workers to access and interpret research evidence in response to particular problems.[3] The aim of ARIF is to provide timely access to, and advice on, existing reviews of research. Details of previous enquiries, together with sources used to answer them, are placed on the ARIF website:

http://www.hsrc.org.uk/links/arif/ arifhome.htm

I.4   THE INTERNET

In addition to databases listed above, which are all commercially available, there are several databases of interest to health service staff that can be accessed free of charge via the Internet. Current examples include:

- the European Clearing House on Health Systems Reforms;
- Outcomes Literature and Outcomes Activity Databases from the Nuffield Institute for Health at the University of Leeds;
- the NHS EED, HTA and DARE databases from the NHS CRD at the University of York;
- the databases of the English National Board for Nursing, Midwifery and Health Visiting, the Health Development Agency (HDA) and the Health Education Board for Scotland.

For an up-to-date listing of free Internet health databases, complete with hypertext links, the reader is referred to the Trawling the Net resource guide at:

http://www.shef.ac.uk/~scharr/ir/trawling.html

The more significant of these databases are described in more detail below.

I.4.1 Turning Research Into Practice (TRIP) database

The TRIP database is a meta-search engine that searches across 61 sites of high-quality information. At present, there are over 17 000 links to high-quality sources of evidence, such as *Bandolier* and Cochrane Reviews.
http://www.tripdatabase.com/

I.4.2 NHS Economic Evaluation Database

The NHS Economic Evaluation Database (NHS EED) is a database of structured abstracts of economic evaluations of healthcare interventions. Cost-benefit analyses, cost-effectiveness analyses and cost-utility analyses are identified from a variety of sources and assessed according to set quality criteria. Detailed structured abstracts are produced. The database can be accessed via:
http://nhscrd.york.ac.uk/Welcome.html
As from Issue 1 2000, it is also available in The Cochrane Library (see I.2.1).

I.4.3 Health Technology Assessment Database

The Health Technology Assessment (HTA) Database, mounted by the NHS CRD at the University of York, contains abstracts produced by the International Network of Agencies for Health Technology Assessment (INAHTA) and other healthcare technology agencies. The database can be accessed via:
http://nhscrd.york.ac.uk/

I.4.4 Health Technology Assessment Agencies

Several organisations have been set up world-wide to assess the impact of new health technologies. Many of them have websites, with the option of downloading full reports or executive summaries. A starting point is the resource guide at:
http://www.shef.ac.uk/~scharr/ir/htaorg.html
However, for searchable details of work in progress, try the INAHTA Work in Progress on the New Zealand Health Technology Assessment website:
http://nzhta.chmeds.ac.nz/inahta/inahta.htm

I.4.5 Medical Search Engines

I.4.5.1 OMNI

OMNI is a gateway to Internet resources in medicine, biomedicine, allied health, health management, and related topics. The aim is to provide comprehensive coverage of the UK resources in this area, and access to the best resources world-wide. A process of selection, evaluation and description ensures that the collection is continuously updated. As at July 2000, it contains 4579 links to high-quality resources.
http://omni.ac.uk/

I.4.5.2 CliniWeb

The aim of CliniWeb is to provide quick and easy access to biomedical information on the World Wide Web. The focus is on information that would be used by healthcare profession students and practitioners. Information has been organised using the Medical Subject Headings (MeSH) disease and anatomy classifications, with rapid access provided by both searching and browsing.
http://www.ohsu.edu/cliniweb/

I.4.5.3 Medfinder

Medfinder, describing itself as the World Wide Web's Medical Librarian, is a very precise search engine which uses clinical terms to retrieve pre-selected, manually indexed materials on a broad range of conditions. It also allows searches for images, ECGs and X-rays:
http://www.netmedicine.com/medfinder.htm

I.4.5.4 Healthfinder

A rich source of health information established by the US Government.
http://www.healthfinder.gov/default.htm

References

1. DEEKS, J., GLANVILLE, J. and SHELDON, T. (1996) *Undertaking systematic reviews of effectiveness: Guidelines for those carrying out or commissioning reviews*. NHS CRD Report No.4. NHS CRD Publications, York.
2. NAYLOR C.D. (1995) *Grey zones of clinical practice: some limits to evidence-based medicine*. Lancet 345: 840–2.
3. HYDE, C. (1996) *Active research dissemination in the West Midlands*. J. Clin. Effectiveness 1: 30.

Further reading

BOOTH, A. (1996) *In search of the evidence: informing effective practice*. J. Clin. Effectiveness 1 (1): 25–29.

BOOTH, A. (1998) *Following the evidence trail: EBHC on the Internet*. Information on the Internet (1): 4–5.

BOOTH, A. (1998) *Information about health technology assessment*. Evidence-Based Health Policy and Management June: 2: 30–1.

CHALMERS, I. and ALTMAN, D.G. (1995) *Systematic Reviews*. BMJ Publications, London.

GLANVILLE, J. (1998) *Where's the evidence? How to find clinical effectiveness information*. Clinical Performance and Quality Health Care 6(1):44–48.

GLANVILLE, J., HAINES, M., and AUSTON, I. (1998) *Finding information on clinical effectiveness*. Br. Med. J. 317: 200–3.

GLANVILLE, J., HAINES, M., and AUSTON, I. (1998) *Sources of information on clinical effectiveness and methods of dissemination*. In: HAINES, A. and DONALD, A. (Eds). *Getting Research Findings into Practice*. pp 19–26. BMJ Publications, London.

TRINDADE, E., TOPFER, L.A. and De GIUSTI, M. (1998) *Internet information sources for the identification of emerging health technologies: a starting point*. Int. J. Technology Assessment in Health Care 14: 644–51

FILTERING THE EVIDENCE

II.1. RESOURCE OVERVIEW

Sources of evidence can be divided into:

- those that are *pre-filtered*, i.e. strict inclusion and quality criteria are applied before materials are added to a resource (e.g. The Cochrane Library, DARE and NHS EED);
- those that contain a broad range of materials of varying quality, typically hundreds of thousands of records, and subsequently need to be filtered (*post-filtered*) to identify higher quality materials (e.g. MEDLINE and other bibliographic databases).

In the latter case, optimal search strategies are devised from methodological terms or from various publication types (e.g. meta-analysis or clinical trial) and combined with a subject search.

These search strategies, commonly known as *filters*, are ideally constructed experimentally by combining and evaluating numerous permutations of candidate terms. However, the considerable logistics involved have led to an increasing number of empirically derived filters, lacking the authority and wider applicability of their research-based counterparts, but, nevertheless, useful tools in limiting search results to high-grade materials. Finally, filters for retrieval of diagnosis, aetiology, prognosis and therapy studies, for reviews, economic evaluations or guidelines or for outcome studies have been developed in a number of variations, for example, as 'one-line' filters, as high-, low- and mid-range sensitivity and specificity strategies, and as comprehensive strategies used to compile databases such as the Cochrane Clinical Trials Register, DARE or NHS EED.

II.2   RESOURCES

II.2.1 PubMed Clinical Queries Interface

This specialised search service is intended for clinicians, and has built-in search 'filters' based largely upon work from McMaster University.[1] Four study categories – therapy, diagnosis, aetiology, prognosis – are provided, and the user may indicate whether they wish their search to be more sensitive (i.e. include most relevant articles and probably some less relevant ones) or more specific (i.e. include mostly relevant articles but probably omit a few): http://www.ncbi.nlm.nih.gov/PubMed/clinical.html

II.2.2 SUMSearch

SUMSearch (formerly SmartSearch) is an experimental interface provided by the Society for General Internal Medicine in the USA. It allows you to specify the nature of your question (diagnosis, therapy, etc.) and then automatically to filter the more rigorous articles from general articles on the subject. This resource uses the PubMed version of MEDLINE, as well as providing one-stop access to important resources such as the Database of Abstracts of Reviews of Effectiveness, the National Guideline Clearinghouse and the Merck Manual. http://badgett.uthscsa.edu/cgi-bin/sumsearch.exe

II.2.3. Institute of Health Sciences (IHS) Library Filters

This guide contains tried and tested search strategies to identify systematic review and RCT literature on MEDLINE. It also lists methodological search filters to assist the retrieval of sound clinical studies that deal with diagnosis, prognosis, therapy, aetiology, guidelines, treatment outcomes, and evidence-based healthcare methods. The filters are in both Ovid and SilverPlatter MEDLINE versions and can be downloaded for use on a local machine: http://www.ihs.ox.ac.uk/library/filters.html

II.3   THE INTERNET

Several organisations have provided websites hosting
documentation to support the use of search filters:

* NHS Centre for Reviews and Dissemination – Search
  Strategy to Identify Reviews and Meta-analyses in
  MEDLINE and CINAHL
  http://www.york.ac.uk/inst/crd/search.htm
* North Thames Regional Library Service – Evidence
  Strategies
  http://www.nthames-health.tpmde.ac.uk/
  evidence_strategies/index.htm
* University of Alberta – EBM Tool Kit
  http://www.med.ualberta.ca/ebm/main.htm
* University of Rochester – Evidence-based Filters for
  Ovid MEDLINE
  http://www.urmc.rochester.edu:80/Miner/Educ/
  Expertsearch.html

Reference

1. HAYNES, R.B. et al. (1994) *Developing optimal search strategies for
   detecting clinically sound studies in MEDLINE.* J. Am. Med. Inform. Assoc.
   1: 447–58.

Further reading

How to harness MEDLINE:

McKIBBON, K.A. and WALKER, C.J. (1994) *Beyond ACP Journal Club : how to
harness MEDLINE for diagnosis problems [Editorial].* ACP Journal Club
Sep–Oct: A10 (Ann. Intern. Med. 121, Suppl. 2).

McKIBBON, K.A. and WALKER-DILKS, C.J. (1994) *Beyond ACP Journal Club:
how to harness MEDLINE for therapy problems [Editorial]* ACP Journal
Club Jul–Aug 121:Suppl. 1: A10–12. [Published erratum appears in ACP
Journal Club Nov–Dec: 121(3): A11.]

McKIBBON, K.A. and WALKER-DILKS, C.J. (1994) *Beyond ACP Journal Club:
how to harness MEDLINE to solve clinical problems [Editorial].* ACP Journal
Club Mar–Apr: A10–12 (Ann. Intern. Med. 120, Suppl. 2).

McKIBBON, K.A. and WALKER-DILKS, C.J. (1994) *Beyond ACP Journal Club:
how to harness MEDLINE for diagnostic problems [Editorial].* ACP Journal
Club 121: Suppl. 2: A10–12.

McKIBBON, K.A., WALKER-DILKS, C.J., WILCZYNSKI, N.L. et al. (1996)
*Beyond ACP Journal Club: how to harness MEDLINE for review articles
[Editorial].* ACP Journal Club May–Jun: A12–13.

WALKER-DILKS, C.J., McKIBBON, K.A., HAINES, R.B. and WILCZYNSKI,
N. (1995) *Beyond ACP Journal Club: how to harness MEDLINE for prognosis
problems [Editorial].* ACP Journal Club Jul–Aug: A12–14 (Ann. Intern.
Med. 123, Suppl. 1).

WALKER-DILKS, C.J., McKIBBON, K.A. and HAINES, R.B. (1994) *Beyond
ACP Journal Club: how to harness MEDLINE for etiology problems
[Editorial].* ACP Journal Club Nov–Dec: A10–11 (Ann. Intern. Med. 121,
Suppl. 3).

Other items

BOYNTON, J., GLANVILLE, J., McDAID, D. and LEFEBVRE, C. (1998) *Identifying systematic reviews in MEDLINE: developing an objective approach to search strategy design.* J. Information Science 24: 137–57.

DICKERSIN, K., SCHERER, R. and LEFEBVRE, C. (1994) *Identifying relevant studies for systematic reviews.* Br. Med. J. 309: 1286–91.

HUNT, D.L. and McKIBBON, K.A. (1997) *Locating and appraising systematic reviews.* Ann. Intern. Med. 126: 532–8.

LEFEBVRE, C. (1994) *The Cochrane Collaboration: the role of the UK Cochrane Centre in identifying the evidence.* Health Libraries Review 11: 235–42. [For searches to identify RCTs.]

McDONALD, S.J., LEFEBVRE, C., and CLARKE, M.J. (1996) *Identifying reports of controlled trials in the BMJ and Lancet.* Br. Med. J. 313: 1116–17.

McKIBBON, K.A. and WALKER, C.J. (1993) *Panning for applied clinical research gold.* Online July; 105–8.

McKIBBON, K.A. and WALKER-DILKS, C. (1995) *Evidence-based health care for librarians : panning for gold. How to apply research methodology to search for therapy, diagnosis, etiology, prognosis, review, and meta-analysis articles.* Ontario Health Information Research Unit, McMaster University, Ontario.

McKIBBON, K.A., WILCZYNSKI, N.L. and WALKER-DILKS, C.J. (1996) *How to search for and find evidence about therapy.* Evidence-Based Medicine 1: 70–2.

APPRAISING THE EVIDENCE

There are typically four main ingredients in the process of critical appraisal of research literature.

1. The originating *problem or scenario* that acts as a context for the appraisal of the evidence.
2. The evidence itself, either a *primary research study* or an *integrative systematic review.*
3. An appropriate *checklist* with which to assess the validity, reliability, and applicability of the candidate article.
4. The *product of appraisal,* whether it be an evidence-based digest, a critical commentary or a critically appraised topic (CAT). These products can either be in the form of a commentary on a specific article, as in an evidence-based journal (such as *Evidence-based Healthcare*), or it can be a summary and brief synthesis of several articles that address a specific clinical question.

Additional materials that assist in the critical appraisal process include calculators for the various clinically useful measures of effectiveness (such as odds ratios, NNTs), glossaries of terms, and teaching aids for explaining unfamiliar concepts.

III.2   RESOURCES

III.2.1 ACP Journal Club

The ACP Journal Club was the pioneer for a growing genre of secondary journals that provide a one-page structured abstract and commentary for major journal articles that have been selected for their clinical importance and methodological rigour. Published bi-monthly by the

American College of Physicians, the exclusive focus of this publication is internal medicine. It covers original research studies and reviews, describing important advances in the understanding of treatment, prevention, diagnosis, cause, prognosis, and economics.
http://www.acponline.org/journals/acpjc/jcmenu.htm

III.2.2 *Bandolier*

Bandolier is a monthly journal that contains 'bullets' of evidence-based medicine, hence its title. Access to *Bandolier* on the Internet is free of charge, and a printed version is made freely available within the NHS through distribution by Regional R&D Departments. Two cumulative volumes containing issues published to date are also available. Further details are available from the *Bandolier* website:
http://www.jr2.ox.ac.uk:80/Bandolier/

III.2.3 Clinical Evidence

Clinical Evidence is a compendium of the best available research findings on common and important clinical questions, which is updated and expanded every six months. The first issue is available in book format. *Clinical Evidence* is published jointly by the BMJ Publishing Group and the American College of Physicians. Sample pages are available from the website at:
http://www.bmjpg.com/evid99/index.html

III.2.4 Evidence-Based Health Care Workbook and CD-ROM

An open-learning resource – interactive CD-ROM with workbook – has been produced by the Critical Appraisal Skills Programme (CASP) and Finding the Evidence Workshop (CASPFew) teams to assist health professionals in accessing and using the best available evidence in their area of practice. The CD-ROM includes many interactive features such as a glossary, additional material dealing with statistics, and links to key Internet sites. It can be ordered from Update Software Ltd, Summertown Pavilion, Middle Way, Oxford OX2 7LG (tel: 01865 513902; e-mail: info@update.co.uk) or visit:
http://cebm.jr2.ox.ac.uk/casp/home3.html

A paper-based resource of five separate units featuring practical activities and case-studies has also been produced (new edition available from Autumn 2000). For details contact CASP, The Institute of Health Sciences, Old Road, Oxford OX3 7LG (tel: 01865 226968).

III.2.5 *Evidence-based Healthcare*

This secondary journal was formerly known as *Evidence-based Health Policy & Management*. The principal purpose of *Evidence-based Healthcare* is to provide managers with the best evidence available about the financing, organisation, and delivery of healthcare. The aim is to promote access to the best possible evidence for those who make decisions about groups and populations in order to inform their judgement.
http://www.ihs.ox.ac.uk/ebhc/index.html

III.2.6 *Evidence-Based Medicine*

Published bi-monthly, the purpose of *Evidence-Based Medicine* is to survey at least 70 international medical journals to identify the key research papers that are scientifically valid and relevant to practice. These articles are selected according to scientific criteria and only those papers with a direct message for practice are included. *Evidence-Based Medicine* also provides more informative structured abstracts of articles alongside commentaries on those articles which make clear the importance of the papers. Finally, this important secondary journal supplies educational material for teaching evidence-based medicine. In addition to internal medicine, it covers the major specialties, including general surgery, paediatrics, obstetrics, gynaecology, psychiatry, general practice, anaesthesiology and ophthalmology. Details are available from the BMJ Publishing Group's website:
http://www.bmjpg.com/data/ebm.htm

III.2.7 *Evidence-Based Mental Health*

The purpose of *Evidence-Based Mental Health* is to alert clinicians working in the field of mental health to important and clinically relevant advances in treatment (including specific interventions and systems of care), diagnosis, aetiology, prognosis/outcome research, quality improvement, continuing education, and economic evaluation. *Evidence-Based Mental Health* covers a broad range of mental health problems including those experienced by adults, children, older adults, people with

learning disabilities, people with head injuries, people who have drug and alcohol problems, people with personality disorders, and individuals who have developed psychiatric and psychological problems as a result of trauma or of physical health problems. An excellent and comprehensive website can be found at:
http://www.psychiatry.ox.ac.uk/cebmh/journal/

III.2.8 *Evidence-Based Nursing*

Evidence-Based Nursing gives access to the best research related to nursing, and provides regular updates of the most important new evidence within nursing. *Evidence-Based Nursing* facilitates implementation of the evidence as expert commentators put every article into a clinical context and draw out the key research findings. Every edition of *Evidence-Based Nursing* contains 24 different summaries covering a wide variety of nursing-related issues.
http://www.bmjpg.com/data/ebn.htm

III.2.9 CAT-Maker

CAT-Maker is a software package developed and marketed by the NHS R&D Centre for Evidence-Based Medicine, Oxford. It is purpose-designed to handle the production of brief critical appraisal summaries that address specific clinical questions. These summaries are known as critically appraised topics or CATs.[1,2] CAT-Makers assist in important clinical calculations, and in the storage of questions, search strategies, and appraisals while generating a file that can be formatted and printed using a word processor.
http://cebm.jr2.ox.ac.uk/docs/catbank.html

III.3 ORGANISATIONS

III.3.1 NHS R&D Centre for Evidence-Based Medicine

The NHS R&D Centre for Evidence-Based Medicine at the John Radcliffe Hospital in Oxford was the first of several similar centres around the UK, the broad aims of which are to promote an evidence-based approach, and to provide support and resources to anyone who wants to make use of

them. A comprehensive website with detailed information
and teaching materials is available at:
http://cebm.jr2.ox.ac.uk/

III.3.2 Centre for Evidence-Based Child Health

The Centre for Evidence-Based Child Health at the Institute
of Child Health, London, is part of a national network of
centres for evidence-based healthcare. The overall aim of
the Centre is to increase the provision of effective and
efficient child healthcare through an educational
programme for health professionals. Introductory seminars,
short courses, MSc modules, workshops for groups in the
workplace, and training secondments are being offered to
paediatricians, nurses, general practitioners, healthcare
purchasers, and others involved in child health.
http://www.ich.bpmf.ac.uk/ebm/ebm.htm

III.3.3 Centre for Evidence Based Mental Health

The website contains a range of resources to promote and
support the teaching and practice of evidence-based mental
healthcare:

- OXAMWEB (a comprehensive list of links to evidence-
  based mental health websites);
- toolkit of teaching resources, including examples of
  scenarios used in the teaching of evidence-based practice
  in mental health;
- details of the secondary journal – *Evidence-Based Mental
  Health*;
- details of forthcoming workshops and conferences;
- details of how to join the centre or subscribe to their
  mailing list: http://www.psychiatry.ox.ac.uk/cebmh/

III.3.4. Centre for Evidence-Based Nursing

The two principal aims of the Centre for Evidence-Based
Nursing are:

- to work with nurses in practice, other researchers, nurse
  educators, and managers to identify evidence-based
  practice through primary research and systematic
  reviews;
- to promote the uptake of evidence into practice through
  education and implementation activities in areas of
  nursing where good evidence is available.

The Centre is also conducting research into factors that promote and impede the implementation of evidence-based practice: http://www.york.ac.uk/depts/hstd/centres/evidence/ev-intro.htm

III.3.5 Critical Appraisal Skills Programme

The Critical Appraisal Skills Programme (CASP) was established in the UK with the aim of helping health service decision-makers, and those who seek to influence the decision-makers, to develop evidence management skills, i.e. to find, critically appraise and change practice in line with evidence of effectiveness. The acquisition and use of these skills promote the delivery of evidence-based healthcare. At the heart of CASP's work is a cascade of half-day workshops at which participants learn by embarking on an interactive journey. CASP introduces people to the ideas of evidence-based healthcare and, through critical appraisal of systematic reviews, introduces people to the related ideas of the Cochrane Collaboration. CASP has also developed an interactive CD-ROM, which can be used in conjunction with workshops, video-conferencing, as a stand-alone package, or to reinforce learning, thereby taking these skills to a wider audience and giving opportunities for independent practice or learning.
http://www.phru.org/casp/

III.3.6 North Thames Research Appraisal Group

The North Thames Research Appraisal Group (NTRAG) is an education and training consultancy consisting of a group of researchers, academics, clinicians, and other healthcare professionals who are interested in promoting evidence-based healthcare. The means by which they achieve this goal is through the design and delivery of a wide range of critical appraisal workshops and related activities. In addition to delivering an annual programme of critical appraisal skills workshops covering nine topic areas, NTRAG staff and tutors also work with NHS Trusts, health authorities and other NHS organisations around the country to create short-course programmes tailored specifically to local requirements. These activities are generally delivered on-site, enabling educational content to be linked directly to local patient and service-delivery priorities. It is possible to contact NTRAG at: ntrag@unl.ac.uk

III.4 THE INTERNET

III.4.1 EBM Tool Kit

Not to be confused with the resource produced by the NHS R&D Centre for Evidence-Based Medicine which has a similar name, the EBM Tool Kit is a Canadian-based collection of resources to support the practice of evidence-based medicine. It includes appraisal checklists, methodological filters, and other User Guide-associated resources:
http://www.med.ualberta.ca/ebm/ebm.htm

III.4.2 Journal Club on the Web

This website is an experiment in implementing an online, interactive general medical 'journal club' at which articles from the recent medical literature are periodically summarised and appraised and readers' comments are posted. The articles are primarily in the field of adult internal medicine, and mainly from the *New England Journal of Medicine, Annals of Internal Medicine, Journal of the American Medical Association* and *The Lancet*.
http://www.journalclub.org/

III.4.3 Journal of Family Practice Patient Oriented Evidence that Matters (POEMs)

The POEMs feature is designed to support the evidence-based practice of medicine. Each month, they review over 80 journals to identify the eight articles with patient-oriented outcomes that have the greatest potential to change the way primary care clinicians practise. These articles are then critically appraised by expert family physicians, educators, and pharmacologists.
http://www.infopoems.com/POEMs/poems_home.htm

References

1. LEE, H.N., SAUVE, J.S., FARKOUH, M.E. and SACKETT, D.L. (1993) *The critically appraised topic: a standardised aid for the presentation and storage of evidence-based medicine*. Clinical Research 41: 543A.
2. SAUVE, S., LEE, H.N., MEADE, M.O., LANG, J.D., FARKOUH, M., COOK, D.J. and SACKETT, D.L. (1995) *The critically appraised topic: a practical approach to learning critical appraisal*. Ann. Roy. Soc. Phys. Surg. Canada 28: 396–8.

Further reading

Users' Guides to the Medical Literature (JAMA)

The Evidence Based Medicine Working Group, a group of clinicians at McMaster University and colleagues across North America, has created a set of guides which are published in the *Journal of the American Medical Association (JAMA)*. The aim of the series is to assist clinicians to keep up-to-date in their clinical discipline and to find the best way to manage a particular clinical problem. The Users' Guides put much emphasis on integrative studies, including systematic overviews, practice guidelines, decision analysis, and economic analysis. They introduce strategies for searching the medical literature efficiently. A complete list of the published guides, together with their full bibliographic references, is available at:
http://www.shef.ac.uk/~scharr/ir/userg.html

Centres for Health Evidence.net have produced Users' Guides to Evidence-Based Practice based on the Users' Guides to the Medical Literature, which are available at:
http://www.cche.net/principles/content_all.asp

GUYATT, G., RENNIE D. and THE EVIDENCE BASED MEDICINE WORKING GROUP *Why Users' Guides?* EBM Working Paper Series. Only available at: http://www.cche.net/principles/content_all.asp

GUYATT, G.H. (1993) *Users' guides to the medical literature.* JAMA 270: 2096–7.

OXMAN, A., SACKETT, D.L. and GUYATT, G.H. (1993) *Users' guides to the medical literature. I. How to get started.* JAMA 270: 2093–5.

GUYATT, G.H., SACKETT, D.L. and COOK, D.J. (1993) *Users' guides to the medical literature. II. How to use an article about therapy or prevention. A. Are the results of the study valid?* JAMA 270: 2598–601.

GUYATT, G.H., SACKETT, D.L. and COOK, D.J. (1994) *Users' guides to the medical literature. II. How to use an article about therapy or prevention. B. What were the results and will they help me in caring for my patients?* JAMA 271: 59–63.

JAESCHKE, R., GUYATT, G. and SACKETT, D.L. (1994) *Users' guides to the medical literature. III. How to use an article about a diagnostic test. A. Are the results of the study valid?* JAMA 271: 389–91.

JAESCHKE, R., GORDON, H., GUYATT, G. and SACKETT, D.L. (1994) *Users' guides to the medical literature. III. How to use an article about a diagnostic test. B. What are the results and will they help me in caring for my patients?* JAMA 271: 703–7.

LEVINE, M., WALTER, S., LEE, H., HAINES, T., HOLBROOK, A. and MOYER, V. (1994) *Users' guides to the medical literature. IV. How to use an article about harm.* JAMA 271: 1615–9.

LAUPACIS, A., WELLS, G., RICHARDSON, S. and TUGWELL, P. (1994) *Users' guides to the medical literature. V. How to use an article about prognosis.* JAMA 272: 234–7.

OXMAN, A.D., COOK, D.J. and GUYATT, G.H. (1994) *Users' guides to the medical literature. VI. How to use an overview.* JAMA 272: 1367–71.

RICHARDSON, W.S. and DETSKY, A.S. (1995) *Users' guides to the medical literature. VII. How to use a Clinical Decision Analysis. A. Are the results of the study valid?* JAMA 273: 1292–5.

RICHARDSON, W.S. and DETSKY, A.S. (1995) *Users' guides to the medical literature. VII. How to use a Clinical Decision Analysis. B. What are the results and will they help me in caring for my patients?* JAMA 273: 1610–13.

HAYWARD, R.S.A., WILSON, M.C., TUNIS, S.R., BASS, E.B. and GUYATT, G. (1995) *Users' guides to the medical literature. VIII. How to use clinical practice guidelines. A. Are the recommendations valid?* JAMA 274: 570–4.

WILSON, M.C., HAYWARD, R.S.A., TUNIS, S.R., BASS, E.B. and GUYATT, G. (1995) *Users' guides to the medical literature. VIII. How to use clinical practice guidelines B. What are the recommendations and will they help you in caring for your patients?* JAMA 274: 1630–2.

GUYATT, G.H., SACKETT, D.L., SINCLAIR, J.C. et al. (1995). *Users' Guides to the medical literature. IX. A Method for Grading Health Care Recommendations.* JAMA 274: 1800–4.

NAYLOR, C.D. and GUYATT, G.H. (1996) *Users' guides to the medical literature. X. How to use an article reporting variations in the outcomes of health services. Evidence-Based Medicine Working Group.* JAMA 275: 554–8.

NAYLOR, C.D. and GUYATT, G.H. (1996) *Users' guides to the medical literature. XI. How to use an article about a clinical utilization review. Evidence-Based Medicine Working Group.* JAMA 275: 1435–9.

GUYATT, G.H., NAYLOR, C.D., JUNIPER, E. et al. (1997) *Users' guides to the medical literature. XII. How to use articles about health-related quality of life. Evidence-Based Medicine Working Group.* JAMA 277: 1232–7.

DRUMMOND, M.F., RICHARDSON, W.S., O'BRIEN, B.J., LEVINE, M. and HEYLAND, D. (1997) *Users' guides to the medical literature. XIII. How to use an article on economic analysis of clinical practice. A. Are the results of the study valid? Evidence-Based Medicine Working Group.* JAMA 277: 1552–7.

O'BRIEN, B.J., HEYLAND, D., RICHARDSON, W.S., LEVINE, M. and DRUMMOND, M.F. (1997) *Users' guides to the medical literature. XIII. How to use an article on economic analysis of clinical practice. B. What are the results and will they help me in caring for my patients? Evidence-Based Medicine Working Group.* JAMA 277: 1802–6. {Published erratum appears in JAMA 1997; 278:1064.]

DANS, A.L., DANS, L.F., GUYATT, G.H. and RICHARDSON, S. (1998) *Users' guides to the Medical Literature. XIV. How to decide on the applicability of clinical trial results to your patient. Evidence Based Medicine Working Group.* JAMA 279: 545–9.

RICHARDSON, W.S., WILSON, M.C., GUYATT, G.H., COOK, D.J. and NISHIKAWA, J. (1999) *Users' guides to the medical literature: XV. How to use an article about disease probability for differential diagnosis.* JAMA 281: 1214–19.

GUYATT, G.H., SINCLAIR, J., COOK, D.J. and GLASZIOU, P. (1999) *Users' guides to the medical literature: XVI. How to use a treatment recommendation.* JAMA 281: 1836–43.

BARRATT, A. IRWIG, L., GLASZIOU, P. et al. (1999) *Users' guides to the medical literature: XVII. How to use guidelines and recommendations about screening.* JAMA 281: 2029.

RANDOLPH, A.G., HAYNES, R.B., WYATT, J.C., COOK, D.J. and GUYATT, G.H. (1999) *Users' guides to the medical literature: XVIII. How to use an article evaluating the clinical impact of a computer-based clinical decision support system.* JAMA 282: 67–74.

BUCHER, H.C., GUYATT, G.H., COOK, D.J., HOLBROOK, A. and McALISTER, F.A. (1999) *Users' guides to the medical literature: XIX. Applying clinical trial results. A. How to use an article measuring the effect of an intervention on surrogate end points.* JAMA 282: 771–8.

McALISTER, F.A., LAUPACIS, A., WELLS, G.A. and SACKETT, D.L. (1999) *Users' guides to the medical literature: XIX. Applying clinical trial results. B. Guidlines for determining whether a drug is exerting (more than) a class effect.* JAMA 282: 1371–7.

McALISTER, F.A., STRAUS, S.E., GUYATT, G.D. and HAYNES, R.B. (2000) *Users' guides to the medical literature: XX. Integrating research evidence with the care of the individual patient.* JAMA 283: 2829–36.

HUNT, D.L., JAESCHKE, R. and McKIBBON, K.A. (2000) *Users' guides to the medical literature: XXI. Using electronic health information resources in evidence-based practice. Evidence-based Medicine Working Group.* JAMA 283: 1875–9.

McGINN, R.G., GUYATT, G.H., WYER, P.C., NAYLOR, C.D., STIELL, I.G. and RICHARDSON, W.S. (2000) *Users' guides to the medical literature: XXII. How to use articles about clinical decision rules.* JAMA 284: 79–84.

GIACOMINI, M.K. and COOK, D.J. (2000) *Users' guides to the medical literature: XXIII. Qualitative research in health care. A. Are the Results of the Study Valid?* JAMA 284: 357–62.

Other Items

BOOTH, A. (1998) *Finding and evaluating sources of evidence.* J. Clin. Effectiveness 2: 113–16.

BURLS, A. and MILNE, R. (1996) *Evaluating the evidence: an introduction.* J. Clin. Effectiveness 1: 59–62.

CRUMP. B.J. and DRUMMOND, M.F. (1993) *Evaluating clinical evidence: A Handbook for Managers.* Longman, Harlow.

DIXON, R. and MUNRO, J. (1997) *Evidence Based Medicine: a Practical Workbook for Clinical Problem Solving.* Butterworth-Heinemann, London.

FAHEY, T., GRIFFITHS, S. and PETERS, T.J. (1995) *Evidence based purchasing: understanding results of clinical trials and systematic reviews.* Br. Med. J. 311: 1056–60.

GREENHALGH, T. (1997) *How to read a paper: the basics of evidence based medicine.* BMJ Publishing Group, London.

MILNE, R., DONALD, A. and CHAMBERS, L. (1995) *Piloting short workshops on the critical appraisal of reviews.* Health Trends 27: 120.

SACKETT, D.L., STRAUS, S.E., RICHARDSON, W.S., ROSENBERG, W. and HAYNES, R.B. (2000) *Evidence-Based Medicine: How to Practice and Teach EBM.* 2nd Edition. Churchill Livingstone, London.

SHELDON, T.A., SONG, F. and DAVEY SMITH, G. (1993) *Critical appraisal of the medical literature: how to assess whether health-care interventions do more good than harm.* In: Drummond, M.F. and Maynard, A. (Eds) *Purchasing and Providing Cost-Effective Health Care.* pp. 31–48. Churchill Livingstone, Edinburgh.

STORING THE EVIDENCE

IV.1 RESOURCE OVERVIEW

The exponential growth of the evidence base in general and the volume of literature required for systematic review activities in particular makes it desirable, if not essential, to use some form of software to manage a paper-based collection and its associated bibliographic references. There are two main options:

1. to use a generic database package such as Access (Microsoft relational database software) or Idealist (a text retrieval package);
2. to purchase specific reference management software.

The former option has the advantages that:

*   software will often already be available on local machines for other unrelated purposes;
*   it can be used to store and organise additional data beyond the brief bibliographic record;
*   there will often be expertise in the use of such packages within an organisation.

However, in general, it is possible to manipulate the data only in the form in which it was originally imported, and the design of import filters for a variety of database sources is both time-consuming and technically complex.

The latter option, which is the focus of this appendix, has the advantages of:

*   the availability of bespoke input and output facilities for source databases and for target journals;
*   utilities for commonly performed functions.

However, it is more limited if one wishes to use the software beyond the prescribed limits for which it was originally designed. A local librarian will often be able to advise on both the suitability and availability of reference management software.

IV.2 RESOURCES

There are four leading reference management packages, all of which have enthusiastic advocates. In a very competitive software market, in which features are continually being added, the consumer should be alert to the current state of each package. The situation has been complicated in recent years with the acquisition of ProCite by Research Information Systems, the developers of Reference Manager and a subsidiary of the Institute of Scientific Information (ISI). At present, both of these packages are being developed side by side. In selecting a reference management package, you should look at the following features:

- the range of databases from which the package can import references;
- the range of journal styles in which references can be exported;
- the interface with popular word-processors;
- technical factors, such as the maximum number of records, the maximum size and the maximum number of databases.

A booklet, entitled 'How to Select Bibliographic Management Software' is available at no charge from Reference Information Systems Inc., Camino Corporate Center, 2355 Camino Vida Roble, Carlsbad, CA 92009, USA.

The four leading reference management packages are described briefly below.

A comparison of the features in EndNote, Procite, and Reference Manager can be found on the World Wide Web at: http/www.biblio-tech.com/html/pbm_features.html

IV.2.1 EndNote

EndNote is marketed by Niles Software Inc. This package is currently at Version 4.0 (released March 2000). A free trial version and up-to-date product information can be found on the World Wide Web at: http://www.niles.com/
In the United Kingdom/Republic of Ireland, contact:

Cherwell Scientific Publishing, Ltd.
The Magdalen Centre
Oxford Science Park
Oxford, OX4 4GA UK
Phone: +44 (0)1865 784800

Fax: +44 (0)1865 784801

e-mail for general information: sales@cherwell.com
e-mail for technical support: endnote@cherwell.com
http://www.cherwell.com/

IV.2.2 PAPYRUS

PAPYRUS is marketed by Research Software Design, 2718 SW Kelly Street, Suite 181, Portland, OR 97201, USA. This package is currently available as Version 7.0 for DOS/Windows and Version 8.0 for the Macintosh. Up-to-date details can be requested from info@rsd.com or found on the World Wide Web at:
http://www.teleport.com/~rsd/

IV.2.3 ProCite

ProCite originated within the library and information sector but has gained wide acceptance among other disciplines. It is currently available as Version 5 for Windows 95/98/2000NT4 and Version 4 for Macintosh. Up-to-date details and a demonstration copy can be found at: http://www.risinc.com/pc/pcdownload.html
Procite Version 4 is reviewed on the World Wide Web at: http://www.biblio-tech.com/html/procite.html

IV.2.4 Reference Manager

Developed within the life sciences community, Reference Manager is currently available as Version 9.5 for Windows 95/98/2000NT4 and as Version 7 for Windows 3.1. A recent addition is a Web interface called Reference Web Poster. Reference Manager is marketed by Reference

Information Systems and a demonstration copy can be found at: http://www.risinc.com/rm/rmdownload.html

Reference Manager Version 8 is reviewed on the World Wide Web at: http://www.biblio-tech.com/html/reference_manager.html

Further reading

COMBS, J. (1996) *ProCite 3.1 for Windows: professional and personal bibliographic reference management from Personal Bibliographic, Inc.* Library Software Review 15: 119–31.

COMBS, J. (1998) *Reference Manager for Windows 95/NT from Research Information Systems.* Library Software Review 17: 219–27.

HANSON, T. (1995) *Bibliographic Software and the Electronic Library.* University of Hertfordshire Press, Hatfield.

NICOLL, L.H., OUELLETTE, T.H., BIRD, D.C., HARPER, J. and KELLEY, J. (1996) *Bibliography database managers – a comparative review.* Comput. Nurs. 14: 45–56.

SATYA-MURTI, S. (2000) *EndNote v.4 Reference Manager 9.0 ProCite 5.0.* JAMA 284: 1581–3.

SHAPLAND, M. (1999) *Evaluation of Reference Management Software* (comparing Papyrus with ProCite, Reference Manager, Endnote, Citation, GetARef, Biblioscape, Library Master, Bibliographica, Scribe, Refs), University of Bristol, 28 July. Available at: http://www.cse.bris.ac.uk/~ccmjs/rmeval99.htm

TAYLOR, G. (1998) *Surviving the information explosion – Reference Manager version 8.01.* Trends Genet. 14: 41.

IMPLEMENTING THE EVIDENCE

V.1   RESOURCE OVERVIEW

Resources to support implementation of the evidence are, without doubt, the least plentiful of all the stages in the process. Materials can be categorised as:

- those that appraise the evidence for the effectiveness of different implementation methods, for example, the publication Implementing Clinical Practice Guidelines, *Effective Health Care Bulletin*, Volume 1, No.8, 1995;[1]
- those that support a particular project or initiative often characterised by a bewildering array of acronyms such as PACE, PRIMA, PRISE, CHAIN and FACTS.

In the latter case, resources are limited to descriptions or examples of methods, project documentation or newsletters, and published evaluations. The limited lifespan of such examples, and the fact that they have often been conceived as pilot projects of prescribed geographical limits, means that the integration of this corpus of good practice is less advanced than one might expect.

V.2   RESOURCE

V.2.1 Effective Practice and Organisation of Care (EPOC) Database

EPOC is a downloadable Idealist database from the Cochrane Collaboration Effective Practice and Organisation of Care Group (see V.3.2 below) in which are documented experimental studies of the effectiveness of mechanisms for changing behaviour. Owing to the complexity of questions addressed by the EPOC Group, they accept a wider range of study designs than the strict criteria applied to RCTs for other databases produced by The Cochrane Collaboration. http://www.abdn.ac.uk/public_health/hsru/epoc/index. htm

V.3   ORGANISATIONS AND INITIATIVES

V.3.1   Contacts, Help, Advice and Information Network (CHAIN)

The Contacts, Help, Advice and Information Network is a contacts database designed to facilitate links among healthcare professionals, teachers, managers, librarians, IT specialists, researchers, and other professionals working in the health service. CHAIN is a pilot project. The database is available on floppy disk, CD-ROM, and the Internet. It was established in response to a demand from the service for information about 'who is doing what' in evidence-based healthcare and clinical effectiveness. CHAIN is funded through the NHS R&D Programme. The purposes of this network are:

1. to allow healthcare professionals working throughout the NHS to identify and contact people who are active or interested in clinical effectiveness or evidence-based healthcare;
2. to share information on relevant training and events.

The Internet version of CHAIN can be used actively as an online communication tool for health service professionals who share an interest in these subjects. http://www. nthames-health.tpmde.ac.uk/chain/chain.htm

V.3.2   The Cochrane Effective Practice and Organisation of Care (EPOC) Group (formerly known as Cochrane Collaboration on Effective Professional Practice, CCEPP)

The focus of EPOC, one of the Cochrane Collaborative Review Groups, is to undertake reviews of interventions designed to improve professional practice and the delivery of effective health services, including various forms of continuing education, quality assurance, informatics, and financial, organisational and regulatory interventions that can affect the ability of healthcare professionals to deliver services more effectively or efficiently. Interventions that can affect professional practice through patients' influence are also within the scope of EPOC. http://www.abdn. ac.uk/public_health/hsru/epoc/index.htm

V.3.3 Framework for Appropriate Care Throughout Sheffield (FACTS) Project

FACTS is a city-wide project based in Sheffield, with the aim of implementing change in primary care.[2,3] Initial efforts have been targeted at ensuring that heart disease patients receive aspirin. The full text of a report, *Lessons from FACTS*, detailing the methods of the project together with broader implications for the evidence-based change management, is available from their website. http://www.shef.ac.uk/uni/projects/facts/

V.3.4 Promoting Action on Clinical Effectiveness (PACE)

The PACE initiative, which was based on the learning points that arose from the FACTS and GRIPP[4] projects, is organised from the King's Fund in London. There is a network, and sixteen demonstration projects in which the aim is to achieve clinical change for effective healthcare. A progress report[5] is available from their website. http://www.kingsfund.org.uk/pace/evidence.htm

V.3.5 Primary Care Information Management across Anglia (PRIMA)

The PRIMA project ran from March 1997 to March 2000. The aim was to empower primary care workers to deliver effective healthcare in their provider and commissioning roles by furnishing them with the necessary skills to access and use electronic and other information sources. Features included the identification of information-based training needs within a selected group of primary care practices, the creation and implementation of a training scheme aimed at improving the quality of information handling, and the evaluation of the best ways in which information, documents and related services might be delivered to primary care workers:
http://wwwlib.jr2.ox.ac.uk/prima/

V.3.6 Primary Care Sharing the Evidence (PRISE)

The PRISE project ran for two years (ending in February 1998). The aim was to provide timely access to high-quality evidence for GPs and other practice-based professionals. The focus of the project was 12 primary healthcare sites, comprising one dental practice and two GP practices in each of the four counties of the former Oxford Region. The goal was to achieve a better understanding of the mechanisms and skills that will enable primary healthcare teams to provide high-quality care based on the best evidence available. A final report was circulated widely to general practices, libraries, and public health departments. It is also available to download from the PRISE website: http://libsun1.jr2.ox.ac.uk/prise/

V.4   THE INTERNET

V.4.1 Implementation and Change in the Health Service

This is a sub-site of the Turning Research Into Practice (TRIP) initiative. It provides a summary of between 5 and 10 articles on changing clinical practice each month. It also includes other useful Internet links on implementation and change.
http://www.gwent.nhs.gov.uk/trip/ic/I&C.html

References

1. NHS CENTRE FOR REVIEWS AND DISSEMINATION and NUFFIELD INSTITUTE FOR HEALTH (1995) *Implementing Clinical Practice Guidelines: can guidelines be used to improve clinical practice?* Effective Health Care Bulletin, Volume 1, No. 8. University of Leeds, Leeds.
2. EVE, R., GOLTON, I., HODGKIN, P. et al. (1996) *Beyond guidelines: promoting clinical change in the real world.* J. Management Med. 10: 16–25.
3. HODGKIN, P., EVE, R., GOLTON, I. et al. (1996) *Changing clinical behaviour on a city-wide scale: lessons from the FACTS project.* J. Clinical Effectiveness 1: 8–10.
4. ANGLIA AND OXFORD REGIONAL HEALTH AUTHORITY (1994) *Getting research into Practice and Purchasing (GRIPP), Four Counties Approach. Resource Pack.* Anglia and Oxford RHA, Oxford.
5. DUNNING, M., ABI-AAD, G., GILBERT, D., GILLAM, S. and LIVETT, H. (1998) *Turning Evidence Into Everyday Practice.* King's Fund Publishing, London.

Further Reading

ANONYMOUS (1995) *Promoting the implementation of research findings in the NHS.* NAHAT Briefing November; 89. NAHAT, Birmingham.

APPLEBY, J., WALSHE, K. and HAM, C. (1995) *Acting on the evidence: a review of clinical effectiveness, sources of information, dissemination and implementation.* NAHAT Research Paper 17. NAHAT, Birmingham.

BATSTONE, G. and EDWARDS, M. (1996) *Professional roles in promoting evidence-based practice.* Br. J. Health Care Management 2: 144–7.

BUDD, J. and DAWSON, S. (1994) *Influencing Clinical Practice: Implementation of R&D Results.* Management School, Imperial College, London.

DAVIS, D.A., THOMSON, M.A., OXMAN, A.D. et al. (1995) *Changing physician performance: A systematic review of the effect of continuing medical education strategies.* JAMA 274: 700–5.

DAVIS, P and HOWDEN-CHAPMAN, P. (1996) *Translating research findings into health policy.* Soc. Sci. Med. 43: 865–72.

DOPSON, S., MANT, J. and HICKS, N. (1994) *Getting research into practice: facing the issues.* J. Management Med. 8: 4–12.

DUNNING, M., McCQUAY, H. and MILNE, R. (1994) *Getting a GRiP.* Health Service Journal Apr 24; 104 (5400): 24–5.

DUNN, E.V., NORTON, P.G., STEWART, M., TUDIVER, F. and BASS, M.J. (1994) *Disseminating research/changing practice. Research Methods in Primary Care*, Volume 6. Sage, London.

NHS CENTRE FOR REVIEWS AND DISSEMINATION (1999) *Getting Evidence into Practice.* Effective Health Care Bulletin, Volume 5, Number 1. University of York, York.

HAINES, A. and DONALD, A.(Eds) (1998) *Getting research findings into practice.* BMJ Publications, London.

HAINES, A. and JONES, R. (1994) *Implementing findings of research.* Br. Med. J. 308: 1489–92.

HARRISON, S. (1994) *Knowledge into practice: what's the problem?* J. Management Med. 8: 9–16.

HAYNES, R.B., HAYWARD, R.S.A. and LOMAS, J. (1995) *Bridges between healthcare research evidence and clinical practice.* J. Am. Med. Informatics Assoc. 2: 342–50.

IBBOTSON, S.L., LONG, A.F., SHELDON, T.A. et al. (1993). *An initial evaluation of effective health care bulletins as instruments of effective dissemination.* J. Management Med. 7: 48–57.

OXMAN, A.D., THOMSON, M.A., DAVIS, D.A. et al. (1995) *No magic bullets: a systematic review of 102 trials of interventions to help health care professionals deliver services more effectively or efficiently.* Can. Med. Assoc. J. 153: 1423–31.

ROGERS, E.M. (1995) *Diffusion of innovations.* 4th Edition. Free Press, New York.

STOCKING, B. (1995) *Why research findings are not used by commissions – and what can be done about it.* J. Public Health Med. 17: 380–2.

WALSHE, K. and HAM, C. (1997) *Acting on the evidence: progress in the NHS.* NHS Confederation, Birmingham.

WILLIAMSON, P. (1992) *From dissemination to use: management and organisational barriers to the application of health services research findings.* Health Bull. 50: 78–86.

Page numbers in *italics* refer to boxes and tables, and those in **bold** type to figures.